HEALTH CARE SYSTEM AND HOSPITAL ADMINISTRATION

3

HEALTH POLICY AND PROGRAMMES

HEALTH CARE SYSTEM AND HOSPITAL ADMINISTRATION

3

HEALTH POLICY AND PROGRAMMES

DR. S.L. GOEL

Professor of Public Administration (Retd.),
Panjab University, Chandigarh
Editor, Indian Journal of Public Administration, IIPA, New Delhi
Former Member, UGC, Former Member Distance Education Council
Former Member All India Board of Management, AICTE
Member, Executive Council, IIPA, New Delhi.
Former Vice-President, IIPA, New Delhi.
Emeritus Fellow, University Grants Commission
Former Director, State Bank of India (Local Board) Chandigarh
Former Director, National Horticulture Board, Ministry of Agriculture,
Government of India, New Delhi.

DEEP & DEEP PUBLICATIONS PVT. LTD.

F-159, Rajouri Garden, New Delhi-110027

HEALTH CARE SYSTEM AND HOSPITAL ADMINISTRATION
Vol. 3—Health Policy and Programmes

ISBN 978-81-8450-193-3 (Vol. 3)
ISBN 978-81-8450-198-8 (Set)

Typeset by S.S. COMPOSERS
3190, Mohindra Park, Shakur Basti, Delhi-110034.

Printed in India at MAYUR ENTERPRISES
WZ Plot No. 3, Gujjar Market, Tihar Village, New Delhi-110018.

Published by DEEP & DEEP PUBLICATIONS PVT. LTD.
F-159, Rajouri Garden, New Delhi-110027.
Phones: 25435369, 25440916
E-mail: ddpbooks@yahoo.co.in • ddpubs@gmail.com
Showroom:
2/13, Ansari Road, Daryaganj, New Delhi-110002 • Telefax: 23245122

Contents

Preface

Promotion of health is basic to national progress. Nothing could be of greater significance than the health of the people in terms of resources for socio-economic development. In spite of this realization, the people living in the developing world and especially 70 percent of them who live in rural areas have little or no access to modern medicine and health care. Inevitably this results in morbidity and high rate of mortality from preventable diseases. This state of hopelessness and frustration among the people is not because of the lack of professional knowledge or competence but due to poor administration of health services. Administration can provide the means whereby the most effective use can be made of the knowledge and skills of the personnel responsible for the health care delivery system. The benefits of modern science and technology can reach the people only if such services are properly planned and effectively implemented.

Inspite of the importance of health policies and programme designed to provide better health service to people especially in rural areas, urban slums and tribal areas, there is less impact of National Health.

This National Health Policy 2002 envisages a key role for the Central Government in designing national programmes with the active participation of the State Governments. Also, the Policy ensures the provisioning of financial resources, in addition to technical support, monitoring and evaluation at the national level by the Centre. However, to optimize the utilization of the public health infrastructure at the primary level, NHP-2002 envisages the gradual convergence of all health programmes under a single field administration. Vertical programmes for control of major diseases like TB, Malaria, HIV/AIDS, as also the RCH and Universal Immunization Programmes, would need to be continued till moderate levels of prevalence are reached. The integration of the programmes will bring about a desirable optimisation of outcomes through a convergence of all public health inputs. The Policy also envisages that programme implementation be effected through autonomous bodies at State and district levels. The interventions of State Health Departments may be limited to the overall monitoring of the achievement of programme targets and other technical aspects. The relative distancing of the programme implementation from the State Health Departments will give the project team greater operational flexibility. Also, the presence of State Government officials, social activists, private health professionals and MLAs/MPs on the management boards of the autonomous bodies will facilitate well-informed decision-making.

The Policy also highlights the need for developing the capacity within the State Public Health Administration for scientific designing of public health projects, suited to the local situation. The Policy envisages that apart from the exclusive staff in a vertical structure for the disease control programmes, all rural health staff should be available for the entire gamut of public health activities at the decentralized level, irrespective of whether these activities relate to national programmes or other public health initiatives. It would be for the Head of the District Health Administration to allocate the time of the rural health staff between the various programmes, depending on the local need. NHP-2002 recognizes that to implement such a change, not only would the public health administrators be required to change their mindset, but the rural health staff would need to be trained and reoriented.

Goals to be Achieved by 2000-2015

Goal	Year
Eradicate Polio and Yaws	2005
Eliminate Leprosy	2005
Eliminate Kala Azar	2010
Eliminate Lymphatic Filariasis	2015
Achieve Zero-level growth of HIV/AIDS	2007
Reduced Mortality by 50% on account of TB, Malaria and other Vector and water borne diseases	2010
Reduce Prevalence of Blindness to 0.5%	2010
Reduce IMR to 30/1000 and MMR to 100/Lakh	2010
Increase utilization of public health facilities from current level of <20% to >75%	2010
Establish an integrated system of surveillance, National Health Accounts and Health Statistics	2005
Increase health expenditure by Government as a % of GDP from the existing 0.9% to 2.0%	2010
Increase share of Central Grants to Constitute at least 25% of total health spending	2010
Increase State Sector Health spending from 5.5% to 7% of the budget	2005
Further increase to 8%	2010

Source: National Health Policy, 2002.

This volume concentrates on Communicable and Non-Communicable diseases.

Communicable diseases continue to constitute the major public health problem. In spite of increased efforts to control Malaria, the morbidity and mortality due to the disease appear to be on the increase in most of the countries. The region is free from small-pox. However, tuberculosis, cholera and diarrhoeal diseases have been the cause of concern. Besides, sexually transmitted diseases pose a serious challenge to the region.

Communicable diseases were mainly responsible for high mortality and morbidity and an immediate need of control and eradication of these diseases. Malnutrition, which is a more serious scourge than hunger, is, to a certain extent, caused by ignorance and faulty food habits, though largely it may be due to depressing poverty. According to Dr. Mahler:

Non-communicable diseases in India are prevalent like cardiovascular diseases, cancer, drug addiction, mental diseases and radiological hazards are emerging as significant health problems. UNICEF, WHO study has nicely analysed the health problems in developing countries. It was stated:

> "The principal causes of mortality in the developing world are malnutrition, vector borne diseases, gastrointestinal diseases, and respiratory diseases—themselves the result of poverty, squalor and ignorance. To them must be added the disease of mothers related to deprivation, unregulated fertility, and exhaustion, with their effects on the unborn and new born child. These conditions are linked with social problems such as overwork among women, unemployment among the young, population growth and urbanization; and their solution calls for an integrated effort in which the health services have a major role to play."

Some countries in the Region are in a phase of prolonged epidemiological transition, a period in which the health problems of the affluent and the not-so-affluent societies co-exist. Thus, these countries will have to bear a double burden of disease: Communicable diseases associated with poverty, over-population and deprivation arising out of malnutrition, ignorance, and crowded and unhygienic living conditions, compounded by non-communicable diseases (NCDs) such as ischaemic heart disease, high blood pressure, cancer and diabetes associated with affluence, stress, changes in lifestyles and dietary habits and longer life span.

It is important to realize that, globally, non-communicable diseases are emerging as the leading cause of death in developing regions. At present, the risk of death from NCDs during adulthood (15-60 years) is considerably higher in the developing world, including South-East Asia, than in the established market economies. Cardiovascular diseases, cancer, diabetes and mental disorders are some of the major diseases which contribute increasingly to morbidity and mortality.

The health needs of the elderly must be kept in mind as societies evolve. The rate of increase in the number of people older than 65 years is occurring faster in middle and low-income countries than in advanced industrialized nations. Although the elderly in many countries enjoy better health, population ageing is often accompanied by increases in non-communicable diseases and mental health problems.

New, Emerging and Re-emerging Diseases

Together with the new, emerging and re-emerging diseases, health problems arising out of population growth, poverty, urbanization, speed of travel and environmental degradation are the most important threats to the Region in the 21st century. Infectious diseases like tuberculosis, diarrhoeal diseases and malaria have been dominant in the Region and it is likely that most of them will remain prevalent well into the 21st century. Compounding the problem is the emergence of drug-resistant strains of tuberculosis, gonococcal infections and malaria in addition to new diseases like cholera, and HIV/AIDS.

If the current trends continue into the next century, tuberculosis will remain a serious public health problem. Malaria and cholera will remain prevalent and the newly-emerging viral haemorrhagic fevers will cause local epidemics. There will be a return of plague and epidemics of yellow fever and widespread epidemics of HIV/AIDS in the countries of the Indian sub-continent. Recurring outbreaks of dengue haemorrhagic fever in India is a cause for concern

In this volume Health Policy and Programmes divided into 16 chapters, we have tried to cover communicable and non-communicable diseases and how to overcome them. Chapters 1 and 2 deal with Health Policy and Projects aimed at elimination of diseases and provision of health services and quality of life to the people. Chapter 3 deals with Vector Borne Diseases covering six diseases and integrated surveillance programmes. Chapters 4 and 5 examine National Tuberculosis and Blindness Control Programme. Chapter 6 examines the serious problems of HIV/AIDS. Chapters 7 and 8 deal with mental health and Retardation and Cancer Control Programme. Chapter 9 deals with Diabetes, Cardio-Vascular Diseases and Stroke Programme. Chapters 9, 10, 11 and 12 deal with Nutrition, Oral Health and Occupational Health followed by Chapters 13, 14, 15 and 16 dealing with the health of Women, Youth, Children and Elderly.

It is self-evident that in a country as large as India, which has a wide variety of socio-economic settings, national health programme have to be designed with enough flexibility to permit the state public health administration to craft their own programme package according to their needs. Also, the implementation of the national health programme can only be carried out through the State Governments, e.g. decentralized public health machinery. Since, for various reasons, the responsibility of the Central Government in funding additional public health services will continue over a period of time, the role of the Central Government in designing broad-based public health initiatives will inevitably continue. Moreover, it has been observed that the technical and managerial expertise for designing large-span public health programmes exists with the Central Government in a considerable degree; this expertise can be gainfully utilized in designing national health programmes for implementation in varying socio-economic settings in the States. With this background, the

NHP-2002 attempts to define the role of the Central Government and the State Governments in the public health sector of the country.

Over the last decade or so, the Government has relied upon a 'vertical' implementational structure for the major disease control programmes. Through this, the system has been able to make a substantial dent in reducing the burden of specific diseases. However, such an organisational structure, which requires independent manpower for each disease programme, is extremely expensive and difficult to sustain. Over a long time-range, 'vertical' structures may only be affordable for those diseases which offer a reasonable possibility of elimination or eradication in a foreseeable time-span.

In any developing country with inadequate availability of health services, the requirement of expertise in the areas of 'public health' and 'family medicine' is markedly more than the expertise required for other clinical specialities. In India, the situation is that public health expertise is non-existent in the private health sector, and far short of requirement in the public health sector. Also, the current curriculum in the graduate/post-graduate courses is outdated and unrelated to contemporary community needs. In respect of 'family medicine', it needs to be noted that the more talented medical graduates generally seek specialization in clinical disciplines, while the remaining go into general practice. While the availability of post-graduate educational facilities is 50 percent of the total number of qualifying graduates each year, and can be considered adequate, the distribution of the disciplines in the post-graduate training facilities is overwhelmingly in favour of clinical specializations. NHP-2002 examines the possible means for ensuring adequate availability of personnel with specialization in the 'public health' and 'family medicine' disciplines, to discharge the public health responsibilities in the country.

What is needed is to lay emphasis on emerging and thrust areas to keep the medical science knowledge and delivery of health services as per the needs of the people. It is hoped that this book on "Health Care System and Hospital Administration—Health Policy and Programmes" would make a modest contribution to the knowledge and existing literature in this expanding field. Besides, this would help the academicians, national health officials, public health administrators, medical research workers and the policy-makers and planners in the proper understanding of health care delivery system. I will consider my labour well rewarded if the findings of the study are translated to provide decent health care to the millions of people living in rural areas, urban slums and tribal areas. Comments and suggestions from the readers would always be welcome.

Chandigarh S.L. GOEL

CHAPTER 1

Policy-making for Health Administration

"It is hard enough to design public policies and programs that look good on paper. It is harder still to formulate in words and slogans that resonate pleasingly in the ears of political leaders and the constituencies to which they are responsive. And it is excruciatingly hard to implement them in a way that pleases anyone at all, including the supposed beneficiaries or clients"

—*Eugene Bardach*

NATURE AND SIGNIFICANCE

Policies may be thought of as the main system which provides the framework for the accomplishment of intended objectives. Formulation of policies involves making explicit, the various assumptions which are made with respect to the basic premises needs and the priorities and allocating the finances accordingly. Besides, policies are intended to spell out the parameters in the context of which organisational decisions are to be made. Policy is very essential in administration, for it gives a concrete shape to the political and social objectives which the government lays down in the form of laws, rules, regulations, etc. Davis states: "A policy is basically a statement either expressed or implied of those principles and rules that are set-up by executive leadership as guides and constraints for the organisation's thought and action. Its principle purpose is to enable executive leadership to relate properly the organisation's work to its objectives."

Policies may be looked upon as general guides to action. They may be verbal, written or implied. They set the overall boundaries for action by individuals or groups in an organisational setting. They indicate the framework within which executives may make decisions for the performance of organisational action. According to Ishwar Dayal: "Policy prescribes the aims, the objectives, the targets that would be used to achieve the objectives. Operationally, the policy statement, in this sense, must specify the expected results, the measures for achieving them and mechanism or method with which the results are expected to be achieved. ". . . Policy formulation refers to that aspect of administration which is concerned with defining the objective and determining the choice of action. Decision-making refers to the process by which this policy is determined."[1]

The public policies may be written or unwritten, explicit or implicit. Important polices of the government are often clearly expressed in a written form. Generally Public policies are formally adopted by the government authorities. However, there are public policies embodied only in a set of practices, conventions and precedents. According to Koontz and O'Donnell, written policy is preferable, as:

> "It builds on proved decisions of the past conserving executive energy for new decisions: it creates an atmosphere in which individual actions may be taken with confidence; it speeds administration by reducing repetition to routine; it supports consistency of endeavour across a large group through the years; it stabilizes the enterprise; it frees the top management so that more creative considerations can be given to the problem of today and the new programme of tomorrow."

Public policy management in India is in the stage of infancy. The ongoing process of the integration of the Indian society is providing a rigour to the art and science of public policy management in India.[2] A sound public policy management is expected to contribute to both the country's political stability and its efforts to bring about the much desired socio-economic transformation.[3]

DEFINITION OF HEALTH POLICY

The health policy of a country generally provides a broad framework of decisions for guiding the health interventions which are useful to its population in improving their health, reducing the gap between health status of different classes in the society and positively contribute to the quality of life. It aims at making sure that health services are integrated, accessible and affordable to all people and are carried out with active involvement of the population. The health policy is guided by the economic, socio-cultural history of a country, its techno-scientific and intellectual development, its political system, constitutional commitments and overall goals for national development. In a country like ours, issues of population, education, poverty, patterns of occupation, consumption and production, environment sanitation and health are so closely inter-connected that none of these can be considered in isolation for designing a meaningful policy for national development. Health policy thus involves, taking a 'holistic perspective' of the current and future health care needs of the population as well as providing the context, contents, objectives, guidelines, strategies and time-frame for achieving the desired goals of health development.

From a managerial perspective, health policy is closely related to 'mission', 'vision' and 'outcomes' and it helps the programme managers to convert the 'aspirations' reflected in the policy to 'operational' entities through planning, organising, implementing, monitoring and evaluation of different programmes. The link and matching between health policy formulation process and programme operations is crucial for achieving effectiveness in programme management and policy goals as well as for ensuring clarity between the 'means' and 'ends' in the policy framework. Any policy on health care system (which is a sub-system of the overall socio-economic system of the country) can not be designed and implemented independently without taking into consideration the inter-sectoral variables which influence and affect the health situation. Further health care being a multi-disciplinary subject reflecting epidemiological, technological, managerial, social and political dimensions, requires inputs from different disciplines and high degree of competence for health policy and programme management.[4]

The aim of health policy is to secure a fundamental change in health status of people to help break the circle of poverty encircling the masses in the developing world and liberate the population to secure the change that they have chosen and in which they participate. It includes the decisions on medical education, health facilities, health coverage, medical research, choice of systems of medicine, etc. It also includes the decisions as regards the relative role of the government, the private and voluntary agencies in the promotion of health care. The health policy must be made with relevance to the time dimension. It can be a long-term policy, e.g., provision of comprehensive health care to all by the year 2020, or a medium-term, e.g., providing elementary care to all by 2010, or immediate, i.e. covering half the population by 2008 and so on.

In the developing world, there is no comprehensive health policy encompassing all the components affecting the health status of the people. There are piece-meal policy decisions about a particular aspect of health care administration. Besides, there is no continuity in the formulation of health policy because of the change of political leadership. Ministry of Health and Family Welfare and the State Health Departments must come out with a Health Policy which can provide a decent health care to all especially the people living in rural areas, urban slums and the tribal areas in 21st century.

The objectives of the policy of health care delivery system are described as under:

1. To provide universal coverage and enable the whole population to have access to the type of services best suited to their state of health, richness or disablement.
2. To provide comprehensive, preventive, curative and

rehabilitative health services for whoever requires them, without financial or other bars and making the best possible use of the available scientific and technological knowledge.

3. To reduce the cost of treatment, giving priority to primary care and services of a preventive and ambulatory type and reserving hospital treatment for those who need it. The hospital standard should correspond to the average standard of living of the population covered.
4. To decentralize health care through a system of levels of care designed so that each person enters the system through the level best equipped to provide the form of treatment most suited to his individual needs and that all services, from the primary up to the specialized level, are accessible to whoever needs them through an information and referral system.
5. To organize the "health team", composed of professional, technical and auxiliary staff in various disciplines who assume responsibility for the health of the community, acting individually at different levels but with their activities coordinated through an effective system of communication and supervision.

Relationship between Policy-making and Planning (Refer Chart 1.1)

Planning and policy-making are inter-related. Policy determines the principle for action and planning provides the instrument for the application of policy and review. Policy decisions are needed in the planning process and in defining its goals and limitations

Therefore, planners who ignore policy only jeopardize the good results of their endeavours. On the other hand, a planning process has various possible feedback effects on policy. For example:

(a) it requires explicit policy statements, thus bringing certain subjects to the political arena;
(b) it should reflect the rationale of the policies, show how they can be implemented, and indicate their financial and other implications;
(c) it provides the policy-making with instruments for dialogue, coordination, mobilisation of resources; and continuity of action; and
(d) its impact on the national situation should influence future policy-making.[5]

The Executive Board of WHO has stated (Health for All, Series No. 2, p. 14) that:

"National policies, strategies and plans of action form a continuum, and there are no sharp dividing lines between them. ..."A national

CHART 1.1

Relationship between Policy and Plan

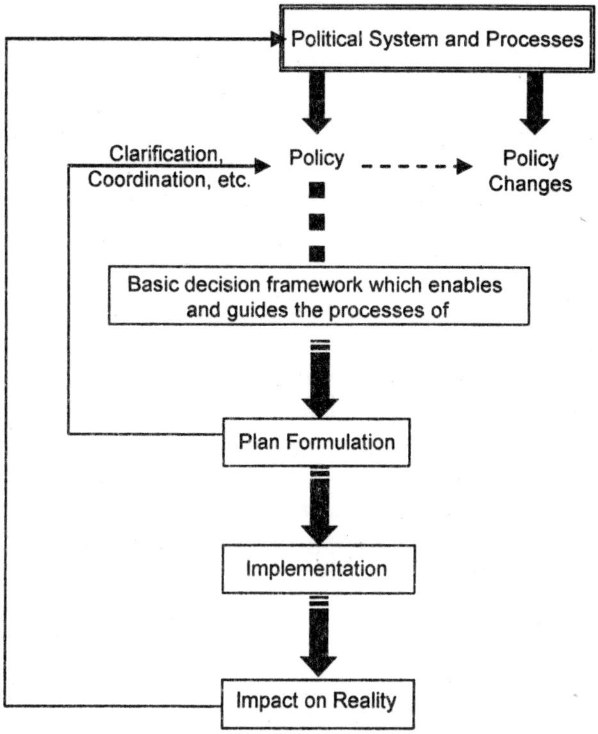

health policy is an expression of goals for improving the health situation, the priorities among those goals, and the main direction for attaining them. A national strategy, which should be based on the national health policy, includes the broad lines of action required in all sectors involved to give effect to that policy. A national plan of action is a broad inter-sectoral master plan for attaining the national health goals through implementation of this strategy. It indicates what has to be done, who has to do it, during what time frame and with what resources. It is a framework leading to more detailed programming, budgeting, implementation and evaluation."

Relationship between Policy-making and Decision-making

Policy-making and planning involve decisions. Decision-making is the core of policy formulation and planning. Man has been performing the act of taking decisions ever since he became a social animal but a scientific study of these actions is of a very recent origin. During World War II, some studies led to the theory of decisions. Today, the process of decision-making has become the essence of any productive activity. It is an act of intelligence, will and precision. B. Govemay suggests that there are a minimum of four elements which when put together result in a decision:

(a) There must be choice.
(b) The choice must be conscious.
(c) The choice must be oriented by various purposes.
(d) The choice must lead to an action.

It is essential to understand the meaning and art of decision-making to formulate scientific and sound health policies. Webster's dictionary defines decision-making as 'the art of determining in one's own mind upon an opinion or courses of actions'. According to Brooke Groves, "Decision-making is the selection from two or more reasonable possibilities of a course that will, at the time and under the circumstances, provide the suitable solution of the problem at hand." It is essential for the policy-makers to keep in mind the five steps mentioned below while taking decisions.

Thus we see that decision-making is an important constituent of the processes of policy-making and planning as the decisions weave individual choices into a web of relationship which constitute a policy. According to Herbert A. Simon, decision-making comprises three principal phases: (i) finding occasion. . . for making a decision; (ii) finding possible courses of action; and (iii) choosing among courses of action. The first phase has been described as intelligence activity, the second phase as design activity, and the third phase as choice activity. This analysis of the process of decision-making has special reference for the policy-makers and planners in the Government as they are to ensure that the policies based on such decisions are not only correct and just but must also appear to be correct and just to the people at large.

PARAMETERS OF POLICY-MAKING

Policy-making must be done to suit the legal, social, economic and political framework prevailing in a country. Policy-making must be in consonance with the constitutional system and structure of the government and administrative apparatus. Besides, policy-making to be effective must be broadly acceptable to the people as we know that ultimate sovereignty rests with the people. Effective policy formulation can help organisations to respond to and react to the changes in the environment-establish environment linkages. Linkages are points of interactions with the environment. These can be classified into four categories-enabling, functional, normative and diffused linkages. Enabling linkages ensure and protect the organisational authority to operate its access to resource and its power to achieve results. Since political constraints are neither permanent nor inseparable, there is urgency in adopting policies designed to optimize the positive contributions of political support as well as minimize and mitigate the harmful effects of partisan interferences. The job of functional linkages is to link the policies with the task environment, i.e. help in achieving cooperation and coordination among allied agencies. Diffused linkages ensure that the policies must reach the beneficiaries through mass media and personal contact. The art of developing common understanding among people through policies is vital to bring about changes of attitudes and behaviour through users participation. Normative linkages attempt to fit the policies into the value system. Besides, the policies must try to change the norms with the cooperation of the people to induce socio-economic changes.

According to Christopher Pollit and others, the following are essential characteristics of Public Policy:

1. Policies are process of decision-making and activity. They customarily involve a series of decisions taken over an extended period of time—an exercise of power and rationality.
2. The process of decision-making takes place mainly though not exclusively, within a framework of prescribed organisational roles. In the case of public policy, these roles are those constituting a series of formal institutions with special legal characteristics. They are the institutions of the state.
3. Policies commonly involve exchanges of information resources, discussions, bargaining, etc. without and within the state agencies, with a variety of 'external' interest groups. The content, closeness and timing of these interactions is an important subject for empirical investigation.
4. Not all decisions are part of 'Policy' but only those which are of a strategic (in the military sense) or guideline nature.
5. Policy is directed at the increasing probability of occurrence of desired stakes of the world in the future.
6. The state institutions, which claim responsibility for public policies, almost invariably legitimatize their activities by claiming that their policies are in general (public) interest rather than favouring any group, section or individual.

Our concern for formulation of a national health policy dates back to pre-independence period and owes its origin to the National Planning Committee (NPC) of 1938 set-up by the Indian National Congress, which set-up a sub-committee on National Health under the chairmanship of Colonel S.S. Sokhey to assess the health situation and health service in the country and recommend measures for their improvement. The Report submitted in 1940, among others recommended the need for an integration of curative and preventive functions of health services under a single State Agency, maintenance of the health of the people was the responsibility of the State, training of community health workers with emphasis on first aid and simple-medical treatment, social implications of medical and public health, people-oriented health services, etc. It as suggested that practitioners of Ayurveda and Unani systems should be integrated with the State Health

System after giving them scientific training. Other aspects highlighted in the report were nutrition, expansion of medical education and research, production of drugs, etc. Prior to the adoption of National Health Policy in 1983, the following Committees were set-up at different times not only to identify the health and health-related issues but also suggest remedial actions for improvements in health services and health care delivery system in the country.[6]

I. Bhore Committee (1943-46)

Taking into consideration the findings of interim report of National Planning Committee on Health (1940) and being dissatisfied with the then health care system in meeting the health problems of the community, particularly of rural population, in 1943, the then British Government appointed the "Health Survey and Development Committee" with Sir Joseph Bhore as Chairman, to make a survey of the existing health conditions and health organisations and to make recommendations for future development. The recommendations and guidance provided by the Bhore Committee formed the basis for organisation of Basic Health Services in India. The report was submitted to Government in 1946. The Bhore Committee made two types of recommendations:

(a) A comprehensive blue print for the distant future (20 to 40 years)—the smallest service unit was to be Primary Health Unit, serving a population of 10,000 to 20,000;
(b) A short-term scheme covering 2 to 5 years period the emphasis would be on setting up 30 bedded hospitals, one for every two Primary Health Units.

The country-side was the focal point of these recommendations. Other recommendations were:

(i) Formation of Village Health Committee to secure active cooperation and support in the development of health programme.
(ii) Provision for Doctor of future who should be a "Social Doctor" combining both curative and preventive measures.
(iii) Formation of a District Health Board for each district comprising of district health officials and representatives of the public.
(iv) To ensure suitable housing, sanitary surroundings, safe drinking water supply, elimination of unemployment and to lay special emphasis on preventive work.
(v) Intersectoral approach to health services development.

II. Mudaliar Committee (1959-61)

The Government of India, in the Ministry of Health, set-up a Committee on the 12th June, 1959, under the Chairmanship of Dr. A.

Lakshmanswami Mudaliar. Detailed recommendations on these aspects were submitted in 1961. Their salient features were:

(a) Upgrading and strengthening of PHUs.
(b) Strengthening of District Hospitals.
(c) Mobile Service teams for Rural Areas.
(d) Levying of small fee for availing hospital facilities.
(e) Long range health insurance policy for all citizens.
(f) Formation of Central Health Cadre.
(g) Extension of the functions of the University Grants Commission to education in the fields of the Medicine, Engineering, Agriculture and Veterinary Sciences.
(h) Institution of National Programmes for eradication of Malaria, Small Pox, Cholera, Leprosy, Tuberculosis and Filariasis.
(i) Making the Central Council of Health more effective.
(j) Director General of Health Services should enjoy the Status of an Additional Secretary.

III. Chadha Committee (1963)

In April 1963, a special Committee was constituted by the Government of India under the Chairmanship of Director General of Health Services, Dr. M.S. Chadha, to go into the details of the requirements of primary health centres, their planning, the necessary priority required. according to the 'needs of the maintenance phase of Malaria Eradication Programme' and also for other health activities and the manner in which the technical and supervisory staff of the NMEP organisation should be utilised after malaria eradication has been achieved. The committee considered that the maintenance was the responsibility of the general health services, which should be adequately strengthened, particularly the rural health services. Vigilance through medical institutions (government or non-government) must be developed. Multi-purpose domicialiary health services should be developed for all health programmes, including malaria, small-pox, control of other communicable diseases, health education, etc.

IV. Mukherjee Committee (1966-67)

The Central Council of Health, at its meeting on the 31st December 1965, in Madras, appointed a Committee under the Chainnanship of Union Health Secretary to undertake the review of Family Planning Programme and its strategy. The Committee recommended strengthening of the administrative set-up at all levels from the Primary Health Units to the State Headquarters. It also recommended delinking of malaria maintenance activities from Family Planning Programme, so that the latter could receive undivided attention of its staff and could be carried through as a crash mass programme.

Jain Committee: This study group undertook a study of working of different classes of hospitals in the country with a view to improve the standards of medical care and developing sound guidelines for the future expansion of the hospital service as well as review of the working of the Central Government Health Scheme, its progress and performance and made suggestions for improvements and reduction in Government liability.

V. Kartar Singh Committee (1972-73)

In pursuance of the recommendations made by the Executive Committee of the Central Family Planning Council, the Government of India constituted a committee in October 1972, which recommended that:

(a) Multi-purpose workers for the delivery of health, family planning and nutrition services to the rural communities are both feasible and desirable.
(b) To begin with, one Male Health Worker (Muiti-purpose) should be available for a population of six to seven thousands.
(c) Atleast one Female Health Worker (ANM) should be available for a population of ten to twelve thousands.
(d) Each PHC should ultimately serve 50,000 population and should have 16 sub-centres spread over its area.
(e) Training for all workers engaged in the field of health, family planning and nutrition should be integrated.

VI. Shrivastava Committee (1974-75)

The Government of India, in 1974, formed a Committee on 'Medical Education and Support Manpower under the Chairmanship of Dr. J.B. Shrivastava. The Committee submitted its detailed report in 1975 and made specific recommendations for the initiation of the following major programmes for immediate action:

(a) Organisation of the basic health services (including nutrition, health education and family planning) within the community itself and training the personnel needed for the purpose.
(b) Organisation of an economic and efficient programme or health services to bridge the community with the first level referral centre, viz. the PHC (including the strengthening of the PHC itself).
(c) The creation of a National Referral Services Complex by the development of proper linkages between the PHC and higher level referral and service centres.
(d) To create the necessary administrative and financial machinery for the re-organisation of the entire programme of medical and health education from the point of view of the objectives and needs of the proposed programme of national health services.

VII. National Health Policy Document (1983)

The major directions laid down in the Seventh National Health Policy Document (1983) are:

- Provision of universal and comprehensive primary health care services with special emphasis on the preventive, promotive and rehabilitative aspects.
- Securing small family norms through efforts and moving towards the goal of population stabilisation and enunciation of a national population policy.
- To formulate a National Medical and Health Education Policy for health manpower development and to ensure that personnel at all levels are socially motivated to adopt community health approach.
- To decentralise the primary health care system by restructuring the health care services to promote community participation and linking it with a systematic back-up support of referral services at secondary and tertiary levels.
- Integrally linking the health education and extension activities with primary health care services.
- Transferring simple health care knowledge, skills and appropriate technology to community, so that majority of common health actions could be handled effectively by the community.
- Mobilizing untapped health resources and encouraging investment by private sector, NGOs, and voluntary bodies to establish curative services, wherein all affluent sectors could be looked after by paying for the services.
- To remove the existing regional imbalances and to provide services within the reach of all, whether residing in the rural or the urban areas.
- Assist in the enlargement of the services being provided by private voluntary organisations active in the health field, specially those which seek to serve the needs of the rural areas and the urban slums.
- The entire approach to health manpower development should ensure their functioning as a "Health Team." To integrate the services of ISM practitioners at the appropriate levels, within specified areas of responsibility and functioning in the over-all health care delivery system, specially with regard to the preventive, promotive and public health care aspects.

Thus, the Health Priorities, Needs and Major Tasks identified by the National Health Policy in 1983 were:

- Provision of primary health care with special emphasis on the preventive, promotive and rehabilitative aspects.
- Reorganisation of curative services to prevent, control and treat diseases.

- Restructuring of medical and health education as per national health priorities and needs.
- Re-orientation of existing health personnel.
- Integration of the indigenous and modern systems.
- Utilisation of practitioners of indigenous and other system of medicine in health care.
- Provision of maternal and child health including immunization programme.
- Ensuring adequate nutrition to all especially those in rural and urban slums.
- Prevention of food adulteration and maintenance.
- Nationwide health education programme with appropriate communication strategies and approaches to health information in easily understandable form, to motivate development of an attitude for healthy living.
- Establishment of an effective health information system.
- Building-up sound technological and manufacturing capability in the field of drugs, vaccine, biomedical equipments, etc.
- Introduction of health insurance scheme on a statewise basis.
- Working towards a unified, comprehensive legislation in health field.
- Conducting medical research to aim at balanced development of basic, clinical and problems oriented operational research.
- Ensuring effective coordination between health and its more intimately related sectors.
- Monitoring and periodically reviewing the success of the effort made and results achieved.[7]

VIII. National Health Policy-2002

The main objective of the policy is to achieve an acceptable standard of good health amongst the general population of the country and increase access to the decentralized public health system by establishing new infrastructure in deficient areas, and by upgrading the infrastructure in the existing institutions. Salient features of the policy are as follows:

(i) Increase health sector expenditure to 6 per cent of GDP with 2 per cent of GDP being contributed as public health investment by the year 2010.

(ii) Increased allocation of 55 per cent of the total public health investment for the primary health sector; the secondary and tertiary health sectors being targeted for 35 per cent and 10 per cent respectively.

(iii) Key role for the Central Government in designing national programmes with the active participation of the State Governments. The Policy ensures the provisioning of financial resources in addition to technical support, monitoring and evaluation at the national level by the Centre.

(iv) Apart from the exclusive staff in a vertical structure for the disease control programmes, all rural health staff would be available for the entire gamut of public health activities at the decentralized level.

(v) Revival of the Primary Health System by providing some essential drugs under Central Government funding through the decentralized health system. Provisioning of essential drugs at the public health service centre would create a demand for other professional services also from the local population.

(vi) More frequent in service training of public health medical personnel at the level of medical officers as well as paramedics.

(vii) Expand the pool of medical practitioners to include a cadre of licentiates of medical practice, as also practitioners of Indian systems of Medicine and Homoeopathy.

(viii) Implementation of public health programmes through local self-government institutions and decentralize the implementation of the programmes to such institutions by 2005.

(ix) Minimal statutory norms for the deployment of doctors and nurses in medical institutions.

(x) Setting up of a Medical Grants Commission for funding new Government Medical and Dental Colleges in different parts of the country.

(xi) Modify the existing curriculum.

(xii) Enable fresh graduates to contribute effectively to the providing of primary health services as the physician of first contact.

(xiii) Raise the proportion of post-graduate seats in public health and family medicine discipline in medical training institutions to 114th of the earmarked seats.

(xiv) Improvement in the ratio of nurses vis-à-vis doctors/beds.

(xv) Improving the skill-level of nurses and increasing the ratio of degree holding nurses *vis-a-vis* diploma holding nurses.

(xvi) Need for basing treatment regimens, in both the public and private domain on a limited number of essential drugs of a generic nature.

(xvii) At least 50% of the requirement of vaccines/sera to be sourced from public sector institutions to ensure uninterrupted supply of vaccines at an affordable price.

(xviii) Setting up of an organized urban primary health care structure.

(xix) Funding for the urban primary health system to be jointly borne by the local self-government institutions and State and Central Governments.

(xx) Established of fully-equipped 'hub-spoke' trauma care networks in large urban agglomerations to reduce accident mortality.

(xxi) Inter-personal communication of information and folk and other traditional media to bring about behavioural change.

(xxii) Association of PRIs/NGOs/Trusts in IEC activities.

(xxiii) Increase in government-funded health research to a level of 1 per cent of the total health spending by 2005; and thereafter, up to 2 per cent by 2010.

(xxiv) Enactment of suitable legislation for regulating minimum infrastructure and quality standards in clinical establishments/ medical institutions by 2003.

(xxv) Encourage setting up of private insurance instruments for increasing the scope of the coverage of the secondary and tertiary sector under private health insurance packages.

(xxvi) Disease control programmes should earmark at least 10% of the budget in respect of identified programme components, to be exclusively implemented through NGOs.

Government of India and State Governments, through their Health and Family Planning Ministries/Departments bring out Annual reports and statistical analysis, which indicate the past reviews, current status and future projections of health status of the population as well as administrative issues impinging on various programmes. Karnataka State Gazetteer, Part II, Government of Karnataka (1990), Department of Health and Family Welfare Status Report (1989-90), Government of Karnataka (2002), Towards a More Efficient Social Development in Karnataka State, State Planning Board, are all useful in getting factual information about Karnataka.

SUGGESTIONS TO IMPROVE POLICY-MAKING

Before this new policy is adopted, it is suggested that the general administrators and health experts should keep in mind the genuine-health needs of the people and motivate the political actors to formulate balanced health policy based on scientific methods. The health administrators must keep the following facts in mind to frame effective, efficient and relevant health policies.

1. Policies should be made in Consonance with the Objectives

By goal or objective is meant the end towards which action is directed. Since a policy is a guidance for action, it is reasonable to expect that a policy indicates the direction towards which action is guided, either explicitly or implicitly. For this reason, students of policy sciences often define public policies as a programme of goals and objectives.

2. Absence of Contradictions and Inconsistencies

It is necessary for public administrators to help in making policies purposeful and goal-oriented, and to assist in defining goals and objectives clearly, in making them concrete and also quantifiable if possible and in removing, to the extent possible, any contradictions and inconsistencies.

3. Temporal Dimensions

The modern world is rapidly changing. So, our policies must not remain constant but should change with the change in times. A UN report suggests the following three points:

(a) It is a well-known fact that a public policy, in order to be effective, must not be too little or too late;
(b) Time sequence is an essential part of a successful policy. An effective policy should comprise not only what government should do but also when to do one thing after another. Timing is often an essential factor for the success or failure of a policy; and
(c) Synchronization is another timing element. Something, for example, what is required is not only that action '2' should follow action '1' but also that action '3' should be taken at the same time as action as '1'.[8]

4. Feasibility, Probability and Possibility

Policies which are not based on the technical, economic, administrative and perhaps also proposed political feasibility should be avoided unless. it is the specific wish of the policy-makers to adopt such policies. It is important to note that feasibility, probability and possibility are all relative terms. If the policy-makers have reason to believe that what they plan will change the circumstances in favour of the planned objectives, then they are justified in the planning for what may appear to be 'Improbable' or even 'Impossible' to the experts who assume that the circumstances will remain constant. For the developing countries, estimates by experts on feasibility, probability and possibility are often poorly informed guess-work, in part owing to lack of sufficient or decisive evidence and in part owing to a high degree of uncertainty. In a UN document which warns against 'paper planning' and blind commitments to the blatantly impossible, it is stated that:

> "From the previous extremes of seeking the impossible, the planners may go so far in emphasizing the possible that they will think mainly of short-run feasibility. In this effort, they will often be encouraged by economists who have become accustomed to fighting utopia with myopia, that is with 'hard nosed' calculations of small benefits that might be obtained quickly. The result can easily be that instead of planning for the impossible, they will focus upon most possible and feasible of all, namely, the inevitable. This is the fallacy of epiphenomenal planning. Here the main advantage is that the planners can take credit for any minor progress is that might have taken place."[9]

5. Relevant Forecasts and Projections

According to a UN report, "Forecasting and projections are important for public policy-making mainly for two reasons. First, as just indicated, policy is a guidance for action that lies necessarily in the future. Therefore, no rational approach to policy-making is possible without some basis for making assumptions about the future. Forecasting and projection can assist policy-makers in this respect. Secondly, public policies should be used, if at all possible, to avoid crisis rather than to meet crisis and may have to devote most of its resources to crisis management. At the same time, a government which is under constant pressure from immediate crisis may not be able to devote its attention and resources in order to prevent the recurrence of crisis. This is a vicious circle which a government should break, and it can succeed in doing so only by assigning suitable priority to forecasting the future."

6. Appropriate Administrative Machinery

Within the central policy cluster there should also be special arrangement for ensuring that appropriate administrative machinery is established for:

(a) policy and plan implementation,
(b) reporting and feedback,
(c) evaluation and control, and
(d) the adjustment and revision of policies, plans and programmes.

This would ensure effective relationships between policy formulation and policy implementation.[10]

7. Understanding the Implication of Policy

Policies must be interpreted and explained, to all members of the organisation. What people do not understand they cannot use correctly and are likely to distrust. Therefore, there is a need to explain it to all persons to whom it applies.

8. Environmental Considerations

Policy is based on actual information or factual data which can be collected from a number of sources by applying different methods. But, before the data can be changed into a policy, many factors have to be taken into consideration e.g., policies must be made in accordance with the provisions of the constitution and the laws enacted by the legislature; these must also be made in accordance with the social, political, cultural, economic and ethical environment prevailing in the country; these must also be linked with the agencies interested in the same policy to have maximum utility and effectiveness; these must also be made in accordance with the opinion of the public otherwise they (the people) would not cooperate with the government in their execution.

Five Dimensions of National Health Policy (See Chart 1.2)

Dr. Karan Singh has rightly said that, "if the nation wants a first class health care service with special emphasis on nutrition and child health and the combating of communicable diseases, it will have to readjust its priorities so that adequate inputs are made available during the current and subsequent periods."

Perhaps never before the need to reassess our priorities was as great as it is today. The formulation of realistic and scientific health policy based upon our realistic assessment understanding of our health needs and problems and approaches to deal with them will go a long way towards better planning of health services, however meagre may be our resources.

While reviewing the national health policies the following issues need consideration:

CHART 1.2

Five Dimensions of National Health Policy

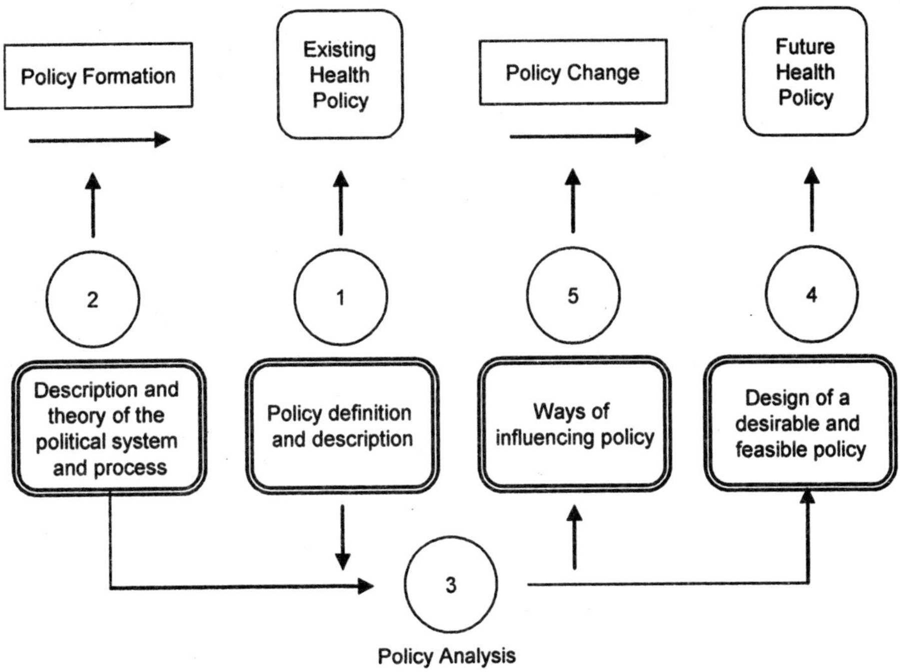

1. Geographical coverage of the population with at least all the essential components of primary health care and the corresponding referral system.
2. A system of financing health care ensuring that all strata of society have an equal opportunity to avail themselves of such care.
3. Coverage of particular population groups, such as mothers and children, working women, school children, workers, and the elderly, and any particular risk group.

4. Preferential allocation of health resources to under-privileged population groups.
5. Facilities available.
6. Rational referred system.
7. Improvement of the human environment by progressive providing safe drinking-water to the whole population, building up waste disposal system, and ensuring clean air.
8. Improvement of communicable and non-communicable diseases.
9. Securing adequate food production and supply and proper nutrition.
10. Community mobilization in planning and development, including promotion of collective responsibility for the health and health care of the community and its constituent families and individuals.
11. Relevant health technologies.
12. Development of human and financial resources for health. Besides, the existing national health policy has not laid down any programme of action like National Policy on education. There is no mechanism to monitor the implementation of health policy. There are a number of the deficiencies in the existing national health policy. The government of India should appoint a team to review the existing National health policy and suggest the New policy based on actual and perceived needs of the people. This can be examined at various levels before sending it to Parliament for their comments, discussion and approval. A health policy for 21st century should not be designed by tinkering the current health policy here and there, but should be designed afresh to take into account the past performance and potential problems to be encountered in the 21st century. Ninth Five Year Plan has made a modest plan to improve upon the targets fixed in National Health Policy upto the year ending 2000. However, there is a need to formulate new health policy to suit the changed circumstances in new millennium.

POLICY-MAKING IN NEW MILLENNIUM

Policy-making is getting complicated, as the number of variables impinging on Policy-making is becoming increasingly complex. This can be attributed to an increase in the magnitude and direction of various impinging factors. Besides, globalisation, privatization and competitiveness have made policy-making more difficult. How can we cope with this complex situation? How can we make a reliable policy? The answer is to make use of information technology the way the business is being done by organisations.

Modern technology has the potentiality to make available to the policy-makers the knowledge in a comprehensive and intelligent manner.

With the proliferation of information technology and electronic access to information, the availability and accessibility of information has undergone profound change. E-mail, inter-net, world wide web (www) and easy access to remote data base, we now have new opportunities to find information at a press of the computer key. The administrators can make use of this rich data in policy formulation. While modern technology opens the doors, it does not compel us to enter. We have to use various technologies, keeping in view availability, accessibility, acceptability, validity, quality, specificity and sensitivity. There is a lot of potentiality in new technology for policy-makers.

Let us illustrate, the policy-making in health. A new discipline "Health Telematics" has emerged based on modern information technology.

Dr. Prakrom Vuthipongse, Permanent Secretary, Ministry of Public Health, Thailand in the Inter-country Workshop on Tele Medicine for Health Development in 21st century from 30th March-3 April 1998 at Bangkok said that as a decision-maker he was aware of the advancement in today's technology, especially in its applications which will help to bring better quality of health care to people in remote and rural areas in cost effective manner. He also said that the initiation of Tele Medicine in the Ministry of Public Health has emerged from the fact that, in remote and rural areas, there has been maldistribution of medical specialities, resulting in poor health care services. He expected the work—hope to come up with fruitful recommendations on regional and national plans of action as well as on inter-country cooperation.

Health Telematics is defined as a composite term for health-relate activities, services and systems carried out over a distance by means of information and communications technologies for the purpose of global health promotion, disease control and health care, as well as education, management and research for health.

The policies for developing the Health Telematics infrastructure can be categorized as under:

(a) *Technological policies*: Deal with the definition of technological standards for hardware, software, management and communications.
(b) *Resources policies*: Address the issues of human and material resources.
(c) *Financial policies*: Identify the sources of finance.

Health Telematics raises certain ethical issues, such as the acceptability of transmitting personal information across cultural boundaries; young doctors setting professionally affected, and the confidentiality of the relationship between the patient and the treating doctor. Full cooperation of the medical and paramedical staff involved, as well as patients is essential. Even in the most advanced form, Health Telematics might not provide a blanket solution for each situation. There would be cases where human intervention is needed. It also raises concern on widening the gap between the poor and the privileged.

The following services are likely to be provided through the Tele Medicine system:

- Medical consultation
- Tele radiology
- Tele cardiology
- Tele pathology
- Distance learning
- Administrative meetings
- Voice and data network
- Internet
- Local call system among the project sites.

Machiavelli said in a famous remark—"There is nothing more difficult to take in hand, more perilous to conduct, more uncertain in its success than to take the lead in the introduction of a new order of things."[10]

However, we must keep in mind the limitations of modern technology, modern technology can provide us tools but we must have the expertise to make use of these tools. Human mind still remains the super computer to control all these tools. R.K. Sapru rightly stresses that processing of information has two components—one that involves merely the communications of verbal, visual or printed facts, and the second that involves evaluation of the information. Distortions can be introduced at one or both these stages. The quality of information needs to be judged on the basis of the degree of distortions introduced at different stage. In the case of the human mind, such a system of quality control has proved elusive so far even though the need is obvious and pressing. Policy-making is a continues process and not a one time activity.[11]

Beneath the drafting of all constitutions is the awareness that change is the law of nature, and as in any other sphere of life, so in the affairs of the state, things cannot remain stationary. It is not given to anyone, however gifted he may be, to foresee the shape of things as they will be after some years, much less after some decades. No constitutional expert, no political philosopher, no man in active public life can pierce through the visage of time and lift the veil of the future to know beforehand the problems which are going to beset the nation and prescribe solution of those problems.[12]

Notes and References

1. Ishwar Dayal, "Organisation for Public Policy in government", a paper submitted to the Seventeenth Conference of the Indian Institute of Public Administration, 30 Oct., 1973.
2. Q.U. Khan, "A model of Public Policy Implementation Process", *Indian Journal of Public Administration*, Vol. 33, No. 1, January-March 1987, pp. 31-39.

3. K.D. Madan, K. Diesh, Ashok Pradhan and C. Chandra Sekharan, Policy-making in Government, New Delhi, Publication Division, 1982, pp. 1-11.
4. Prof. Madhu S. Mishra, "Health Policy and Management of Health Care Delivery Services in India", *Public Health in India: Five Decades*, Vol. I, p. 11
5. WHO: *WHO Chronicle*, November 1977, pp. 441-48.
6. Prof. Madhu S. Mishra, "Health Policy and Management of Health Care Delivery Services in India", *Public Health in India: Five Decades*, Vol. I, p. 11
7. Prof. Madhu S. Mishra, "Health Policy and Management of Health Care Delivery Services in India", *Public Health in India: Five Decades*, Vol. I, p. 20-21
8. Quoted in Waldo, Ideas and Issues in Public Administration, p. 71.
9. UN: The Administration of National Development Planning Report of a meeting of Experts (ST/TAD/M/32) Paras.
10. *Ibid.*
11. R.K. Sapru, Coping with an Information overload, *The Daily Tribune*, 27th March, 2000.
12. Justice, H.R. Khanna, Sardar Patel Memorial Lecture, 1977.

2

CHAPTER

Planning and Management of Health Project

PROJECTS CONSTITUTE IMPORTANT TOOLS IN THE PROCESS OF DEVELOPMENT

A. Meaning, Nature and Characteristics of Health Projects

Health administration. whether in developed or developing countries. is facing administrative and managerial problems in providing total health care to their population. Health policy planning consists primarily in developing long and medium-term health goals and criteria. Health programme planning is that part of planning process that aims at selecting the best out of a number of health alternatives. Health project planning is primarily concerned with the building up of an operational capacity in order to produce the services considered necessary for the achievement of the strategic objectives. The success of the achievement of health goals depends to a great extent upon the success of the implementation of projects. This is the most neglected area in the developing countries. The success of our Five Year Plans and Annual Plans depend to a substantial extent upon the effective project management. In the developing countries, projects are neither properly prepared nor implemented, resulting in the wastage of resources. Before we discuss the procedures for the formulation and implementation of the health projects, let us first of all, define the terms programme and project.

Definition of Programme

Webster's seventh new collegiate dictionary defines, "Programme" as a brief outline of the order to be pursued or the subjects embraced." In one of the U.N. publications, Professor Egbert de Vries takes the programme to mean, "a form of organized social activity with a specific objective, limited in space and time. It often consists of an inter-related group of projects and usually is limited to one more organisation and activities."[1]

In the Field of Health. Programme is Considered to Be "Changes in the output of the health system such as the provision of medical care, environmental health, and other health services-these being considered as operating services or programme."[2]

Definition of a Project

As stated in a UN publication entitled Manual on Economic Development, Project is defined as "the compilation of data which will enable an appraisal be made of the economic advantages and disadvantages attendant upon the allocation of country's resources to the production of specific goals and services."[3]

It further states that the projects are "a link in the process of successive approximations involved in the technique of programming and an important element in the flexibility and continuous revision of the programme.[4]

As stated in a Health Project Management Manual issued by WHO, a health project is a:

"temporary intensive effort to set-up and put into operation a new or revised service (or programme) that will it is believed, result in the education of specified health and health-related problems. This intensive effort takes the form of a coordinated set of activities with well-defined objectives and target dates for their achievement. Once the project objectives have been achieved—once the service or programme is set-up the project team disbands, leaving the service to operate on its own."[5]

A 'project' is defined as "the specification and accomplishment, within a given period, of a related set of activities that will result in a measurable change in a health system's capacity to improve the health status of a community."[6]

Characteristics

From these definitions, we can locate the characteristics which are common to all projects. A project aims at specific goals and purposes. Secondly, it is a time-bound activity. Thirdly, it requires cooperation and coordination with other projects to achieve the goals of the plan. A project may be small or wide; limited or comprehensive in nature and space. It may be set-up with purely indigenous resources or with the help of bilateral agencies or with the help of multilateral technical assistance. The most important health projects in the developing countries like India are provided by the WHO. The term 'Project' is used in the following discussion as a generic concept. No attempt is made to classify the projects into different categories or to specify the unique administrative requirements of different types of projects. The emphasis on the common administrative elements of project, irrespective of their size, sector or substance. Their administrative elements should, *mutatis mutandis,* apply to all projects. Recent examples of Projects started in India are Reproductive and Child health (RCH), Cancer Control Programme, Diabetic Control Programme. The health experts must learn the art and science of project management to make the health programmes a success. We are getting a large number of projects from South-East Asia Regional Office of World Health Organisation, World Bank, USAID and many other sources. All these projects are of great significance and their resources must be used profitably. A relevant trend has been to encourage technical cooperation among developing countries (TCDC). It is the process through which developing countries can share their development capacities, i.e. ideas practised and resources so as to make possible a sustained and continuous economic and social growth through their joint efforts. After an early period of philanthropy and paternalism, international action towards development switched to the idea of technical assistance. During the last decade, this approach evolved to a rather subtle and new dimension, described as "technical cooperation", based upon the dual principles of self-reliance and cooperation among nations. From the idea of 'help' or 'aid', we have moved to the idea of cooperation. D.R. Ferreria, Chief of Human Resources at the Washington Headquarters of WHO's Region of the Americas has rightly said: "But although attitudes have changed the whole process of cooperation is hampered in its development by the rigidity of bureaucratic procedures. The mobilisation of resources alone, while easily definable in terms of time and quality of specialist and the number of recipient country trainees, all too often results in a dissertation of the real needs. Thus, a tendency arises to perpetuate the need for high cost resident or long-term international consultants. Conversely, the piece-meal approach of scattering extremely limited resources in a broad and superficial coverage of almost any health-related field often jeopardizes the major goal of solving relevant priority problems." He further adds that:

> "Development that is based on local potentials and on interchanges among countries of similar technological capacity can be promoted through international technical cooperation in the following ways: By elaborating development plans and strategies including feasibility studies, pre-transfer research and the collection of information and basic ways;
>
> - By creating, adapting and diffusing, appropriate technology;
> - By creating an institutional infrastructure; and
> - By formulating and carrying out experimental programmes with innovative and multi-disciplinary approaches."

Here, we would be concentrating mostly on the administrative implications of the technical assistance provided through the South-East Asia Regional Office of the World Health Organisation to its member-states. The observations are valid for all types of external assistance in the field of Health.

All the technical assistance provided by these international organisations take the form of projects. A written request from the Government concerned is the firm basis of Planning and implementing a project.

B. Steps Involved in Project Management

Origin of a Project

Projects usually do not emerge themselves. The motivation and decision to set-up a health project mostly emerge within the health organisations at various levels. Sometimes, bilateral and multilateral agencies ask the health organisation to set-up a project. The impetus to set-up a project can come from the political parties, pressure groups, interest groups or can emerge from the research. evaluation or studies conducted by the universities and training institutions. Before the project may take birth, it is necessary to ensure that the project is:

(a) according to the health policy of the country;
(b) able to meet the priority needs of the people;
(c) linked properly with the objectives and goals of health planning;
(d) fitted into the overall economic and social development of the country;
(e) properly linked with projects in the allied area; and
(f) able to achieve useful and permanent results.

There must also be sufficient administrative capability and financial resources to continue the programme after the termination of the project. All these factors are very important in order to conceive a sound health project. Lack of well conceived projects retard the Implementation of development projects. Most of the schemes in the field of health management come under this category. For example, in India, the policies regarding centrally sponsored projects originate from the Union Government. The State governments adopt these projects as these are cent per cent aided by the Union Government, without taking into consideration the above-mentioned facts. This results in great wastage of human and material resources. J.M. Kitchulu, while outlining the phases of life cycle of a project says: "The need of carrying out detailed planning is being increasingly recognized but there are still cases where projects are being approved without essential steps regarding all stages of preparation and scrutiny being undertaken in the pre-construction stage. This has resulted in the formulation of

Incompletely conceived plans and estimates and thus has led to unsound decisions on projects size, scope, location and product mix."[7]

The effective project choice would enhance the value of plans as well. As stated in a UN publication, "The availability of well-conceived projects and the institution of work on their formulation simultaneously with the institution of the formulation of plans will improve their implementability. By the time a plan is finalized and improved enough projects should be available to go in the implementation phases."[8]

Project Formulation

Project formulation becomes a large and complex task after a positive decision has been taken on a project idea. We have to spell out here all the input in a comprehensive form. The manual of Health Project Management lists nine steps required for the project formulation (see Chart 2.1). In step 1, i.e. preparation of project formulation. The health organisation appoints a team to formulate the project. A term of reference, including time dimension, expected results, resources and problems is decided upon. The team obtains the necessary data required for the concerned project. Steps 2 and 3, relating to situation analysis. may be done simultaneously or one after the other. In Step 2, i.e. analysis of Organisational Situation: a clear picture of the organisational environment is worked out, description of the relevant organisation and agencies, their decision-making process, past experiences relating to the success or failure of the project, need of current or future levels of the resources for the project, etc. the team should concentrate on producing reasonable and informative summaries. In Step 3 Analysing the health socio-economic and demography situation, the present and future analysis is done of the health situation, the socio-economic situation, and the demographic situation. In precise terms, we can say that it may be useful to group the problems into the following categories:

1. Environmental factors—lack of safe water and over crowding, prevalence of mosquitoes or other pests.
2. General or ill-defined conditions—malnutrition. accidents, etc.
3. Not well defined conditions—malaria. measles., etc.
4. General symptoms—fever, respiratory difficulties.
5. Results of health conditions—temporary disability—permanent impairment, deaths.
6. Health service difficulties—excess or under utilization of health services, critical resource shortages, poor staff performance.
7. Socio-economic factors—that contribute or are influenced by health problems, low family income, illiteracy, cultural or religious habits, etc.

In Step 4, Analysis and projection of the problems', we define the problems and projection of the future situation which is worked out on the assumption that existing trends continue without changes in the relevant systems and their policies.

CHART 2.1

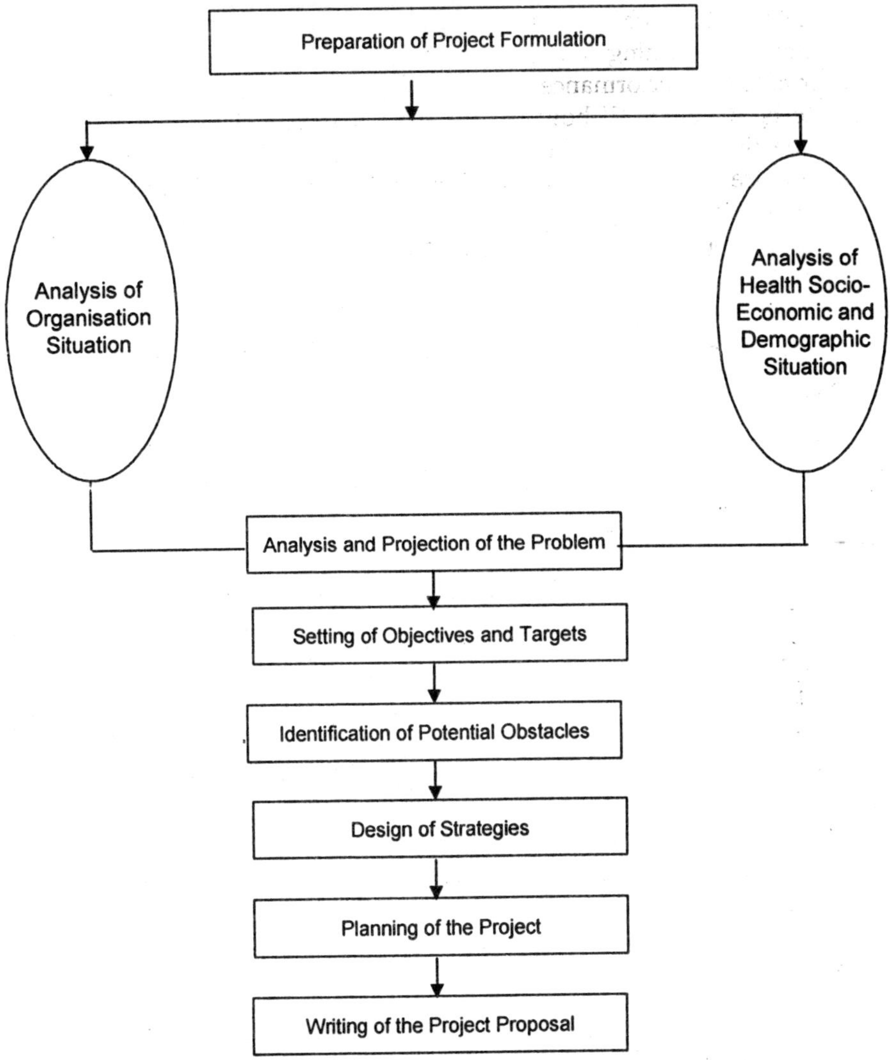

In Step 5, 'Setting the objectives and targets', entails a statement of the problem-reduction to be achieved through the project and translating them into the kind and magnitude of services (operational targets) that would have to be provided at various stages in the future in order to reach the objectives.

In Step 6, 'Identification of potential obstacle', an attempt is made to predict the potential obstacles that might stand In the way of reaching the operational targets established in Step 5.

In Step 7, 'Design of Strategies' the key sub-steps involved are the establishment of explicit criteria of strategy design, the selection of flexible strategies, the assessment of their implications in costs and resources requirements, and the revision of the targets and strategies under consideration in the light of assessment.

In Step 8, 'Planning the Project', the team decides an organisational design for efficient performance. The thinking of the team shifts here from 'what is to be developed?' how it is to be developed?

In the final Step 9, 'Writing the Project Proposal', the products of earlier steps are re-examined, synthesised and documented in the form of a project proposal.

In this whole process, the details would differ from country to country:

(1) In situations where such planning has not taken place, the formulation procedures provide useful guidance and support to such planning as part of project formulation.
(2) In situations in which such higher-level planning has taken place, the analytical and general design steps would be considerably, shortened and more specific in content than the procedures now indicates."[9]

TABLE 2.1

Aspects	*Basic Questions*
1. Technical	1. Is the project sound form the technical and engineering point of view ?
2. Economic	1. Is the project in a sector of high priority?
	2. Is the project likely to contribute to the development of that sector?
3. Financial	1. Is the enterprise to construct and operate the project financially sound?
	2. What financing will be needed to bring facility into operation and from what sources ?
	3. What will be the probable operational costs and revenues, prospective liquidity and rate of return?
4. Commerical	1. Have adequate arrangements been made for the supply of goods and services needed for construction?
	2. Have adequate arrangements been made for the supply of inputs needed in the operaton?
5. Organisational	1. Is the organisation proposed to carry out and to operate the project likely to be successful ?

	2.	Would outside help be needed ?
	3.	Are prospective controls adequate?
6. Managerial	1.	What is the quality of the proposed management ? Is it likely to be adequate to ensure performance not inferior to that to be expected from the appraisal?
7. Social	1.	What are the changes caused by the project in the behavioral pattern, and the attitude in the population?
	2	What are the attitudes of the population towards the projects?
	3.	Does the projects require specific elements of social change?
8. Environmental	1.	Does the project cause pollution?
	2.	Does the project disturb the equilibrium of ecology?
	3.	Does the project fit into the enviornment

After the project has been formulated, there is a need to examine its soundness. J.P. Gupta feels that in the appraisal of a project, the following questions need to be answered.[10] (see Table 2.1)

Project planning has to be more scientific and approval procedure more realistic to ensure that avoidable time and cost overruns are much less frequent. The approval procedure should be linked with early completion of incomplete projects and sustainability of project output. Because of the unrealistic approval procedure, many of the projects are delayed. At the other extreme, less stringent approval procedures encourage a tendency to get too many projects cleared without the requisite financial resources in sight. There is, thus, a need for striking a balance between these extremes. It is important to ensure that rigour in appraisal and planning does not itself become a cause of delay because of repetitive and multi-level examination of technical and economic data. Strict time-tables need to be laid down for completion of the approval processes and preliminary work. Similarly, strict financial procedures should be formulated for eliminating projects, which do not have financial backing.

The lesson learnt from the experience of executing thousands of development schemes during the last forty years can be briefly summarised as follows:

- There is inadequate analysis of available information during programme formulations. This happens primarily, because there is no established mechanism through which the programme agencies can have ready access to the relevant information regarding the target groups/areas or the findings of evaluation studies. As a result, avoidable errors at the planning stage creep in. For example, in a programme designed for the empowerment of rural women, the basic and well known fact that most rural women, in India are illiterate was not explicitly considered while formulating the operational rules and designing the delivery system.

- The operational cost of some programmes tends to be abnormally high, partly because of redundant and ineffective administration and partly due to other inadequacies in planning and implementation.
- The general approach in implementation is "top-down" and "target-oriented." Some physical and financial targets are sought to be achieved in most programmes. However, evaluation studies by the Planning Commission reveal that the fulfilment of these targets does not necessarily ensure that the programme objectives are being met. In many anti-poverty programmes though the targeted number of families/beneficiaries/districts/ villages have been covered and the allotted money spent, such programmes have failed in making the desired impact on the well-being of the beneficiaries. The implementing agencies are often more concerned with the mere fulfilment of targets assigned to them than with the actual flow of benefits to the target groups.
- Formulation of a multiplicity of programmes in an area of social concern without any specific thrusts can lead to several problems. Available resources are spread too thinly across a large number of projects leading to sub-optimal projects outcome.
- For some programmes separate implementing agencies are created, whereas these are actually implemented by the existing line departments, who work independently for different components of a programme. This results in lack of focus on target groups, wastage of resources and lack of coordination among the line departments. The creation of such agencies without the necessary institutional changes makes them redundant and affects the implementation and operation of programmes.

Lack accountability of the implementing agencies either to the Government or to the people has been the single major cause for diversion of funds in development programmes. Several social sector programmes are formulated without addressing the question of sustainability of benefits. The most distressing part of financing of the development projects and programme under the Five Year Plan regime has been the failure to ensure timely and adequate flow of funds to the implementing agencies.

The essential ingredients of people's participation for self-development, as revealed in the success stories, are assessment of local resources and local level planning, sensitizing people and building local organisations for collective actions and an umbrella support mechanism to facilitate people's development actions. If these processes and mechanisms are to be multiplied on a wider scale: these will have to be institutionalized. The multiplication process requires a major political commitment by the State to provide the necessary political space and a policy framework for a sensitive support mechanism. This will call for, among other things, simplification of ground rules that would facilitate participation of grass roots level organisations in the development process, bringing about flexibility and dynamism among the providers of public services, and orienting the judicial system for speedy disposal of disputes and be sensitive to the needs of the disadvantaged people.

Project Implementation (See Chart 2.2)

Proper implementation of the project is vital and great attention and energy are required to ensure this. In this context, India's Planning Commission said:

'The success of the Plan will rest very largely on the efficiency with which it is implemented." The purpose of implementation is to ensure that the project activities have been completed on schedules and within a budget, and that there are favourable conditions to maintain the desired changes generated by the project after the project as such is terminated. Project implementation steps are repetitive ones and each project manager will have to adopt the procedures according to his own set-up depending upon the nature of the project and the organisation structures. The steps of implementation, i.e. from 10-16 have been discussed in the Health Project Management Manual, which are described below: (Chart 2.2)

CHART 2.2

Steps in Project Management

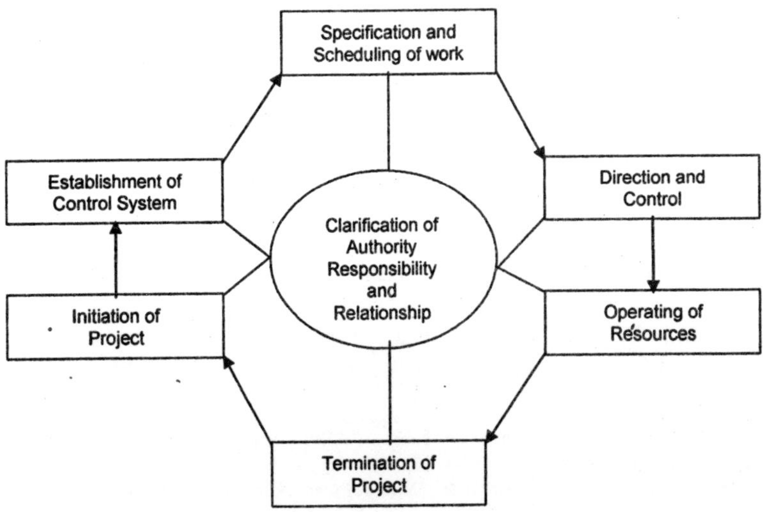

Evaluation of Projects

All development projects undertaken need to be evaluated for the results they have achieved or failed to achieve. Careful evaluation is the backbone of all projects. It is indispensable as a guarantee of effective use of resources, and of accountability for their use. Evaluation of results achieved in a project is required in order to benefit fully from the experience. Evaluation would be futile unless it is carried out in a systematic and coordinated fashion with clearly defined objectives and consistent procedures applied by competent evaluators. Barnabas contends that "to be most effective, evaluation must not be made merely of physical achievements but also of the cost of such achievements."[11]

Evaluation can be effective only if we have well designed format to secure timely, regular and dependable information on the performance of projects. Thus a reporting system is essential. Most of the health projects operating at the Union, State and local levels can be classified into two categories:

(a) Indigenous projects., i.e. projects run without any bilateral or multilateral technical assistance.
(b) Projects assisted through bilateral or multilateral technical assistance.

Such a step ensures the following inherent advantages:

- It would aid in Project Management and control throughout the duration of the Project.
- It would help to ensure compliance with user community objectives before implementation.
- Process of systems design would be evaluated at all stages to aid in improving effectiveness of the Design Teams.
- Cost savings would be realized by modifying systems through evaluation before, rather than after implementation.
- Evaluation would help to ensure that proper design procedures and policies were being carried out.*

Ninth Five Year Plan has also suggested the need for monitoring and Evaluation. The need for an effective monitoring and evaluation (M & E) system was felt as early as in the First Plan itself. The First Plan document stated that "with increased investment on development, more attention to systematic assessment and evaluation of the results from public expenditure was necessary. With every important programme, provision should always be made for the assessment of results. Inspite of considerable development

---

* Gary/Green and Robert T. Kein, "After Implementation, What's Next ? Evaluation", *Journal of Systems Management*, Vol. 34, No. 9, Issue No. 269, Sept. 1983, Association for Systems Management, Cleveland, Chill.

in economic and social sciences, our knowledge of human motivation and social processes is but limited. We cannot always say for certain that a given set of causes will produce a particular, clearly definable, set of results and none other." The Second Plan document emphasized the need for a strong M & E system for building up a strong development administration, training of personnel, informing and educating the public and organizing a sound system of planning based as much on the participation of the people at each level as on the best technical, economic and statistical information available. As a review of the past Plan performance revealed gaps in achievement in various areas of development, the need for a strong M & E system only got reinforced in subsequent Plan documents. over time and elaborate monitoring and evaluation mechanism has been built for efficient development administration and a large number of institutions for training in public administration at the Centre and State level have been created. While the M & E system has proved its utility in development administration, it is not as effective as it should be. The scope and nature of development programmes have been undergoing changes and the interaction between a programme and its environment is becoming increasingly complex. The government now operates under increasing financial and competitive pressures. The M & E system has not shown the necessary dynamism to cope with these changes and complexities. The Working Group on Monitoring and Information System of the Seventh Five Year Plan identified the following programs:

- Ineffectiveness in identifying/reducing likely delays and problems;
- Large data gaps, delays in data generation and transmission, inadequate data;
- Analysis, feedback not reaching proper users;
- Inadequate information on interlinked projects.
- Information difficult to retrieve in the absence of data bank;
- Information not reflecting the true picture;
- More emphasis on reporting than on action; and
- Inadequate use of monitored information in decision-making

We shall now examine these projects to find out the causes of unsatisfactory performance and their solutions.

C. Working of Projects

We are analysing here the management of health projects, i.e. from the planning to implementation and evaluation. Every health project is affected by the capacity and morale of persons associated with it. No single factor by itself determines the success or failure of a project; a combination of several adverse factors may, however, injure and wreck it. In the field of health, a large number of projects have proved failure. This was indicated and accepted by all the persons who were interviewed. All were of the view that some radical changes and innovations were required to manage the health projects efficiently. Let us examine critically the factors which have been responsible for the total or partial failure of the health project. The writer contacted different persons to rank the causes of unsatisfactory working of health projects on the basis of their preferences. The persons interviewed were selected on random basis. These causes were framed on the basis of the study of the official records, discussion with health experts and persons connected with the formulation and implementation of health projects. The causes have been arranged accordingly:

(1) Lack of training and motivation on the part of the persons associated with the project formulation.
(2) Absence of well-designed health information system to provide reliable and timely information for the formulation of health projects.
(3) Poor linkages among the allied projects.
(4) Lack of clarity among the personnel responsible for the implementation of health projects.
(5) Projects under the centrally sponsored schemes are not adapted but adopted.
(6) Absence of full involvement of the beneficiaries in the formulation and implementation of projects.
(7) Absence of any satisfactory monitoring system to measure the regulated performance during implementation.
(8) Lack of proper follow-up after the termination of the project.
(9) Health projects not dovetailed with health policy. health plans and programmes.
(10) Unscientific manpower planning-insufficient utilization of project personnel.
(11) Lack of clarification of authority, responsibilities and relationship.
(12) Irregular supply of inputs of right quality impede the smooth progress of the project.
(13) No reservoir of any cumulative implementation experience of the completed projects in the past.
(14) Faulty and cumbersome administrative procedure. Let us now discuss in detail each of these factors.
(15) No correlation between need, resources and use.

I. Lack of Training and Motivation of the Project Formulation Team

Most of the persons associated with the project formulation have neither the requisite skill nor the necessary aptitude to formulate the health project in consonance with the goals of the project. In developing countries, people are appointed to work in the project formulation team on the basis of their status and not on the basis of their capability and interest. Besides. it is understood in these countries that any general administrator can take up formulation of a project. This assumption in this age of specialization and sophistication does not hold good. Project formulation is an art which must be learnt and developed. Secondly, it requires hard work and motivation. Even the best trained persons are of no use if they do not possess high morale—a socio-psychological situation in which men and women voluntarily work on a chosen field because of their intellectual satisfaction. The trained persons with high morale can be very successful in the management of health projects. It has been rightly mentioned that. "Project formulation can be characterized in two words—hard work. The fact that logical sequence of steps is outlined, some of which utilize techniques of systems analysis and modern management. This should not mislead the reader into thinking that this is a quick and easy method for producing bullet-proof proposals. A good deal of information must be reviewed. structured and manipulated. A great deal of thinking must be done by intelligent. experienced and practical people for this method to yield its full benefits. This being said. it is felt that the formulation method has features that can help ensure that reasonable proposals for Improving the state of health of a given population can be produced in a reasonable amount of time through the concentrated efforts of a handful of dedicated people."[12]

Before implementing the health project it would be better to arrange a workshop to provide training for the persons responsible for this task. In such a workshop, potential difficulties may be analysed and solutions may be found to solve such difficulties. The workshop should not be convened into a classroom situation. but should encourage active participation so that participants get sufficient training and motivation to handle the project.

2. Absence of Well-Designed Health Information System to Provide Reliable and Timely Information

Health and vital statistics are the bricks and mortar of health Planning, policy-making and project management. In the field of health management there are no well-designed information systems to cater to the needs of planners and administrators. We have the statistical sections in the health directorates but without any pre-designed system of information. It is important to utilize existing data and documents profitably. In the developing countries, more information is available from a variety of sources than can be used effectively. It is very important to select the most reliable and relevant data from among the many overlapping sources. The information system, key to health project management planning, implementation and evaluation should produce statistical information which is:

(a) relevant to the needs;
(b) sufficiently reliable to serve the purpose for which it is collected;
(c) usable-it is better to collect less information of sufficient reliability than to collect a mass of data of unsatisfactory quality; and

(d) comparable, i.e. uniformity of health statistics system in terms of its organisational structure and the scope and contents of the data collected.

The quality of data needed for the different stages of the health project management—formulation, implementation, evaluation would be different. Hence, a system of health information may be designed in collaboration and cooperation between the planners, project managers, administrators and the health statisticians.

As stated in a UN publication:

(a) The system should generate information that is available in time and is designed to be readily usable for decision-making.
(b) It should establish both financial and performance accountability.
(c) It should have a format that will facilitate its use for more than one purpose.
(d) It should provide each echelon with the information it needs."[13]

3. Poor Linkages Among file Allied Projects

In a particular geographical or functional area. a number of projects are being implemented to improve the standard of living of the people, most of these projects are complimentary and supplementary. Because of the poor coordination among the various departments at the state level, the projects are implemented in the area without developing linkages with each other. It was mentioned in the Draft Plan (1978-83) that inadequate attention to inter-linkages, the lack of systems approach and poor monitoring and evaluation feed-back systems are the major problems in this area identified in the previous plans. For example, the projects of adult education can be of great significance for any health project.[14] Every health project can serve its clients better if they possess functional literacy. A project for the agriculture development to grow more food can be beautifully linked with the health projects on nutrition. Population control has many dimensions and needs the cooperation of many agencies. Thus, there is a need of area planning and developing an integrated area approach where different projects may develop linkages to have optimum benefit. This can be nicely explained with the help of the operations of the Central Government Health Scheme (CGHS). This scheme has been extended to a number of public undertakings, semi-government organisations, autonomous bodies on payment of full contributions. Similarly, seven undertakings outside Delhi have allowed the Central Government employees to receive medical treatment on payment in the hospital run by them. The Estimates Committee is of the view that,

"There should be integrated planning in the setting up of medical facilities by the government and the public undertakings so that there is no duplication and overlapping. Thus, there is a need of area planning and developing an integrated area approach where different projects may develop linkages to have optimum benefit."

4. *Personnel Responsible for the Implementation of Health Projects not Clear about their Role*

In most of the developing countries, there is a dichotomy between the personnel responsible for the formulation and the personnel responsible for the implementation of the health projects. The latter are not clear about the implications of the project. Because of lack of Identity. they develop low morale resulting in poor management. It was mentioned by a number of persons working on various projects that they were thrown into the fields. "to operate the projects without proper briefing about the project and its rationale in the total health system. Besides, the supervisors, at the headquarters, never guide us about our role in the project."

Furthermore, the persons are transferred during the operation of the project resulting in the induction of new untrained persons. There has been hardly any project where the persons appointed in the beginning of the project implementation had continued till the termination of the project. Thus, there is a great need of the involvement of the persons associated with the implementation of the projects at some stage of the formulation to appraise them of the full implications of the project. Besides, they must be briefed properly and recurrent guidance may be provided to keep them rightly informed. This will develop a good rapport between the formulation and implementation of the projects.[15]

5. *Projects under the Centrally-Sponsored Schemes are not Adapted but Adopted*

There are a large number of projects in the field of health and family welfare administration which are sponsored by the Union Government (India). States get 100 percent reimbursement on such schemes. The schemes designed by the Centre cannot suit all the areas equally well. The administrative machinery and inputs of the projects must be designed by the State governments according to the ecological conditions existing in that area. For example, the family planning projects must be adjusted according to the needs of the area. What is happening is that the structure devised by the Union Government for the implementation of the projects is adopted by the State government. This becomes the main cause of the failure of a number of projects.

6. *Absence of the Full Involvement of the Beneficiaries in the Formulation and Implementation of Projects*

Health projects are manned by and meant for human beings. The success or failure of the projects ultimately depends upon the acceptance of these projects by the people. If the people are not taken into confidence during formulation and implementation of projects, these would be less successful. People's participation can enhance the chances of success of the projects. Most of the beneficiaries; contacted by the writer were of the view that beneficiaries are not treated as equal partners in the process of formulation and implementation of projects. The failure of the scheme, e.g. primary health centres, multi-purpose workers, etc. is because of the absence of identity of the people with these projects. It is essential for the health experts in the developing countries to motivate and encourage the people to participate in the formulation and implementation of projects. Although people's participation in affairs governing their lives dates back to the beginning of human society, the concept has taken a new dimension as societies have grown in size and complexity. This is partly because the management has become more and more a specialized enterprise, an area for technocrats and trained general administrators and political leaders. Although they officially advocate and preach people's involvement, in practice they bring them into the picture only after the major decisions have been made. Hence they often leave the ordinary citizens to follow their pre-determined paths. Peter Berger agrees with this contention when he says that "the overwhelming majority of these people have little or no opportunity to influence policy, and their perspectives on the situation are systematically ignored by almost all theorists. For them the problem of development is one of the everyday life."[16]

This is very serious in the field of health projects. The health projects are generally concentrated in cities to benefit the vested interests and urban population. This imbalance can be corrected if the people are involved. We must encourage the setting up of new health projects to benefit the rural people and involve them actively to ensure lasting and permanent benefits. Once the people take the initiative and responsibility to look after their health, we have won more than half the battle.

Local communities are treated as passive participants in improvement and bettering of their lives. Most of the project personnel working in the villages return to the cities after their duty hours. The villagers cannot make their views known to them in cities. The result is lack of communication among them. When the project fails it is intentionally ascribed to the obstinacy, fatalism, illiteracy or apparent irrationality of the poor people. The potential for community involvement has been seriously underestimated. We must encourage people's participation through all methods to promote development.

7. *Absence of Satisfactory Monitoring System to measure the Regulated Performance During Implementation*

Most of the health projects are never completed within the budgeted resources and fixed time schedules. It has become a normal feature to extend the life of the project resulting in the wastage of huge financial resources. It clearly indicates the weakness of the controlling mechanism. Project control is the managerial function that helps the managers to keep the project functioning as scheduled. It is possible only if the realistic advance targets of output are fixed before implementation. This is not being done as is evident from the perusal of most of the projects studied.

Monitoring, if properly designed, can help the managers in keeping the process of implementation as scheduled. The project performance is compared at different intervals of times with the control indicators. Whenever deviations are located, cause of deviations are examined and solutions are found to correct the deviations. The following are the general causes of deviation:

(1) Excessive optimism on the part of the project planners, resulting in unrealistic estimates in respect to the time, funds. Manpower or other resources required to do an activity—the possibility of achieving expected results.
(2) Unforeseen resistance from or changes in the environment of the project (natural disaster, political changes).
(3) Decisions at higher managerial levels to change the planned resources inputs of the project e.g.. (change of a staff member).
(4) Inefficient administrative procedures.

If there is any unavoidable deviation beyond the control of the project authorities, we can think of alternative proposals immediately without wasting the future resources. If such timely action is taken, the developing countries can be sure of the success of the projects. More safely designing the control system means specifying who reports what to whom and when.

Seven Five Year Plan observes the important features of Monitoring the primary responsibility of monitoring lies with the agency entrusted with the execution of programme/project.

- The monitoring responsibility cannot be entrusted to a single individual. It must be a group effort.
- Monitoring should not be construed as a mistrust or a direct interference in the functioning of an organisation.
- Monitoring team should have the motto of furnishing fearless, honest and business like reports.
- Monitoring to be effective and a dynamic force pre-supposes a firm commitment, involvement and team spirit from all concerned.
- Monitoring and scheduling being inter-dependent should have a close rapport with each other.
- In relatively small projects, it would be advisable if both these functions are performed by one body known as scheduler or monitor.
- The scope of monitoring need not be confined to top management. Instead, information in a filtered form may flow from the field to the highest authorities pinpointing critical areas at the appropriate levels.
- Monitoring team should be manned by those who are talented, trained and have the aptitude in the art of monitoring. Suitable

environment also needs to be created so that the personnel get job satisfaction and their future is not at stake.

- The time interval of measuring progress should be in direct proportion (appropriate) to the phenomenon being studied.
- Information reports may be made available to those who can really facilitate in influencing a timely action on them.

In the case of monitoring of complex projects, renowned Project Management Companies may be engaged who have vast experience of project execution and also keep a band of specialists from all disciplines with them. The Seventh Plan document has also stressed the need for developing management consultancy to play its role in quick and economical execution of projects.

8. Lack of Proper Follow-up after the Completion of the Project

It has been observed generally that the programmes are generally shelved on one pretext or the other after the termination of the project. There is a great fan fare when the project is set-up but it would be of no use if the projects; do not continue and convert into permanent on going activities. For example, many projects on health education were terminated without becoming a part and parcel of the life of the community. In the case of Malaria Control Programme, many projects were initiated. After their completion, there was slackness resulting in the resurgence of malaria. Sometimes, this situation emerges because of the change of political leadership. Political leaders are more interested to develop those projects which can make them popular in the eyes of the people rather than looking to their permanent impact. Thus, many health projects come up not because of the priority health sole needs of the people but because of political expediency. These projects die after premature deaths or are wound up after some time wasting the scarce resources. There is a great need to improve the capability, ethos, perception and attitudes of the political elite so that they can take correct decisions in the ultimate interest of the people. Gabriel A. Almoud defines political development in terms of performance capabilities. To him political development is, "the acquisition of new capability, in the sense of a specialized role structure and differentiated orientations which together give a political system of possibility of responding efficiently and more or less autonomously to new range of problems."[17]

Thus, "a political system is said to be developing when there is an increase in its ability to sustain successfully and continuously new types of social goals and creation of new types of organisations."[18]

There is also a possibility that resources may not be budgeted for the continuation of the project after the plan period. Many of the centrally-sponsored schemes in India continue only till the aid is coming from the Union Government. After the aid is stopped, these projects are wound up. It is important to see that the projects are not only formulated and implemented scientifically but should also continue to benefit the people.

9. Health Projects not Dovetailed with Health Policy, Health Plans and Programmes

Health projects are not the outcome of health plans and programmes resulting in the poor impact on the total development. Where policy objectives have been clearly defined, health programme planning can be substantially improved by moving form piecemeal ad hoc decision to a more comprehensive and scientific approach, which provides an opportunity to formulate health programmes and select health development projects with greater coherence and effectiveness. The boundaries between phases of planning may be flexible, as indicated by the shaded area, and each phase is linked to all others by the feed-back of information. The loop suggests that the planning process is interactive and cyclical in nature. (See Chart 2.4)

CHART 2.3

10. Initiation of the Project

All the preparations are made for the starting of the project, obtaining approval for the project proposal.

11. Specifying and Scheduling the Work

Projecting the details of work and deciding what tasks are to be done by whom, and when.

12. Clarifying Authority, Responsibility and Relationships

Obtaining agreement as to who is responsible for ensuring that the work gets done, distributing decision-making authority among the project team and the existing organisational units, and establishing formal lines of communication.

13. Obtaining Resources

Obtaining the funds. manpower, supplies, and equipment necessary for doing the project activities.

14. Establishing the Control System

Determining what information is necessary for project control, identifying sources of such Information, and setting up reporting systems for the project.

15. Directing and Controlling

Motivating project, staff executing project activities, obtaining information for control, and taking corrective action as necessary.

16. Terminating the Project

Handing over responsibilities to existing organisational units, reassigning staff, and preparing the final report. The implementation machinery can resort to modern methods of management to achieve desired results.

CHART 2.4

Hierarchy of Goals	Relationship (Feedback) Between Planning Phases	Planning Phase	Outcome
Goals	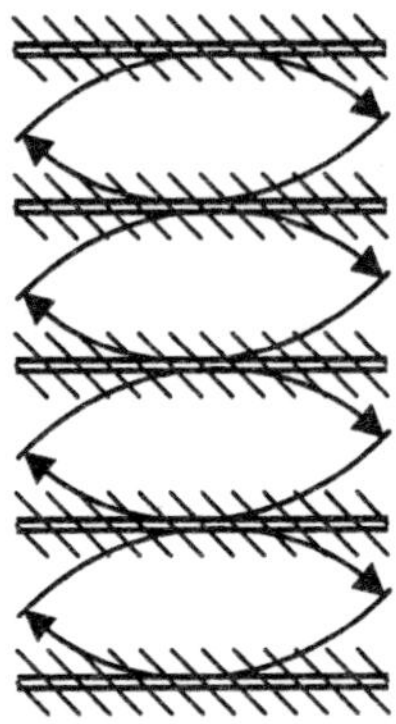		
Policy Objectives		Health Policy Planning	Health Policy Plan
Strategic Objectives		Health Programme Planning	Health Programme Proposal
Operational Objectives		Operational Health Planning	Health Project Proposal
Input (Resources)			

10. Unscientific Manpower Planning: Insufficient Utilization of Project Personnel

The success of the project depends upon the quality and quantity of personnel associated with it. It was observed that in many projects, the projects personnel have their utilization time as low as 20 per cent. This is highly serious as the resources are being consumed by the establishment rather than invested in the welfare of the people. Because of the absence of manpower planning, personnel of the project utilized very little time. People in the area remarked about the workers appointed to motivate people to adopt family planning norm. "They are not available at all. They rarely devote any time for this work. They remain away from their work."

It is essential to see through proper manpower planning that only needed persons are appointed and they are utilised to ensure full benefits. These projects should aim at achieving an increase in the overall cost productivity, efficiency and effectiveness. The projects should be so-administered as to lead to overall improvement in its performance. Let us examine a case to illustrate our viewpoints. The Pasteur Institute of Southern India, Coonoor, has been able to produce only 4.61 1akh trivalent doses of vaccine from December 1966 to May 1973 in a span of about 6+ years while the annual capacity was 12.5 lakh doses. The average annual production works out to only 6 per cent of the capacity of the unit. Besides the cost of production at this Institute comes to about 50 paise per dose while the cost of imported vaccine comes to only about 15 paise. There are many other problems in the institute. Two studies were conducted by a senior official of the Indian Council of Medical Research and by a team of officers of the Council, the National Institute of Communicable Disease. Directorate General of Health Services and the Drug Controller. The following reported facts were responsible for the unsatisfactory state of affairs:

(a) Lack of cooperation and rapport and a complete breakdown of human and personal relationships between the personnel of the production unit and the Director of the Institute.
(b) Carelessness on the part of middle-level supervisory staff in coordinating the activities of the unit.
(c) Absence of the long range plan of work, non-fixation of targets of production, non-assignment of responsibilities and the absence of frequent and regular checks.
(d) Non-availability of trained middle-level staff.
(e) A complete breakdown of the measures that would ensure sterility in the production chamber.
(f) Inadequate maintenance of equipment and records.[19]

The Public Accounts Committee was of the view that "Effective supervision and prompt remedial measures have been inadequate if not altogether non-existent. Since the technical aspects of production Imperatively call for constant scrutiny, the committee cannot countenance such lapses in the production of a sophisticated vaccine. They desire that the responsibility be fixed for the non-observance of even the basic, elementary requirements of successful production."[20] All these facts must be kept in mind while implementing the health projects,

11. Lack of Clarification of Authority, Responsibility and Relationships

In the developing world, the persons responsible for implementation of tile project do not work as a team as there is no clarification of authority, responsibility and relationships among them, i.e. the roles of the various participants are not often mutually understood. This results in friction and disputes. It becomes very difficult for them to devote their whole attention to the project.

In some of the projects, it was found that the lower levels of staff do not really understand the nature of their duties *vis-a-vis* their supervisors. In such a situation, they become indolent and inefficient. It is, therefore, necessary that the team members should know their duties and relationship between their respective authority and responsibility. One of the persons associated with a particular project went to the extent of saying that "Since the last six months, he is not clear of his responsibilities. He has been appointed without any briefing. He is doing negligible work. The project must clearly define the duties of the manager of the project and the staff. This would help in fixing the responsibilities of the person if something goes wrong. Besides, the project staff, as far as possible, must be posted for the whole duration of the project and the transfers in between should be avoided."

12. Irregular Supply of Quality Inputs Impede the Smooth Progress of the Project

After the project is formulated, the project manager must ensure the availability of necessary inputs. It has been generally observed that the projects are delayed because of the absence of timely availability of all the inputs simultaneously. In one of the projects, the health personnel had no work to do because of the non-availability of vaccine. Obtaining resources is a process that takes place periodically throughout the life of the project. It was revealed that failure to obtain resources simultaneously in time is the most common cause of delay in implementation. The project manager must begin the process of procuring resources immediately after the formulation stage. Sometimes, the process may be started quite early if the resources are scarce and not easily available. The absence of one resource would innate the cost of the project as the other resources would remain idle. The project manager must take the following steps:

(a) Working with the concerned administrative units in preparing a time table of administrative steps to be taken to obtain the planned resources.
(b) Monitoring this time table to ensure that the administrative steps are being completed in time.
(c) Taking corrective action as and when necessary.[21]

In spite of all these precautions. there is a possibility of not reaching the resources in time. What can be done under such critical situations? Most of the experts indicated that the whole project staff remain idle for months together. This is very serious in big projects. It was observed in the Malaria Control Programme that lack of timely supply of DDT delayed the operation of the projects. Many of the newly created hospitals are unable to provide the necessary services as the requisite staff has not been recruited. During the Fourth Plan period. Central Government Health Scheme planned to cover 16 dispensaries for Bombay, 8 for Kanpur, 12 for Calcutta. The actual dispensaries opened were: 5 for Bombay and 3 each in Kanpur and Calcutta. Similar problems were witnessed with regard to the coverage of families. The slow progress of the extension of the scheme in these cities has been attributed to:

(a) Non-availability of suitable accommodation for housing dispensaries;
(b) The delay in getting financial clearance and acceptance by State Governments for the provisions of specialist. consultation and hospitalization facilities for CGHS beneficiaries; and
(c) Non-availability of medical and para-medical staff caused problem. The Committee considered that with their experience of the scheme in Delhi since 1954, it was expected that the government should have foreseen all these difficulties before planning the extension of CGHS facilities to these cities and should have taken advance action to obviate them. It appears that this was not done.[22]

It was suggested that the project officers may be delegated powers to purchase the inputs locally or employ persons, if the resources are not available from the agency as planned. This would help in maintaining the schedule of the project.

13. Past Experience of the Completed Projects not referred to:

It was a great surprise to learn that there are no records of past experiences in relation to the projects implementation. In hospitals, there is a discussion among the faculty members about the reports of the post mortem to ascertain whether the right type of medicine was administered to the patients and If not, what errors were committed. The location of such errors would help the medical personnel to be more intelligent in the future. One can always learn from the mistakes of others. Some of the project personnel remarked that "they did not know anything about the difficulties encountered by the project personnel and the causes of the failures of the projects undertaken earlier."

It is beneficial to examine how major projects have been managed in the past. It would also be better to identify those approaches which have been most successful. We can keep a record of good and bad points of the past projects and this cumulative experience may be passed on to the present project managers. In this way, many of the difficulties likely to be encountered would vanish.

Frank A. Wilson in his article "Planning for Project Management" in the *Journal of Administration Overseas* (July 1979) has rightly mentioned that, "Disappointing and inefficient project performance is a fact of life, *ex-post* evaluation of existing projects can be the means by which we can systematically seek to analyse the potential for improving project management. Evaluation studies gives the opportunity for developing a greater understanding of the way projects are managed and implemented."

14. Faulty and Cumbersome Administrative Procedures

Whenever a project is formulated, we do not pay much attention to the problems of communication. Coordination, headquarters field relationship, supervision, etc. The purpose of these procedures is to help in the smooth functioning of the project. Without proper procedures, most of the project personnel remain engrossed in preparing unnecessary reports. These procedures should be clarified in the initial stages of the project management, so that no confusion arises later on. If there are already set procedures in a particular organisation, these may be adopted otherwise new procedures may be designed and made known to the project personnel. It must be clear that administrative procedures are an aid to help the efficient functioning of the project. The rigid application of these procedures may result in red-tapism and inefficiency.

The Five Year Plan (1978-83) has also indicated the technical, administrative and managerial problems which affect project efficiency. These are mentioned below:

(a) Inadequate investigation and data collection as a result of which the project appraisal, even when it is sought to be done in a systematic way, has to be come out on the basis of wholly inadequate information, thus leading to wrong investment decisions.
(b) Inadequate detailed planning of projects in terms of their time schedules. input resource requirements and skills needed for project implementation.
(c) Lack of delegation of authority to subordinate organisation levels.
(d) Delays in issuing sanctions, approvals, fund authorizations and releases.
(e) Organisational weaknesses in planning and implementation at various levels.
(f) Lack of specific assignment of responsibility and accountability for results.
(g) Problems of industrial relations and inadequate motivation of personnel, lack of proper career planning and incentives and commitment to results.
(h) Inadequate share of representation of the weaker sections in elected bodies in the village. district and block levels and agencies.[23]

15. No Correlation between Need, Resources and Use (See Table 2.2)

To quote WHO; the allocation, organisation and evaluation of human, technological, financial and physical resources are the principal functions of planning. There are a number of ways in which comparable data on perceived need, resources and use can be combined so as to advance our understanding of their relationships. For this purpose, geographically defined areas can be divided in relation to whether they are above or below the medians for appropriate measures of need, use and resources, provided these are defined uniformly for all the project areas and based on comparable data. Table 2.1 shows a model in which areas can be assigned to one of the eight cells on the basis of their relative balance of need, resources, and use. The assignment depends on the findings for each area being above or below the median level of need, resources, or use for all areas in the set. In this model, for example, a relatively high level resources and a relatively high rate of use in the presence of a relatively high rate of perceived need is defined as balance (Type A). Here, the population's perceived need is reflected in a supply of appropriate combination and in levels of use that indicate neither excess capacity of, nor unmet demand for, a particular resource category. Conversely, a relatively low level of use in the presence of low need, is also regarded as constituting balance (Type H).

A cybernetic model like this would not allow the investment in costly resources to continue longer than is justified by the perceived needs of the population, because the information made available to decision-makers would show them that the use of the services or the application of resources

TABLE 2.2

Model of Relationships between Need, Resources and Use

Use	*High Need*		*Low Need*	
	High	*Low*	*High*	*Low*
High	Type A Balanced Appropriate Allocation of Resources	Type B Compensatory High Productivity of Resources	Type E Unbalanced Overuse of Resources	Type F Unbalanced High Productivity of Resources
Low	Type C Unbalanced Under use of Resources	Type D Unbalanced Underinvest-ment in Resources	Type G Unbalanced Overinvest-ment in Resources	Type H Balanced Appropriate Resources

Note: Needs, resources and use may be defined by any appropriate measures as long they are uniform over all the areas being considered.

Source: WHO, Public Health Paper, 67, p. 80.

has become excessive in relationship to perceived need.

We can improve the management of health projects if we keep these difficulties or problems or obstacles in mind and try to reduce them to negligible proportions. Besides. there is a need of training health project personnel in the art of project management. In the developing world, there is dichotomy between the medical, scientific and the social scientists. The medical personnel may be equipped with the knowledge of social sciences, statistics, etc. to make them understand better the implications of health project management or they may be encouraged to seek the guidance of the experts in the social sciences.

NOTES AND REFERENCES

1. Eiben de Vries, "Programme Formulation and Implementation", in *Administration of Development Programmes and Projects, op. cit.,* p 25.
2. WHO: Technical Report Series, p. 596, p. 51.
3. UN. Manual on Economic Development Projects (UN Publications, Sales No. 58 II, G5), p. xii.
4. *Ibid.,* p. 5.
5. J. Bainoodge and S. Sapine, Health Project Management: A Manual of Procedures for Formulating and Implementing Health Projects, WHO, Geneva, 1974, p. 279.
6. WHO: Technical Report Series, 596, p. 50.
7. J.M. Kitchulu, "Project Management", in V.A. Pai Panandiker, (ed.) *Development Administration in India,* (Delhi, Macmillan, 1974, pp. 83-84).
8. UN, Administration of Development Programmes and Projects: Some major

issues continued. (UN: Publication Sale No. E-71, Ii, H.47), p. 75.

9. WHO, Technical Report Series, 596, p. 54
10. J.P. Gupta, "Priorities Appraisal Planning and Implementation."
11. A.P. Babas. "Reporting Appraisal and Evaluation in Development Administration" in V.A. Pai Panandiker (ed., Development Administration in India, Delhi, Macmillian Company, 1974, pp. 219-20).
12. Health Project Management, *op. cit.*, p. 5.
13. Administration of Development Programme and Projects, *op. cit.*, pp. 85-86.
14. Govt. of India, Planning Commission. Draft Plan (1978-83), p. 13.
15. Lok Sabha Secretariat, Fifth Lok Sabha, Fifty Seventh Report, New Delhi, 1974, p. 18.
16. Peter Berger, Pyramids of Sacrifice, Political Ethics and Social Change, Garden City, New York, Anchor Books, 1976, p. 9.
17. Gabriel, A. Almond, "Political System and Political Change" in *American Behavoural Scientists*, Vol. VI, June 1963, p. 9.
18. Alfred Diamand, "Political Development: Approaches to Theory and Strategy", in Montgomery and Stiffin, (eds.) *Approaches to Development: Politics Administration and Change*, New York, McGraw Hill, 1966, pp. 25-26.
19. Lok Sabha Secretariat, Public Accounts Committee, 5th Lok Sabha, 179th Report, New Delhi, 1976, pp. 41-47.
20. *Ibid.*
21. Health Project Management, *op. cit.*, p. 228.
22. Lok Sabha Secretariat: Estimates Committee, 5th Lok Sabha, Fifty Seventh Report, 1974, New Delhi, p. 15.
23. Govt. of India: Planning Commission, Draft (1978-83), p. 121.

3

CHAPTER

National Vector Borne Disease Control Programme

INTRODUCTION

As per the National Rural Health Mission, GOI, Annual Report, 2006-07 The National Vector Borne Disease Control Programme (NVBDCP) is one of the most comprehensive and multi-faceted public health activities in the country and concerned with prevention and control of vector borne diseases namely Malaria, Filariasis, Kala-azar, Dengue and Japanese Encephalitis (JE). The Directorate of NVBDCP is the nodal agency for planning, policy making and technical guidance and monitoring and evaluation of programme implementation in respect of prevention and control of these vector borne diseases. The States are responsible for planning, implementation and supervision of the programme. The vector borne diseases namely Malaria, Filaria, Japanese Encephalitis, Dengue and Kala-azar are major public health problems in India. Chikungunya fever, that re-emerged as an epidemic outbreak after more than three decades, has added to the problem. The vector borne diseases are complex; since their presence and transmission depends on interaction of numerous ecological, biological, social and economic factors. Increasing travel within and across countries is also responsible for spread of vector borne diseases.

Out of the six vector borne diseases, malaria, filariasis, Japanese Encephalitis, dengue and chikungunya are transmitted by different kinds of vector mosquitoes, while Kala-azar by sand flies. The transmission of vector borne diseases in any area is dependent on frequency of man-vector contact, which is further influenced by various factors including vector density, biting time, etc. Mosquitoes density is directly related with water collection – clean or polluted, i.e. it is dependent on availability of suitable larval habitats.

CHART 3.1

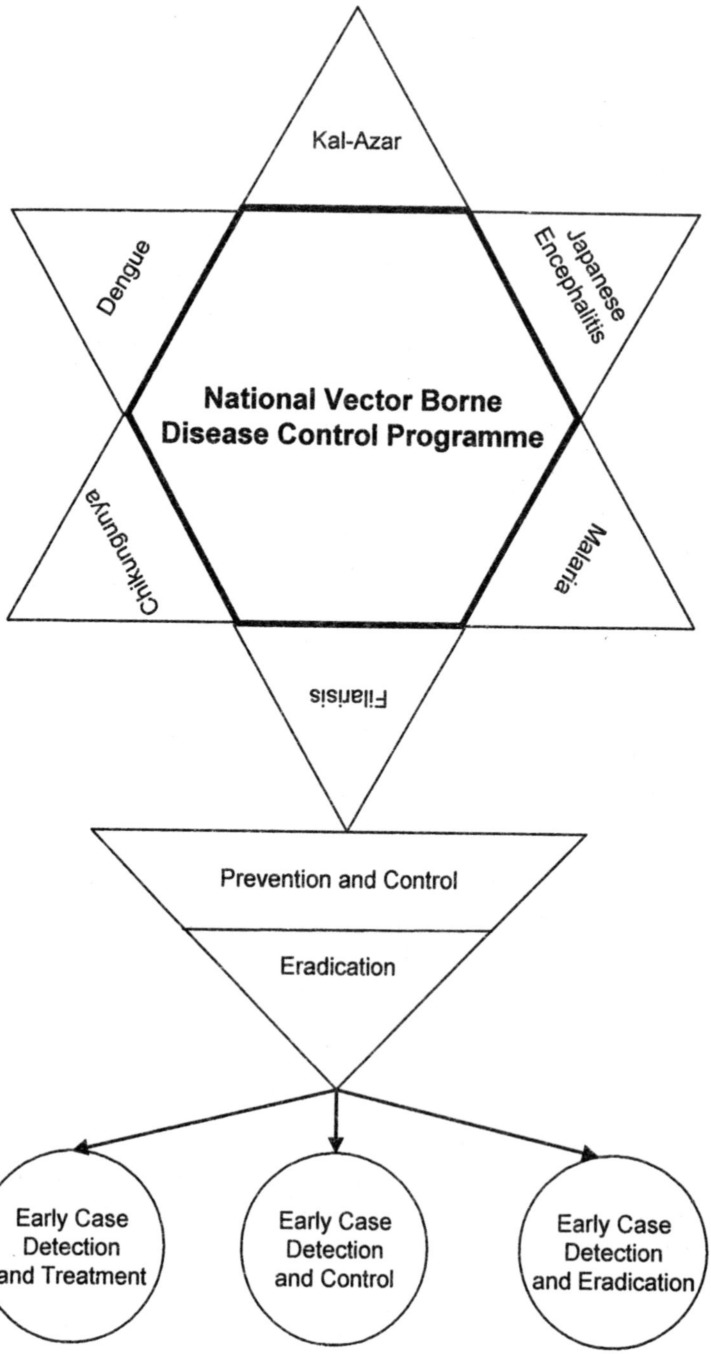
Kal-Azar
Dengue
Japanese Encephalitis
National Vector Borne Disease Control Programme
Chikungunya
Malaria
Filarisis
Prevention and Control
Eradication
Early Case Detection and Treatment
Early Case Detection and Control
Early Case Detection and Eradication

Under NVBDCP, the three pronged strategy for prevention and control of VBDs are: (i) Disease Management including early case detection and complete treatment, strengthening of referral services, epidemic preparedness and rapid response. (ii) Integrated Vector Management (For transmission Risk Reduction) including Indoor Residual Spraying in selected high risk areas, use of Insecticide treated bed nets, use of Larvivorous fish, anti-larval measures in urban areas, source reduction and mirror environmental engineering. (iii) Supportive Interventions including Behaviour Change Communication (BCC), Public-Private Partnership and Inter-sectoral convergence, Human Resource Development through capacity building, Operational research including studies on drug resistance and insecticide susceptibility, Monitoring and evaluation through periodic reviews/field visits and web-based Management System.

I. NATIONAL MALARIA ERADICATION PROGRAMME

Genesis

Nicholas J. White[1] in his article "Watch for the Symptoms" in *World Health*, Oct. 1991 has rightly said that Malaria is the most important of the parasitic diseases that afflict mankind. Whereas many of the other human parasites seems happy to live in relative harmony with their hosts, the parasites of Plasmodium falciparum (one of the four species of malaria) have a tendency to multiply rapidly and in an uncontrolled way in their human hosts, which may prove fatal. The disease is acquired when a biting female anopheline mosquito takes a blood meal. Whilst probing for blood she injects the microscopic parasite which then finds its way to the victim's liver. There it invades a few of the liver cells and develops over a period of one or two weeks. During this period the human host is blissfully unaware of the infection. At the end of this incubation period, the infected liver cells rupture and release a much increased number of parasites into the blood stream, where they rapidly invade the circulating red blood cells. Once inside the red cell, the malaria parasite proceeds to consume the contents of its new home and grow. At the end of a further two days (or three in the case of Plasmodium malaria) the destroyed cell bursts, releasing more parasites which immediately invade more red cells. Thus, the infection expands and within a week the victim begins to feel ill.

In ancient Chinese it was known as "the mother of fevers." Today, it accounts for 300-500 million cases of sickness a year globally and kills over 1.5 million people—possibly as many as 2.7 million—including one million children under five.

In the meantime, there is no prospect of a "quick fix" for malaria. For the foreseeable future at least, malaria control will continue to be a race to stay one step ahead of the emergence of drug-resistant forms of the disease."[2]

Negative Impact of Malaria on Socio-Economic Development

Malaria has been a worldwide disease and primary public health problem in tropical and sub-tropical countries. It has played an important role in world history throughout the ages. Adversely affecting the progress of nations and it has been the decisive factor in many wars. For centuries, it directly or indirectly accounted for approximately half the morbidity of the human race. It is a chronic invalidating disease which does not directly kill a high percentage of its victims. The mortality being only about one per cent, but it is often a major cause of infant mortality.[3] Its insidious debilitating effect had led to an increased number of deaths from other causes and shortened the life-expectancy in the past. Even today, some of its adverse effects on health continue to some extent. The large number of victims of repeated attacks of malaria become physical wrecks with low efficiency and work potential. Its stunning effect on the physical and mental development of the various categories in the affected communities, races and nations is felt to this day. Osler's of trepeated dictum that malaria was probably the greatest single destroyer of the human race was no exaggeration.[4] Wherever it exists, human progress is retarded or inhibited. The development of many potentially fertile areas of the world is barred by its presence; other areas in which human activities encouraged the breeding of anopheline mosquitoes that carry the disease had to be abandoned.[5]

History is full of instances where the execution of large scale construction or irrigation projects has been impeded or even given up due to the ravages of malaria. The construction of Panama Canal is a case in point. Similarly in India, e.g., in Bombay, the outbreak of malaria hampered the construction of the Alexandra Dock, while in Uttar Pradesh (India), the Sarda Canal Head Works suffered through the same cause.[6] Christopher, a careful observer, wrote in 1926:

> "Whether from the point of view of enhanced mortality, sickness and individual suffering or from the effect of preventing natural increase and sapping of the vitality of populations, or the paralysing effect on industry and exploitation of the mineral or other natural wealth of the country, or in the direct loss to Government in a variety of ways, malaria is universally recognised as the most important sanitary problem with which India has to cop."[7]

In India, malaria has long been recognised as the biggest and most important public health problem. Sinton estimated in 1935 that at least a hundred million people suffered from malaria each year with about a million deaths. In 1947, just after the partition, it was estimated that no fewer than 75 million persons suffered from it each year and during epidemic years, the toll was twice as much or even more. It claimed a greater number of deaths every year than any other disease. It has been calculated that approximately half of the five and a half million annual deaths in India from all causes were accounted for by fevers and nearly one-third of the fever deaths were directly attributable to malaria. Besides, a large number of persons debilitated by malaria fell easy victims to other diseases."[8]

Apart from the high annual morbidity and mortality, malaria has been responsible for untold sickness and suffering. It was one of the greatest obstacles to the development of the natural resources of the country. The economic loss to the nation due to malaria was thus incalculable and ran into hundreds of crores of rupees every year. In his conservative estimate of the annual financial loss to the country due to malaria, Sinton arrived at the figures of Rs. 1,000 crores. He stated:

> "It constitutes one of the most important causes of economic misfortune engendering poverty, diminishing the quality and quantity of food supply, lowering the physical and intellectual standards of the nation and hampering increased prosperity and economic progress in every way."[9]

Malaria is not only a major public health problem but also an important obstacle to development. Its spread is linked to specific development policies and actions such as road building, new agricultural settlement and irrigation projects. And in many areas of the world it is a social condition that is closely associated with the development of rural areas and the movement of under-privileged populations.[10]

Activities implemented under the programmes are as follows:

1. Surveillance

Regular fortnightly surveillance (active surveillance) is done by the Health Assistants visiting house to house to screen the fever cases and administer presumptive treatment after collecting blood smears. Passive surveillance is done at the PHCs, Hospitals, Dispensaries, etc. where fever cases visiting the Medical Institutes are screened for Malaria and treated with anti-malarials.

2. Laboratory Services

Laboratory services have been provided at PHC level, District level and State level for examination of blood smears.

3. Radical Treatment

Malaria cases detected are radically treated with anti-malarias F.T.Ds and D.D.Cs have been established.

4. Insecticidal spray

Regular rounds of insecticidal spray operations with DDT, Malathion and synthetic pyrethrioids taken up in areas reporting Annual Parasite incidence per thousand population, API 2 and above and focal spray in areas below API 2.

5. *Entomologial Studies*

The team conducts regular entomological studies to study the prevalence of vector species bionomics and resistance status to the insecticides.

6. *Bio-environmental*

This methods of malaria control is being implemented by introduction of larvivorous fish for control of mosquito breeding and malaria.

For strengthening early case detection and prompt treatment, 4,99,970 Drug Distribution Centres (DDCs), Fever Treatment Depots (FTDs) and Malaria clinics have been established in the country till 2005. This is in addition to the treatment facilities available at the health facilities and hospitals. Anti-malaria drugs and funds for training are provided to them by the Government of India. On an average, nearly 100 million fever cases are examined yearly.

The National Health Policy (2002) has set the goal of reduction in mortality on account of malaria by 50% by 2010 and efficient morbidity control. Reduction of malaria morbidity and mortality is also important to meet the overall objectives of reducing poverty and is included in the Millennium Development Goals (Goal 6 and Target 8). The high risk areas of malaria are largely tribal, difficult, remote and inaccessible, forested and forest fringed with operational difficulties, although risk factors exist in other parts of the country. About 95% of population lives in malaria endemic areas and 80% of malaria burden is confined to 20% of population in high risk areas. [11]

Policy and Implementation of Malaria Eradication Programme

In order to fight this disease a nation-wide malaria control programme was launched in the year 1953. By this programme, we were able to reduce the number of sufferers and also the number of deaths from malaria to a great extent, i.e. reduced the incidence of malaria from 7.5 crores in post-independence period to only one lakh in 1965. The achievements of the control programme were so encouraging that in 1958 it was switched over to an eradication programme. There have been local outbreaks of malaria since 1964 resulting in upsurge of malaria in the country during the past few years. Eradication of malaria does not appear to be possible in the near future with the situation becoming complex due to the changing behaviour of the vectors, malaria parasite and man himself. The Government of India, therefore, changed the goals from 'eradication' to 'control'. In order to tackle the growing incidence of malaria, a Modified Plan of Operation was approved in November 1976. It has been implemented from 1st April 1977. The basic objectives of this plan are:

(1) to prevent deaths due to malaria;
(2) to maintain industrial and farm production by undertaking intensive anti-malaria measures in such area;

(3) to consolidate the achievements attained so far; and
(4) reduction in the period of sickness.

The main features of the Modified Plan of Operation are:

(1) Insecticidal spray operations are undertaken in rural areas which have incidence of 2 or more cases per thousand population.
(2) The Malaria Units are being reorganized to conform to the geographical boundaries of the districts.
(3) For quick examination of blood smears and to provide treatment of positive cases, laboratory services are being decentralised to the Primary Health Centre level.[12]
(4) In order to have entomological studies and to be sure about the choice of appropriate type of insecticide for spray operations. 72 entomological teams have been provided at the zonal level in various parts of the country. Anti-malaria drugs are being made available through agencies like panchayats, school teachers, and in remote areas fever treatment depots are being established. Anti-malarias are also marketed through commercial channels.

The Central Government provides insecticides to the States free of cost and also gives assistance for procuring vehicles. Spray pumps, microscopes, microslides, etc. required under the programmes. Since the implementation of MPO, the malaria incidence has gradually gone down to 1.66 million cases in 1987 as against 6.47 million cases during 1976. Since 1989 onwards, the total incidence has been between two to three million cases per year. During 1996, 3.04 million cases were reported of which 1.18 million were due to Plasmodium falciparum (Pf). During 1997 there was decline in both total malaria and Pf. cases as 2.45 million total cases and 0.92 million cases were recorded. There were 711 malaria deaths reported in 1997 as against 1009 malaria deaths in 1996. In view of the high incidence of malaria and resource constraints in seven north-eastern states cent per cent central assistance is being provided with effect from December 1994, the incidence of malaria is showing a declining trend from very high levels. In the year 1996, there were 3.04 million of malaria cases, out of which 1.18 million were Plasmodium falciparum cases, which declined to 1.82 and 0.81, respectively in the year 2005.[13]

Recent Development

Insecticide Treated Bed Nets: The Directorate is promoting alternative and cost effective vector control measures like Insecticide Treated Bed Nets (ITNs). Guidelines on use of bed nets have been developed and issued to States. Till date, 45,15,000 bed nets have been supplied free or at highly subsidized rates to the high risk areas of endemic states. The priority beneficiaries are below poverty line population in rural and tribal areas.

Synthetic Pyrethroid tablet formulation for individual use for impregnation and re-impregnation of community owned bed nets has been introduced. Schemes on bet net distribution, insecticide impregnation of community owned bed nets have been developed for involvement of NGOs/Faith Based Organisations/Community Based Organisations/Local Self-Governments.[14]

The key elements of the revised strategy include: (i) programme planning and management; (ii) strengthening surveillance; (iii) targeting interventions to populations "at risk" of malaria; (iv) scaling up the control of vivax malaria; (v) increasing the coverage and proper use of insecticide-treated mosquito nets; and (vi) monitoring and evaluation. Integrated vector management (IVM), one of the strategic elements of the revised strategy, requires strong multisectoral involvement to cope with rapid ecological changes.[15]

CRITICAL APPRAISAL

Malaria Eradication Programme, though controlled to a great extent has the tendency of resurgence from time to time. Many factors are responsible for it:

1. Lack of Integration into Development Efforts

Planning studies for malaria eradication are often confined to the malariological aspects and do not fully take into account economic and social factors, including rural development programmes, the nature and location of development project, the habits of the population, migration, trans-humane into and out of the malarious areas, the attitude of the people towards sickness, their ability to appreciate the advantages of disease eradication and their priority needs. Planning teams do not always receive expert advice on economic, sociological and administrative aspects. Many malaria eradication campaigns failed because they were developed prior to the formulation of long-term national health and socio-economic development plans. Some of them have consequently been handicapped by the lack of sustained government support and of active cooperation of government agencies.[16]

2. Lack of Sound Administrative Support

Sound administrative support is obviously of utmost importance for the successful implementation of a malaria eradication programme as the operations have to be carried out not only efficiently but also according to a definite time schedule determined by epidemiological considerations. But even when the general administrative methods and practices have been adequate, the deficiencies have been reflected in the health services and have frequently caused set-backs to malaria eradication.[17] Continuous evaluation of the effect of the operation and availability of adequate logistic support, including transport and equipment, are therefore important.

3. Lack of Effective Leadership and Team Work

The human factor in malaria eradication programmes ranks with, or even surpasses in importance to. planning, administration and operational features.' Effective leadership, training, efficiency, high morale and dedication among the workers have been found to be essential to success. Technical factors such as the physiological resistance of the vector mosquito to insecticides, behavioural, characteristics of the vector such as "excitorepellency" (resistance of vector to insecticide) and the resistance of malarial parasites to drugs have also to be taken into account. Strictly, technical problems are generally limited to about one per cent of the population covered by the eradication programme. The problem areas, however, need prompt attention since they are sources of spreading malaria to regions already freed from the disease.[18]

The reasons for the failure of malaria eradication programme in India are: lack of effective management as well as of technical competence and suitable methods relating to these deficiencies. Dr. Srivastava, former Director-General of Health Services, Government of India, said:

"Studies in depth carried out in India had provided useful information about the reasons for the failure of the malaria eradication programe in some areas. While in three-fourths of the area covered by these operations, the programme had suffered because of the human failures, such as lack of proper logistics, delays in spraying, etc. the failure in others could be attributed to technological reasons such as resistance to insecticides and lack of full knowledge of the epidemiology of malaria and the ecology of the mosquitoes. This aspect needed to be studied by organisations like the WHO. India could undertake necessary research on its own problems in these areas, but similar situations might exist in other countries. WHO might also assist governments which are able to undertake such special studies."[19]

4. Lack of Logistic Support

The Planning Commission, Government of India, conducted a mid-term appraisal of the Fourth Plan in February 1972. It found that in regard to the National Malaria Eradication Programme, there has been a shortfall in the realisation of the target of phasing of malaria eradication units. There have been delays in the supply of insecticides, anti-malarial drugs and replacement of vehicles. There has been inadequate supervision at various levels. Mosquitoes have developed resistance to insecticides.[20]

In Burma, the main reason for the failure of the malaria eradication programme has been the human factor. Dr. V. Kyaw Sen (Burma) said: "In this country, as the earlier efforts at Malaria eradication had not been able to achieve total success, a reorganisation of the staffing had been undertaken; temporary spraymen had been replaced by permanent workers, and the basic health services had been brought to deal with the problem, under the technical guidance of the malaria staff.[21]

SUGGESTIONS

We mention here suggestions to ensure early control and Eradication of Malaria.

1. Strengthen Regional and Local Epidemiological Services

Epidemiological Services can help in controlling the disease. Dr. Hiroshi Nakajima in his Article, "Breakup the fatal cycle of transmission" suggests that every member of the public can use personal protection whenever and wherever the transmission risks are high, and can learn to recognize signs of the disease and seek prompt treatment. Health services can be made available to ensure timely diagnosis and effective treatment. Epidemic warning and control systems can be developed as part of the national epidemiological services. Where malaria is an important obstacle to development, the capacity to control its transmission can be enhanced by strengthening local and regional epidemiological services.[22]

2. Specialised Competence, Both Technical and Administrative

These should always be an attempt to improve technical and administrative competence to contain the disease. Jose Antonio Najera—Morronda in his Article "Malaria control: History shows it is possible" rightly mentioned, "specialized technical competence is essential to the planning of appropriate control measures, as well as to the training and reorienting of health and medical services so as to improve their performance and ensure the health education of the local population."

3. Adapt to Local Situations

There is a need to adapt Malaria eradication strategy depending upon the local facilities and infrastructure. Dr. Elhadi H. Benzerroug and Mrs. Beatrice Elom in their Article, "The World Malaria Situation" suggest the use of drugs, information education and communication activities, and epidemiological surveillance. In all situations, however, the ready access of the affected populations to early diagnosis and treatment of malaria is absolutely necessary.[23]

The participation of local populations and their ability to adopt personal protection measures to prevent transmission will be an essential element. Individual, family and community action could lead to great reduction in the disease.

The fight against malaria requires continuous action at local level. It is therefore vital to integrate it into primary health care activities at the district level, within the framework of the African health development scenario at present being put into effect in the countries of the Region. The success of the struggle for malaria control will also depend on the will and capacity of countries to work out short, medium and long-term plans appropriate to the resources available locally and to the epidemiological pattern of the disease.[24]

4. Coordinate with School Education

In areas with malaria, teachers can play an important role by detecting cases of fever among pupils and referring them to the health worker, who can then take the necessary action. Teachers can also monitor how often students are absent and for how long, and inform the health centre when children are absent more frequently or for longer periods than usual.

Malaria can only be controlled if everyone participates in the light. Why not contact the staff in your nearest health centre or hospital to discuss what you can do together to teach school children about malaria and become partners in controlling the disease.[25]

To achieve the objective of the Eradication of Malaria, a three pronged attack should continue intensively, i.e.

(a) Government efforts;
(b) Peoples' Participaton; and
(c) Research on Malaria.

Unless the three components are effective, our objective will not be achieved. The most important of them all is the active cooperation of the people. It has been mentioned in the Draft Fifth Five Year Plan,

"The cooperation of the public would be actively sought so as to make this a mass programme particularly in the areas where the incidence is high. The programme will be constantly monitored and research stepped up so as to develop more cost-effective methods of control. The programme will continue to receive 100 per cent central assistance."

There is urgent need to investigate systematically the frequency and geographic distribution of chloroquine resistance in Plasmodium falciparum and also in Plasmodium vivax. These may require expert advice from the National Anti-Malaria Programme, but this process must be defined and established by the state health authorities. The State Level Diagnostic and Reference Laboratory may be entrusted with the continued investigations of drug resistance.

It is also necessary to investigate the susceptibility/resistance of Anopheles mosquitoes to the currently used insecticides. Insecticide sprays/fogging to reduce adult mosquito population should not be done 'routinely' but as specifically planned and applied judiciously, in chosen places and times, as the last resort in malaria control. The use of insecticides under health programmes (such as malaria and filariasis control) or under other Departments (such as Agriculture) should be regulated and monitored by the State Health Authorities, through the integrated vector borne diseases programme.[26]

2. Elimination of Lymphatic Filariases

Filariasis is transmitted by mosquito species Culex quinquefasciatus and Mansonia annulfera/M. uniformis. The vector mosquitoes breed in polluted water in drains, cesspits, etc. in areas with adequate drainage, sanitation.[27]

The National Filaria Control Programme was launched in 1955 for the control of filariasis. Activities taken under the programme include: (i) delimitation of the problem in hitherto unsurveyed areas, and (ii) control in urban areas through recurrent anti-larval measures and anti-parasite measures. It is estimated that out of about 428 million people living in known endemic areas, about 113 million urban people are in urban areas and the rest in rural areas. At present, about 48 million urban population is being protected through recurrent anti-larval measures by 206 control units and 199 filaria clinics. Training in filariology is imparted at three Regional Filaria Training and Research Centres situated at Calicut, Rajahmundry and Varanasi under the National Institute of Communicable Diseases of Delhi. During 1997, 14.18 million population in thirteen districts of seven states, namely, Bihar, Uttar Pradesh, West Bengal, Orissa, Andhra Pradesh, Tamil Nadu and Kerala were covered under the revised strategy for filaria control with single dose annual mass drug administration of diethyle carbamazine (DEC). This strategy is to be continued for five years.

Man, with micro-filaria in the blood, is the main reservoir of infection. The disease is not directly transmitted from person to person, but by the bite of many species of mosquitoes which harbour infective larvae. Important vectors are species of Culex, Anopheles, Mansonia and Aedes. The incubation period varies. and micro-filaria appear in the blood after 2-3 months in B. malayi after 6-12 months in W. bancrolti infections.

Low effectiveness of the tools used by control programmes, the chronic nature of the disease, and that it affects mainly the economically weaker sections of communities result in low priority being accorded by governments for the control of lymphatic filariasis.

An inter-country workshop on the control of lymphatic filariasis in South-East Asia was organized in response to World Health Assembly Resolution of 1997 on the elimination of lymphatic filariasis as a public health problem. The workshop recommended that, by the year 2000, all filariasis-endemic countries of the South-East Asia Region should have established national control programmes aimed at reducing the morbidity/prevalence and/or elimination of the infection.[28]

Several important strategic modifications were proposed. These included macro and micro-stratification of endemic areas, and development of local approaches with an emphasis on disease management as an entry point for disease control activities. Since regular doses of DEC had frequently caused adverse reactions, it was recommended that table salt fortified with reduced DEC content be used in the management of Brugia malayi infections. This would reduce the frequency and severity of reactions to DEC, during the Ninth Plan. The strategy for filariasis control includes:

(1) single dose DEC mass therapy once a year in identified 13 districts and selected DEC treatment in filariasis endemic areas;
(2) continuous use of vector control measures;
(3) detection and treatment of micro-filaria carriers, treatment of acute and chronic filariasis; and
(4) IEC for ensuring community awareness and participation in vector control as well as personal protection measures.[29]

The disease is endemic in about 250 districts in 20 States and UTs. The population at risk is over 500 million. Control of lymphatic filariasis is immensely important due to personal trauma of the affected persons and associated social stigma, even though it is not fatal.

The Government of India is signatory to the World Health Assembly Resolution in 1997 for Global Elimination of Lymphatic Filariasis. The National Health Policy (2002) envisages elimination of lymphatic filariasis in India by 2015.

The strategy of lymphatic filariasis elimination is through:

- Annual Mass Drug Administration (MDA) of single dose of December (Diethylcarbamazine citrate) tablets for 5 years or more to the eligible population (except pregnant women, children below 2 years of age and seriously ill persons) to interrupt transmission of the disease,
- Home-based management of lymphoedema cases and up-scaling of hydrocele operations in identified CHCs/District hospitals/ medical colleges, and
- In pursuit of the goals, the Government of India launched nationwide MDA in 2004 in endemic areas as well as home-based morbidity management, scaling up hydrocelectomies in CHCs and PHCs. During the year 2004, 276.2 million population was covered against a target of 390.2 million population giving a coverage rate of 72.6%.

During the year 2005, 243 filaria endemic districts with a population of 554 million were targetted.[30]

The LF programme was reviewed as part of a joint monitoring mission with WHO support in India in February 2007. The important recommendations of the mission included maximization of coverage through supervised administration, identification of new districts on the basis of surveys and use of line-listing of clinical cases. Timely procurement and supply of drugs is another area of concern. Activities like disability alleviation and the scale up of MDA have been slow due to insufficient political commitment and inadequate resource allocation. WHO will seek more partners to increase political commitment, resource mobilization and effective implementation while continuing to provide technical support.[31]

3. National Programme for Elimination of Kala-Azar

Kala-azar is a slow progressing indigenous disease casued by a protozoan parasite Leishmania donovani and spread by sandfly, which breeds in shady, damp and warm places, in cracks and crevices in the soft soil, in masonry and rubble heaps, etc. Therefore, proper sanitation and hygiene are critical to prevent sandfly breeding. The National Health Policy (2002) of GOI has set the goal for elimination of Kala-azar from the country by 2010. The Government has also signed a Memorandum of understanding with Bangladesh and Nepal to eliminate Kal-azar from South-East Asia Region by 2015.

Kala-azar is endemic in 32 districts in Bihar, 4 districts in Jharkhand, 5 districts of Uttar Pradesh and 11 districts of West Bengal (total 52 districts) besides sporadically occurring in a few other areas. An estimated 130 million population is exposed to the risk of Kala-azar in the endemic areas. The disease incidence has come down from 77099 cases in 1992 to 31217 cases in 2005 and confirmed deaths from 1419 in 1992 to 157. However, in recent years (2003 onwards), there is an increasing .trend. In the current year (up to Sep. 2006), 30160 cases and 187 deaths have been reported from the affected States.

To realize the goal of elimination of Kala-azar, the Govt. of India is providing 100% support to endemic States from 2003-04. In June 2005, advisories were sent to the 4 endemic states to review the Kala-azar situation and monitor programme implementation.

Various initiatives planned/undertaken for Kala-azar elimination:

- Clubbing of surveillance for PKDL with Visceral Leishmaniasis case detection as per case definition of Kala-azar and PKDL as delineated in the NVBDCP guidelines.
- Treatment schedule as delineated in NVBDCP guidelines being formulated.
- Defining the criteria of unresponsiveness and switching over to 2nd line of drug.
- Involvement of medical interns, private laboratories and private practitioners in surveillance and treatment.
- Delimitation of the foci of DDT resistance in vector species.
- Study to be initiated on comparative evaluation of IRS, ITN and environmental engineering methods for cost-effectiveness and sustainability of interventions.
- A pilot study to be initiated in two districts of Bihar on side effects of miltefosine.
- Research on use of GIS, role of sibling species in Kala-azar transmission by Rajendra Memorial Regional Institute of Medical Sciences and National Institute of Malaria Research.
- Strengthening of IEC/BCC activities at grassroots.
- Reorientation training of Medical and paramedical personnel in management of Kala-azar.[32]

A household and a health facility survey on kala-azar were conducted in India during 2006. These surveys were conducted by the national programme in India and implementation research was supported by WHO's Special Programme for Research and Training in Tropical Diseases (TDR). The surveys revealed that the problem of kala-azar was 5-10 times greater than the cases reported. It was also observed that 50% or more cases were diagnosed and treated in the private sector. A programme review was conducted in February 2007 by a joint monitoring mission in India. The recommendations of the mission were used in refining the policy and providing strategic direction to the programme in the elimination of the disease.

Guidelines and standard operating procedures for diagnosis, treatment, vector control operations and disease surveillance were developed and finalized by experts and programme managers from the three endemic countries in April 2007 at a meeting organized by WHO in Kolkata, India. Algorithms were developed for diagnosis and complete treatment of kala-azar and reporting formats were finalized. Research on vector control and treatment was supported by the TDR. The progress of these research activities was reported at the Meeting for Analysis of the multi-centre studies on Vector Control and Treatment of Visceral Leishmaniasis, held in Varanasi, India, March-April 2007.

The kala-azar elimination programme would require sustained advocacy, mobilization of resources and capacity development for implementation of strategies and policies. Partnership formed in this area need to be sustained through multi-country efforts coordinated by WHO.[33]

4. Japanese Encephalitis Programe

Japanese Encephalitis (JE) has been reported in the country since mid-fifties. With increasing development of irrigation projects and changing pattern of water resource management there has been a progressive increase in number of States reporting cases of JE in India. Twelve States/UT's have been implementing the recommendations of the Experts Committee on JE control. However, implementation of the strategies for improving clinical management, vector control, disease surveillance and health education has been sub-optimal in most States.[34]

Japanese Encephalitis—a zoonotic disease is transmitted by yet another vector mosquito, mainly belonging to Culex tritaeniorhynchus, Culex vishnui and Culex pseudovishnui group. The transmission cycle is maintained in the nature by animal reservoirs of JE virus like pigs and water birds. Man is the dead end host, i.e. JE is not transmitted from the infected person to others. Outbreaks are common in those areas where there is close interaction between animals/birds and human beings. The vectors of JE breed in large water bodies such as paddy fields. JE has been reported from mainly, Andhra Pradesh, Assam, Bihar, Haryana, Karnataka, Kerala, Maharashtra, Manipur, Tamil Nadu, Uttar Pradesh and West Bengal. The population at risk is about 300 million.

There is no specific cure for this disease, symptomatic and early case management is very important to minimize risk of death and complications. In addition, implementation of such public health measures as, Health Education through different media like radio, TV including cable network, miking, inter-personal communication, etc. for disseminating appropriate message in the community is crucial. The emphasis is given on keeping pigs away from human dwellings or in pigsties particularly during dusk to dawn, which is biting time of vector mosquitoes. Sensitization of the community regarding avoidance of man-mosquito contact by using bed nets and fully covering the body are also advocated. Since early reporting of cases is crucial to avoid any complication and mortaility, the community is given full information about the signs and symptoms as well as availability of health services at health centres/hospitals. Besides, the states are advised fogging with Malathion (Technical) as an outbreak control measures in the affected areas. [35]

In addition, the Government of India has taken further steps to support the states in 2006. The Directorate of National Vecotr Borne Disease control has provided detailed guidelines for the prevention and control of dengue to the affected states. Intensive health education activities through print, electronic and inter-personnel media, outdoor publicity as well as and inter-sectoral collaboration with civil society organisation (NGOs, CBOs/Self-help Groups), PRIs and Municipal bodies have been emphasized, Regular supervision and monitoring is conducted by the programme.

Control measures should be part of the integrated vector borne disease control package, through the general health service. The vector, Aedes aegypti should come under entomological surveillance and control. Objects that collect water such as old types, tins, jars/bottles, coconut shells, etc. need to be disposed off. Water should be changed regularly in water coolers, tanks, vessels, etc. Health education for administrators, medical and paramedical workers and for students and the general public should be given through the mass media. [36]

5. Dengue

Dengue outbreaks have been reported from urban areas from all States. All the four types of dengue virus exists in India. The vector Aedes Aegypti breeds in peridomestic fresh water collections and is found in both urban and rural areas. Analysis of available data from 54 dengue outbreaks between 1954 and 1995 indicate that:

(1) dengue outbreaks occur both in urban and rural areas; and
(2) over the years there has been an increase in reported cases of dengue haemorrhagic fever and dengue shock syndrome.

Diagnostic tests for dengue virus are not readily available in most parts of the country. At present, there is no mechanism for monitoring and surveillance for dengue. During the Ninth Plan efforts are being made to:

(1) establish an organised system of surveillance and monitoring;
(2) strengthen facilities for early diagnosis and prompt treatment; and
(3) intensify IEC efforts to ensure that all households implement peridomestic measures to reduce breeding of Aedes.

Dengue is endemic in 18 states/UTs with the population of about 450 million at risk. In 1967, the country had experienced an outbreak recording a total number of 16517 cases (suspected) and 545 deaths. During the year 2005 again, 12754 and 11985 cases along with 215 and 157 deaths had been reported respectively. During the year 2006, upto 20-11-2006 the reported number of cases and deaths are 10094 and 162, respectively.[37]

Control measures should be part of the intergrated vector borne disease control package, through the general health service. The vector, Aedes aegypti should come under entomological and surveillance and control. Objects that collect water such as old tyres, tins, jars/bottles coconut shells, etc. need to be disposed-off. Water should be changed regularly in water coolers, tanks, vessles, etc. Health education for administrators, medical and paramedical workers and for students and the general public should be given through the mass media.

6. Chikungunya

Chikungunya, a debilitating non-fatal viral illness and also transmitted by Aedes aegypti mosquito has re-emerged in the country after about three decades. It is caused by Chikungunya virus. Humans are considered to be the major source or reservoir of Chikungunya virus for mosquitoes. Therefore, the mosquitoes usually transmit the disease by biting infected persons and then biting others. The infected person cannot spread the infection directly to other person (i.e. it is not contagious disease). Symptoms of Chikungunya fever are most often clinically indistinguishable from those observed in dengue fever. However, unlike dengue, hemorrhagic manifestations are rare and shock is not observed in Chikungunya virus infection. Currently, the reported number of Chikungunya *suspected cases* upto 31.10.2006 in the country is *1.37 million*. The number of confirmed cases reported from 12 States/UTs stand at 1689 cases on 02.11.2006. There are no reported deaths directly related to Chikungunya. The affected states reporting confirmed cases are: *Andhra Pradesh, Karnataka, Maharashtra, Tamil Nadu, Madhya Pradesh, Gujarat, Kerala, Rajasthan, Goa, Delhi and NCR and Pondicherry.*

Various initiatives undertaken by the MOH and FW, Government of India during the current epidemic outbreak are:

- Continuous monitoring of Chikungunya and Dengue situation right from the first reporting in states.

- Circulation of detailed guidelines and advisories for prevention and control of these diseases to all affected states.
- Launch of Intensive Behaviour Change Communication activities through print, electronic media, interpersonal communication, outdoor publicity as well as inter-sectoral collaboration with civil society organisations (NGOs/CBOs/ Self-Help Groups), PRIs.
- Provision of larvicides, adultcides to affected states.

Identification of Apex Referral institutions and sentinel surveillance centres for diagnosis and regular surveillance.[38]

CONCLUSION

Besides Monitoring and Evaluation, Inter-Sectoral convergence, behavioiur change communication activities for social mobilization, there is a need of capacity building.

The Directorate of NVBDCP has initiated three tier capacity building programme at primary, secondary and tertiary levels to strengthen health care delivery system for prevention and control of vector borne diseases so as to ensure the quality of health manpower development; rational use of drugs, improve timely referral services for appropriate management of severe and complicated cases; provide technical support in outbreak investigations. Guidelines on Integrated training on Vector Borne Disease Control Programme have been circulated to all States/UTs and other stakeholders. Besides training of Private Medical Practitioners and other inter-sectoral partners also being conducted to sensitize them about the National Strategies for VBD control. Specialized trainings for entomologists and laboratory technicians are also being conducted separately. State core team of trainers have already been trained in 24 states. A total of 628 medical college faculties have been trained from 111 Medical Colleges. Besides 169 specialized trainings were conducted at National level through premier institutes, as tertiary level core group of trainer, who are responsible for training at secondary level, i.e. districts wherein 7543 participants were trained.[39]

NOTES AND REFERENCES

1. J. Nicholas White, "Watch for the Symptoms in *World Health*", Sept.-Oct., 1991, p. 9.
2. *World Health*, March-April, 1998, pp. 12-13.
3. E.J. Pampana and P.F. Russel, Malaria—A World Problem (WHO: Geneva, 1955), p. 7.
4. Osler in Birendra Nath Ghosh, A Treatise on Hygiene and Public Health (Culcutta, 1970), p. 445.
5. WHO, First Ten Years of WHO, p. 172.
6. G. Borkar, Health in Independent India (Ministry of Health, Govt. of India, 1961), p. 112.

7. S.R. Christopher in Pampana and Russel, *op. cit.*, p. 7.
8. J.A. Sinton, "What Malaria costs in India, Nationally, Socially and Economically", condensed and reprinted in *Health Bulletin*, 1951, No. 26, GOI, Press, 125.
9. *Ibid.*
10. Bernhard H. Liese, Economic Development and Malaria, in *World Health* Sept-Oct. 1991, p. 28.
11. Ministry of Health and Family Welfare, GOI, Annual Report, 2006-07, p. 66.
12. India, *op. cit.*, pp. 1711-72.
13. Ministry of Health and Family Welfare, GOI, Annual Report, 2006-07, p. 66.
14. Ministry of Health and Family Welfare, GOI, Annual Report, 2006-07, p. 97.
15. The Work of WHO in the South-East Asia Region, Report of the Regional Director, 1 July 2006, p. 7.
16. Official Record of the WHO, 176, p. 114.
17. *Ibid.*
18. WHO, World Health Situation, 1965-68, June 1971, p. 15.
19. 24th Session of WHO Regional Committee for South-East Asia, (New Delhi, No. 1971), p.. 88.
20. The Fourth Plan: Mid-term Appriasal, a Summary, Planning Commission, Govt. of Inida, February 1972, p. 121.
21. 24th Session of WHO Regional Committee for South-East Asia (New Delhi, Nov. 1971), p. 88.
22. Hiroshi Nakajma, "Breaking the fatal cycle of transmission" in *World Health*, Sept.-Oct., p. 3.
23. *World Health*, Sept.-Oct. 1991, p. 5.
24. *Ibid.*, p. 7.
25. *Ibid.*, p. 23.
26. Final Report of The Task Force on Health and Family Welfare, Govt. of Karnataka, April 2001, p. 68.
27. Annual Report of Health and Family Welfare, GOI, Annual Report, 2006-07, p. 69.
28. Ninth Five Year Plan, *op. cit.*, p. 17.
29. Annual Report of Health and Family Welfare, 2006-07, p. 70.
30. The Work of WHO in the South-East Asia Region, Report of the Regional Director, 1st July 2006, p. 14
31. Final Report of The Task Force on Health and Family Welfare, Govt. of Karnataka, April 2001, p. 70
32. The Work of WHO in the South-East Asia Region, Report of the Reigonal Director, 1st July, 2006-07, p. 14.
33. Annual Report, Ministry of Health and Family Welfare, 2006-07, pp. 73-74.
34. Final Report of The Task Force on Health and Family Welfare, Govt. of Karnataka, April 2001, p. 70.
35. National Rural Health Mission, Ministry of Health and Family Welfare, GOI, Annual Report, 2006-07, pp. 73-74.
36. Final Report of The Task Force on Health and Family Welfare, Govt. of Karnataka, April 2001, p. 71.
37. Ministry of Health and Family Welfare, GOI, Annual Report, 2006-07, p. 76.
38. *Ibid.*, pp. 77-78.
39. *Ibid.*, pp. 79-80.

4

CHAPTER

National Tuberculosis Control Programme and National Programme for Control of Blindness

I. NATIONAL TUBERCULOSIS

Recognising the immensity of the burden of disease and numbers of death due to Tuberculosis, the National Tuberculosis Programme (NTP) was established in 1962 based on research proving the effectiveness of domiciliary treatment and on sociological, epidemiological and operations research which established the rationale of passive case detection, the efficacy of sputum microscopy, the expected case load, and the need for integration of the programme into the general health services.[1]

Tuberculosis (TB) is an infectious disease caused by a bacterium, Mycrobacterium tuberculosis. It is spread through the air by a person suffering from TB. A single patient can infect 10 or more people in a year.

In a population of more than 200 lakh in 13 states throughout the country, the quality of diagnosis is dramatically better than that of the previous programme or of private practitioners. Nearly 8 out of 10 patients diagnosed in the programme since 1993 were cured; this cure rate is more than double that of the previous programme.

Tuberculosis is a major public health problem in India. The burden of TRIAL BALANCE in India (Prevalence) as in the year 2000 was 8.5 million total cases of which 3.8 million were bacillary pulmonary cases, 3.9 million abacillary cases and 0.8 million extra-pulmonary cases.

Globally one-fifth of new tuberculosis cases are from India every year. As per the latest estimates every year there are approximately 18 lakh new cases in the country of which approximately 8 lakh are new smear positive infectious cases. An infectious case if not treated on an average infects 10-15 persons in a year. Annual risk of becoming infected with TB is 1.5% and

CHART 4.1

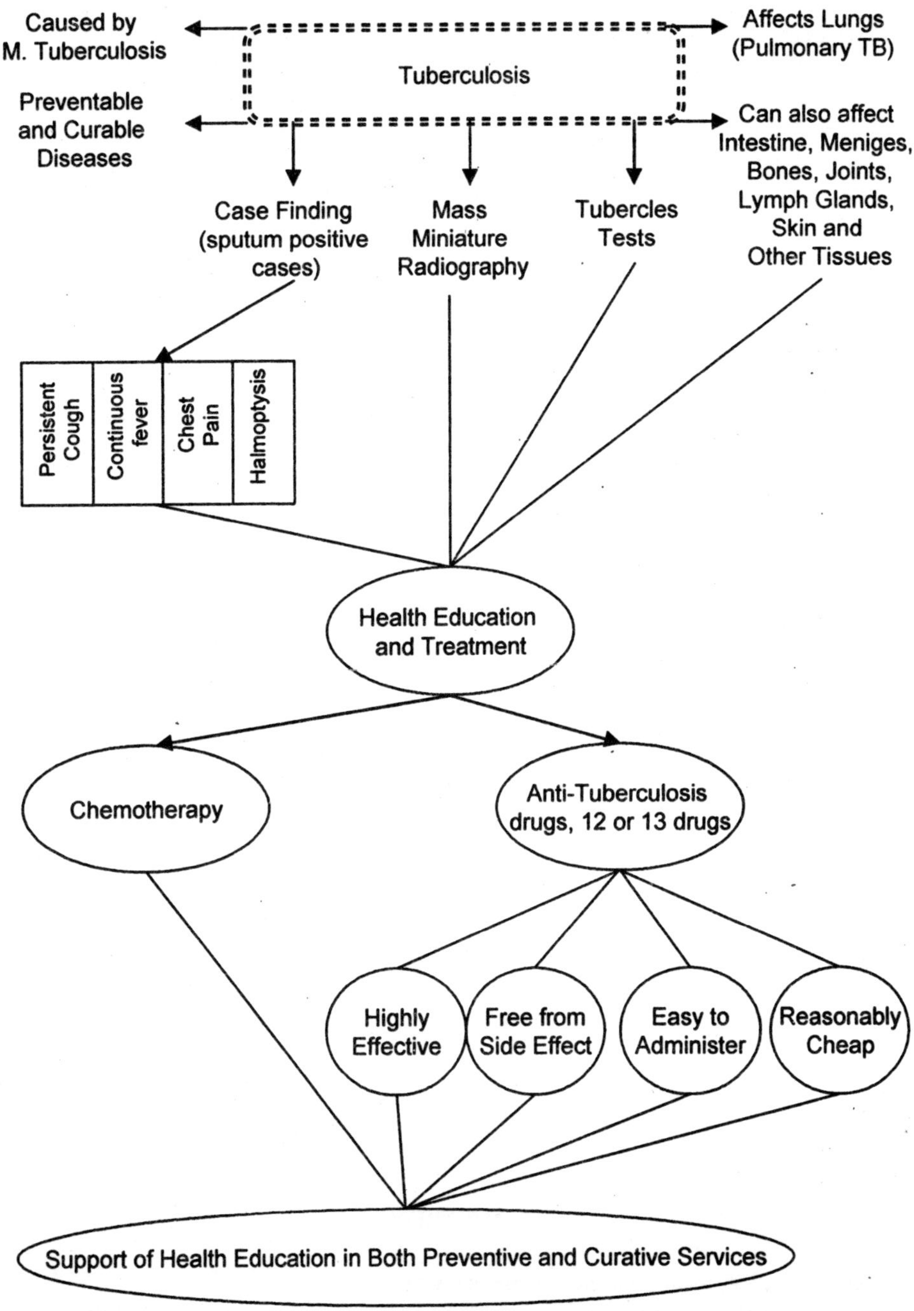
Caused by M. Tuberculosis
Preventable and Curable Diseases
Tuberculosis
Affects Lungs (Pulmonary TB)
Can also affect Intestine, Meniges, Bones, Joints, Lymph Glands, Skin and Other Tissues
Case Finding (sputum positive cases)
Mass Miniature Radiography
Tubercles Tests
Persistent Cough
Continuous fever
Chest Pain
Halmoptysis
Health Education and Treatment
Chemotherapy
Anti-Tuberculosis drugs, 12 or 13 drugs
Highly Effective
Free from Side Effect
Easy to Administer
Reasonably Cheap
Support of Health Education in Both Preventive and Curative Services

once infected there is 10% life-time risk of developing TB disease. Two persons die from TB in India every three minutes, more than 1,000 people every day and almost 3,70,000 every year.[2]

I Directly Observed Treatment, Short-Course (DOTS)

DOTS. known as the Revised National Tuberculosis Control Programme (RNTCP) in India, is a comprehensive strategy for TB control. DOTS is the only strategy which has proven effective in controlling TB on a mass basis. The DOTS strategy is in practice in more than 100 countries. India has adapted and tested DOTS in various parts of the country since 1993, with excellent results.

By March 2006, entire population (1114 million) of the country in all 632 districts had been covered under the Programme.

Achievements of RNTCP

1. Over 55-fold expansion in RNTCP coverage since 1998, leading to total coverage of the country by March 2006. In terms of treatment of patients, RNTCP is the largest programme in the world. Quality of services has been maintained during this rapid expansion.
2. Sound training materials have been developed for all categories of staff. The training materials are modular in content and have been recently revised keeping in view the new developments in RNTCP. Modular trainings ensure uniform standards and avoid possible subjectivity and bias of the trainers.
3. Diagnostic facilities in nearly 11,800 laboratories throughout the country have been established. As a result, the proportions of sputum positive cases confirmed in the laboratory are double that of the previous programme and are on partnership with international standard. Quality Assurance protocol implemented in all the states.
4. Since its inception, the Programme has initiated over 6.30 million patients on treatment, thus saving nearly 11.33 lakh additional lives.
5. During the year 2005, sputum positive case detection rate of 66% and treatment success rate of 86% was achieved.
6. Treatment success rates have tripled from 25% to 86%. TB death rates have been cut 7-fold from 29% to 4%.[3]

2. DOTS IS A SYSTEMATIC STRATEGY WHICH HAS FIVE COMPONENTS

Political and Administrative Commitment

TB is the leading infectious cause of death among adults. It kills more women than all causes associated with childbirth combined and leaves more orphans than any other infectious disease. And, since TB can be cured and the epidemic reversed, it warrants the topmost priority, which it has been accorded by the Government of India. This priority must be continued and expanded at the state, district and local levels.

Good Quality Diagnosis

Top quality microscopy allows health workers to see the tubercle bacilli which is essential to identify the patients who need treatment the most.

Good Quality Drugs

An uninterrupted supply of good quality anti-TB drugs must be available. In the RNTCP, a box of medications for the entire treatment is earmarked for every patient registered, ensuring the availability of the full course of treatment to the patient, the moment he is registered for treatment. Hence in DOTS, the treatment will never fail for lack of medicine.

The Right Treatment, given in the Right Way

The RNTCP uses the best anti-TB medications available. But unless treatment is made convenient for patients, it will fail. This is why the heart of the DOTS programme is "directly observed treatment" in which a health worker, or another trained person who is not a family member, watches as the patient swallows the anti-TB medicines in their presence.

Systematic Monitoring and Accountability

The programme is accountable for the outcome of every patient treated. The cure rate and other key indicators are monitored at every level of the health system, and if any area is not meeting expectations, supervision is intensified. The RNTCP shifts the responsibility for cure from the patient to the health system.

Tuberculosis is one of India's most serious health problem. Despite a long and distinguished tradition of tuberculosis research in India and the existence of a national programme since 1962, tuberculosis remains an all-too-common cause of illness and death. India accounts for 28% of the global burden of tuberculosis, and every day, more than 1,000 people die from tuberculosis in India more than 1 person every minute.

Professor John Sbarbaro says that Tuberculosis is a disease both of the individual and of society. Its spread is dependent upon human environment and behaviour. Therefore, it can only be controlled by society. Control will require intense cooperation between the country's government, its medical colleges and private practitioners. India's National Consensus Conference has resulted in an unprecedented commitment by all political parties to make tuberculosis control a reality.

India led the world in advancing knowledge on how to treat tuberculosis. Now it can lead the world in controlling tuberculosis and diminish forever the spectra of multi-drug-resistant tuberculosis. Phyllida

Brown in his Article, "A disease that is alive and kicking" also throws light on the nature of the disease. "Tuberculosis is a terribly debilitating disease and, if untreated, kills around half of those affected. People with TB suffer from weakness and exhaustion, profuse night sweats, chest pain and cough, sometimes with bloody sputum. Occasionally the bacteria spreads to affect other tissues including the bone, bringing further disability."[4]

Extent

It is estimated that 14 million people are suffering from active tuberculosis in India of which 3 to 3.5 million are highly infectious cases. About 0.5 million die of this disease every year. District TB Centres (DTCs) are functioning in 446 districts. TB clinics have been established in big towns and cities. There are 17 TB Training and Demonstration Centres and about 47,600 TB beds in the country. The National TB Control Programme has been accorded high priority by the Government.

The Revised National Tuberculosis Programme (RNTCP) was launched in the country on 26 March 1997. The revised strategy is proposed to be implemented in a phased manner in 102 districts of the country, covering a population of 271 million, with the assistance of World Bank. The RNTCP has been remarkably successful. In a population of more than 200 lakh in 13 states nearly 8 out of 10 patients diagnosed were cured.[5]

Objectives

1. To provide facilities for diagnosis of TB Patients through integrated general health services.
2. To provide optimum treatment nearer to the residence of the patients.
3. To prevent infection, immunization is done by doing BCG Vaccination.
4. Health education to encourage patients through Health Workers, their relatives and village leaders to take full course of treatment.
5. Detection of New TB cases (Sputum positive, X-Ray Suspects and extra pulmonary cases).

3. ESSENTIALS OF REVISED NATIONAL TUBERCULOSIS CONTROL PROGRAMME (RNTCP)

Director General of Health Services, Ministry of Health and family Welfare in its *Bulletin on RNTCP* mentions the following essentials enunciated by Central T.B. Division.

Good Quality Diagnosis

Top quality microscopy allows health workers to see the tubercle bacilli which is essential to identify the patients who need treatment the most.

Good Quality Drugs

An uninterrupted supply of good quality anti-TB drugs must be available. In the RNTCP, a box of medications for the entire treatment is earmarked for every patient registered, ensuring the availability of the full course of treatment to the patient, the moment he is registered for treatment. Hence in DOTS, the treatment will never fail for lack of medicine.

The Right Treatment, given in the Right Way

The RNTCP uses the best anti-TB medications available. But unless treatment is made convenient for patients, it will fail. This is why the heart of the DOTS programme is "directly observed treatment" in which a health worker, or another trained person who is not a family member, watches as the patient swallows the anti-TB medicines in their presence.

Systematic Monitoring and Accountability

The programme is accountable for the outcome of every patient treated. The cure rate and other key indicators are monitored at every level of the health system, and if any area is not meeting expectations, supervision is intensified. The RNTCP shifts the responsibility for cure from the patient to the health system.

Tuberculosis is one of India's most serious health problem. Despite a long and distinguished tradition of tuberculosis research in India and the existence of a national programme since 1962, tuberculosis remains an all-too-common cause of illness and death. India accounts for 28% of the global burden of tuberculosis. And every day, more than 1,000 people die from tuberculosis in India more than 1 person every minute.

Effective implementation of DOTS will save hundreds of thousands of lives in India. DOTS has been deemed one of the most cost-effective health interventions. Each life saved represents a child. mother, or father who will go on to live a productive. TB free. Longer life. Every patient who is cured stops spreading TB. Working together to implement DOTS, we can win the age-old battle against TB.

Physical Performance

Comparative statement of achievements under RNTCP during the last 4 years.

SUGGESTIONS

We may keep the following facts in mind while dealing with Tuberculosis.

TB can be cured inexpensively:

Indicators	2001	2002	2003	2004	2005	Till June 2006
Population coverage, (millions)	450	530	775	947	1080	Entire country covered in March 2006
Cumulative (in millions) Number of cases put on DOTS	471658	622873	906472	1187353	1293083	698114
New smear positive patients put on treatment	185178	245051	358496	465331	506193	277011
Cure rate (expected 85%)	84%	84%	86%	86%	84%	83%
No. of NGOs involved (approx.)	230	410	650	1011	1600	2056

Source: Annual Report, Ministry of Health and Family Welfare, 2006-07, p. 94.

- TB has a cure and treatment is inexpensive.
- TB control is a very cost-effective health intervention, equivalent to that of the well-known childhood immunization programmes.
- Successful treatment requires 6-8 months of consistent, uninterrupted medication.
- Successful treatment demands education and follow-up.
- New, drug-resistant strains of TB are developing because patients are not completing their treatment. These drug-resistant strains are significantly more dangerous to the individual and the community because they are more difficult and more expensive to treat.
- The best way to prevent TB is to cure infectious cases in their early stages in order to prevent transmission to others.
- TB control programmes that treat infectious patients but don't ensure that they are cured risk doing more harm than good. Patients who have incomplete treatment can develop spread drug-resistant TB.[6]

We may also add other suggestions.

I. Early Detection and Action

Dr. Hiroshi Nakajama in his Article, "Tuberculosis: a global Emergency" rightly suggests the best way to prevent the disease is to cure infections cases at an early stage, since this also puts a stop to transmission. Control programmes should ensure that patients are cured completely and should include an education component to raise public awareness of this problem. The BCG vaccination of infants helps to avoid the most serious forms of childhood tuberculosis.[7]

2. Emphasis on Research

We are witnessing limitations of many existing treatments. There is a need of intensifying research to cope with the changing situations. This requires adequate funding and facilities. The more integration and generalization of tuberculosis services we have, the more we need TB specialists not in a technical way but to provide the brains for the tuberculosis control programme of a nation. "If you have too many hands, you need strong brains to get the hands to work rationally."[8]

3. Holistic Approach

It should be planned in a holistic way as to include all perspectives. A comprehensive national tuberculosis programme must be implemented and it must meet four conditions. It must be 'countrywide' that is to say, services must be available to rural as well as urban population. It must be planned on a 'long-term' basis, since new cases will develop from the pool of infected people for two or three generations to come. It must be 'adapted' to the expressed demands of the population; only accessible and effective services will gain public confidence. And it must be 'integrated' into the community health structure so as to meet all the above requirements.[9]

4. Ambulatory Treatment based on Good Supervision

It has been proved beyond doubt that treatment in a hospital or sanatorium offers no medical advantage over ambulatory care and that the most effective and cheapest way of treating patients is by out-patient treatment. It is absolutely useless to squander limited resources on sending cases to hospital. On the other hand, the success of treatment depends fundamentally on the regularity of drug-taking, and this calls for adequate supervision during the whole period of treatment.[10]

5. Combat TB along with other Communicable Diseases

Here is one more illustration that health can only be attained through a combination of diverse measures in the health and other related sectors. These measures have to be applied within communities to deal with the full range of problems whose combined effects ravage the health of people. With the possible exception of smallpox eradication (which had unique features—the exception that proved the rule), attempts to deal with single communicable diseases in ways that were at best parallel and at worst divergent, have proved to be ineffective. There is no escape from the need to deal in a concerted manner with those factors that in the final analysis are common to most of these diseases. This is the rationale for primary health care, accessible to all in a spirit of social equity.[11]

The multi-disciplinary groups of health care workers and scientists working on tuberculosis are energetic and enthusiastic. Politicians can harness this energy and enthusiasm by providing resources to support control programmes as well as funds to answer both operational and basic scientific research questions. Most essential are communication and cooperation between public health practitioners, scientists, the pharmaceutical industry and politicians aimed at developing a cohesive strategy to deal with this international public health challenge.[12]

The world cannot afford to wait. TB is on the rise again, in part because the disease has been neglected by national and international health programmes. Although the greatest number of TB cases are concentrated in Africa, Asia and Latin America, TB cannot be contained by political boundaries or more strict border controls.

Today's world is increasingly interdependent. With fast and accessible travel, migration and immigration, infectious diseases like TB will not be stopped by borders. Over the long-term, only a world-wide, systematic approach can solve this problem. In short, it will be impossible to control tuberculosis in the industrialized nations unless it is sharply reduced a health threat in Africa, Asia and Latin America.[13]

The problem is that tuberculosis is an airborne disease which is virtually impossible to avoid. It is transmitted by bacteria sprayed into the air by coughing or sneezing. Today, large-scale population movements and a massive increase in airline travel have helped to bring tuberculosis out of oblivion to everyone's doorstep.

Dr. Arata Kochi, Director of WHO's Global Tuberculosis Programme, says it is alarming that many countries still do not have effective TB control programmes in place, despite warnings of the global spread of drug-resistant tuberculosis. "We have the medicine and know-how to control TB", he says. "Unfortunately we don't have the magic potion to wake up the world's governments to the seriousness of the TB crisis and get them to take action."[14] Encouraged by the results achieved in the pilot projects, it was decided to extend the strategy in a phased manner during the Ninth Plan period. Assistance from the World Bank has augmented the resources available for the programme during the Ninth Plan period when:

(a) RNTCP will be implemented in 102 districts.
(b) NTCP will be strengthened in 203 short course chemotherapy (SCC) districts as a transitional step to adopt the RNTCP.
(c) Standard regime will be strengthened in the remaining non-SCC districts, and
(d) The Central Institutions, State TB Cells and State TB training Institutions throughout the country will be strengthened.

The targets for the Ninth Plan were:

(i) to enhance case detection to at least 70 percent of the estimated incidence;
(ii) to achieve at least 85% cure rate amongst smear positive patients of Tuberculosis in 102 districts implementing RNTCP and 60% cure rates in 203 SCC districts;
(iii) to reduce the proportion of smear negative detected under the programme to 50% or less of the total cases;

(iv) to improve the aggregate smear positive rate at least to 50%; and

(v) to ensure that the number of TB suspects tested for smear examination is not less than 2.5% of the general OPD attendance of the PHIs and number of smears examined is at least 3 per suspected patient.[15]

RNTCP Phase-II

The RNTCP Phase Ii of the World Bank project has been approved by the Government for the period October 2006 to September 2011 for a total outlay of Rs. 1,156 crore (USD 256.9 million) which includes credit from World Bank of Rs. 765 crore (USD 170 million) and commodity assistance of anti-TB drugs from DFID through WHO for Rs. 287 crores (USD 63.7 million) with balance of Rs. 191 crores (USD 42.5 million) will be given by Government of India. In addition, 427 crores through GFATM (for states of 56 million population in Chhattisgarh, Jharkhand and Uttranchal from the Round 1,110 million population in Bihar and Uttar Pradesh under Round 2) and USAID (for entire 21 million population of Haryana).

The second phase of the RNTCP will consolidate, maintain and further improve the achievements of the first phase. Phase-II of the RNTCP is a step towards achieving the TB-related Millennium Development Goal (MDG) targets. DOTS remains the core strategy. In addition to the ongoing activities, the following new activities have been envisaged in the second phase.

- The scaling up of the State-level Intermediate Referral Laboratories (IRL capacity for nation-wide implementation of External Quality Assessment (EQA) of sputum smear microscopy services and provision of culture and drug sensitivity testing.
- Implementation of DOTS-Plus of multi-drug resistant TB cases will occur in a phased manner.
- Procurement and distribution of paediatric drug boxes for improved care of paediatric cases has been initiated.[16]

Note: With the spread of HIV infection, tuberculosis problem is deteriorating further. More HIV infected individuals die from tuberculosis than from any other cause. In India about 60 percent of the AIDS cases have evidence of active tuberculosis. There is new infection or reactivation of pre-existing tuberculous infection in HIV infected persons. Persons infected with HIV are 25 times more likely to develop active tuberculosis as compared to persons infected with tubercule bacilli alone. Current information suggests that response to chemotherapy for tuberculosis is good.

RECOMMENDATIONS

- Improve effectiveness and outcomes of the programme by strengthening the State Ophthalmic Cell filling up vacancies with qualified dynamic staff, and long-term continuity of Joint Director.
- Ensure accountability of the ophthalmologist and ophthalmic units regarding number and quality of cataract surgery. The epidemiological surveillance system to include ophthalmic conditions.
- Improve access toinf regarding availability of services, especially for the disadvantaged sections. Area specific health promotion regarding eye care, with community participation.
- Integrate school eye screening with health check-up of school age children.
- All Medical College Eye Departments should take up in-reach base hospital programmes.
- All taluk hospitals (upgraded by KHSDP) should be made base hospitals for conventional cataract surgery and be allotted a fixed geographical area.
- All districts should have at least two government base hospitals where intraocular lens (IOL) surgery is available. All post-operative patients should be given individually corrected spectacles.
- The District Medical Officer should coordinate and depute the available surgical manpower to fixed surgical centres on the operation days in the districts.
- Screening the community by the health worker to identify and refer persons at risk of developing glaucoma, to ophthalmologists for evaluation and management.
- Prevention, early diagnosis and intervention in persons liable for corneal opacities causing blindness. Develop eye collection centres, eyebanks and expertise in corneal grafting for the four divisions in government medical college hospitals.
- Establish specialty clinics: glaucoma, vitreo-retinal and corneal grafting centre.
- Improve networking with the voluntary and private sectors.[17]

CONCLUSION

According to Dr. Hiroshi Nakajima, Director-General of the World Health Organisation, it is defined that the best way to prevent the disease is to cure infectious cases at an early stage, since this also puts a stop to transmission. Control programmes should ensure that patients are cured completely and should include an education component to raise public awareness of this problem. The BCG vaccination of infants helps to avoid the most serious forms of childhood tuberculosis.

II. NATIONAL PRGORAMME FOR CONTROL OF BLINDNESS

Need

It is self-evident that eye-sight is an essential function for carrying out the majority of human functions. Any impairment of the functions creates chaos in the life of the persons affected. However, most of blindness today is totally preventable. There are many diseases that can lead to loss of sight, but the most important are—trachoma, xerophthalmia, cataract and on choccriases (river blindness) which are all preventable or curable.

Although blindness in children is relatively un-common, it poses a heavy burden on the individual, and society. These need to be identified at an early date to avoid total blindness. We may keep in mind that blindness is related to socio-economic conditions of the people as well as lack of facilities.

'Foresight prevents blindness' was the slogan chosen by WHO for World Health Day in 1976, when efforts were made around the world to raise public awareness about the problem of preventable blindness.

Two of the commonest problems encountered in developing countries are poverty and ignorance and both of these have a direct bearing on the burden of blindness. Poverty may sometimes be the reason for a family not seeking early treatment for trachoma, or for an elderly person not having a cataract operated on, but more often lack of information, awareness and motivation is the underlying reason.

To this must be added the equally common problem of the physical and social remoteness of the available health services for the rural poor in outlying areas, together with the general shortage of trained personnel and facilities for eye care in most developing countries. It is hardly surprising, therefore, that blindness rates in many of the least developed countries are often as much as 20 times higher than those found in developed countries and that nine out of ten of today's more than 28 million blind people live in developing countries.[18]

Objectives

- To reduce the backlog of blindness through identification and treatment of blind.
- To develop Eye Care facilities in every district.
- To develop human resources for providing Eye Care Services.
- To improve quality of service delivery.
- To secure participation of Voluntary Organisations in eye care.

New Initiatives proposed under the Programme

- A Task force has been set-up to chalk out the strategy for 11th Plan under NPCB.
- Construction of dedicated Eye Wards and Eye Operation

theatres in Districts and Sub-District Hospitals in North-Eastern States, Bihar, J.&K, Himachal Pradesh, Uttarnachal and few other states as per demand.

- Appointment of Ophthalmic Surgeons and Ophthalmic Assistants in new districts in District Hospitals and Sub-District Hospitals.
- Appointment of Ophthalmic Assistants in PHCs/Vision Centres where there are none. (At present Ophthalmic assistant to all available in block level PHC only)
- Appointment of Eye Donation Consellors on contract basis in Eye Banks under Government Sector and NGO Sector.
- Grant-in-Aid for NGOs for management of other Eye diseases other than Cataract like Diabetic, Retrinopathy, Glaucoma, Laser Techniques, Corneal Transplantation, Vitreoeretinal Surgery, Treatment of childhood blindness, etc. of Rs. 750 per case for Cataract/IOL implantation Surgery and 1000 per case of other major Eye Diseases as described above. For North Eastern States Hilly and Desert Areas Rs. 850 for contract and Rs. 800 for other major eye care management is proposed.
- Special attention to clear Cataract Backlog and take care of other eye health care centres from NE states.
- Telemedicine in Ophthalmology (Eye Care Management Information and Communication Network).
- Vitamin A supplementation and M.M.R. Vaccination through DBCS corpus funds as per requirements to take care of Childhood Blindness.
- Setting up of five centres of Excellence for Eye-care services.
- Provision of vehicles to state programme managers and district.
- Programme Managers under NPCB.
- Provision of Computers, fax and photocopier to District Blindness Control Societies under NPCB.
- Involvement of Private practitioners.
- A provision of Rs. 1550 crores has been proposed to implement various activities under the programme.[19]

Magnitude of the Problem of Blindness

Of the total estimated 38 million blind persons (VA<3/60) in the World, 6 million are in India. Two major surveys were conducted to find out prevalence of blindness in the country. The first survey was done by the ICMR on a national sample in 1974 which arrived at a figure of 1.38 per cent prevalence rate for the economically blind. In the second and latest NPCB/WHO survey (1986-89), the prevalence rate increased to 1.49 per cent. This increase could be due to change in age structure and could also be due to mounting backlog.

Genesis and Growth

National Programme for Control of Blindness was launched in the year I976 as a 100% Centrally sponsored programme. Various activities of the programmes include establishment of Regional Institute of Ophthalmology, upgradation of medical colleges and district hospitals and block level Primary Health Centres, development of mobile units, and recruitment of required ophthalmic manpower in eye care units for provision of various ophthalmic services. The programme also extends assistance to voluntary organisations for providing eye care services including cataract operations and eye banking. The goal is to reduce the prevalence of blindness from 1.4% to 0.3% by 2000 A.D.[20] As per survey in 2001-02, prevalence of blindness is estimated to be 1.1 percent. Target of the Tenth Plan was to reduce prevalence of blindness to 0.8 percent by 2007.

Strategy

The four pronged strategy of the programme is:

(a) strengthening service delivery,
(b) developing human resources for eye care,
(c) promoting outreach activities and public awareness, and
(d) developing institutional capacity.

Infrastructure Development

Tertiary Level

At the tertiary level of ophthalmic care, there are eleven Regional Institutes of Ophthalmology including the Apex institute that is. Dr. R.P. Centre in the All India Institute of Medical Sciences, New Delhi. These centres have been established as centres of excellence in the field of eye care. In addition, 82 medical colleges have been upgraded under NPCB. There are 39 medical colleges, which have been designated as training centres for Para-medical Ophthalmic Assistance. So far, 166 eye banks have been developed in the Government and non-government sector.

Regional Institutes of Ophthalmology	16
Upgraded medical colleges	307
PMOA training centres	39
Eye Banks	166

Recently, under the National programme for control of Blindness, the concept of District Blindness Control Societies (DBCS) has been successfully implemented in five pilot districts. Based on the success, as many as 500 DBCS have been formed till date. These societies have multi-disciplinary structure, which has representatives of Government, non-government and private, aimed at decentralising management of ophthalmic services and evolving a partnership among Government, non-government and private sector.

District hospitals equipped	445
DBCSs formed	510

Primary health centres are the basic units in the rural areas. Till date 5440 primary health centres have been provided with ophthalmic equipments and para-medical ophthalmic assistants, have been posted.

Central Mobile Units	80
District Mobile Units	341
PHCs upgraded	5633
PMOAs posted	4881

The number of Cataract operations has increased from 12.19 lakhs in 1985-86 to 49 lakhs in 2005-06.

World Sight Day has been organized all over the country on 12th October, 2006. The theme for this year's World Sight Day was Prevention and Control of Blindness due to Diabetic Retinopathy. A special campaign was organized during the month of October, 2006 to focus attention of public on prevention of blindness due to retinopathy. The main function was organized in Chennai on 19th November, 2006 under the chairmanship of Hon'ble HFM.[21]

Performance of Cataract Surgery: It has been steadily increasing as indicated below:

ISSUES AND PROBLEMS

1. Lack of Education among the masses about the existing facilities:-Need of wide publicity.
2. Shortage of quality Equipment and medicine: Need of strict control to maintain quality.

Year	*Target*	*Achievement*	*Achievement %*	*IOL Implementation %*
2002-03	4000000	3857133	96	77
2003-04	4000000	4197609	105	83
2004-05	4240000	4491154	107	88
2005-06	4513000	4905619	108	90
2006-07*	4500000	3210000	71	90
Total		21253000	20661515	97

* Provisional.

Source: Annual Report, Ministry of Health and Family Welfare, 2006-07, p. 95.

3. Apathy and indifference on the part of health personnel: Need of change of attitudes.
4. Lack of adequate referral services to take care of complications: Need of designing referral services.

SUGGESTIONS

1. Integrate Eye Care as Part of Primary Health Care

The adoption of this concept of integrated delivery of eye care as part of primary health care is a logical step, given the multifactoral causes of blindness and their close relevance to the essential concerns of primary health care, such as safe water and sanitation, food and nutrition, maternal and child health. These approaches are embodied in the primary eye care efforts that are the basic strategies in a number of national programmes for the prevention of blindness.[22]

2. Involve NGO's

The non-governmental sector has not only the potential for a close and useful partnership with governments but also the capacity to innovate in a way that governments cannot do. However, there are many factors which hamper governmental action—financial, political and bureaucratic among others—but do not generally bog down non-governmental programmes, with their greater motivation, flexibility in thought and action and functioning at grassroot level—a built in element of community participation. Thus, the non-governmental sector has the basic potential for a close and meaningful partnership in avowed governmental efforts to achieve Health for All, including eye health.[23]

3. Train Ophthalmic Medical Assistants

India cannot afford the services of specialists at village level. What is the way out? The need is to train medical Assistants. Training ophthalmic medical assistants to provide eye care within the primary health care services has proved effective in reaching the remote areas where over 70 per cent of the population lives. For years to come, until health services reach the stage where sufficient number of eye specialists will be available, the OMAs will make a significant contribution towards eradicating avoidable blindness.[24]

4. Provide Low Cost Spectacles

Overall, we are dealing with a process which moves quite slowly. If we look at the same processes which evolved in the more industrialised countries, we see that it took well over 100 years to make spectacles available on the present enormous scale. So there is every reason to be optimistic that in a much shorter time reasonably priced spectacles can be made available to all who need them and that countries themselves can develop a sound industrial base for their manufacture.[25]

5. Correct Chronic Vitamin-A Deficiency

A chronic deficiency of vitamin-A in the diet leaves millions of children blind for life. To prevent this is a challenge that calls for imagination, dedication and political will.[26]

There are three facets to the programme: emergency prophylaxis by distribution of vitamin-A supplement (200,000 IU capsules); medium-term prophylaxis by vitamin-A enrichment of certain foods; and lastly, long-tenD prophylaxis by improving dietary intakes of the vitamin. Nutritional education, better use of existing foods, and development of new dietary resources rich in vitamin-A are essential features of this long-term approach.[27]

It is a primary obligation of the Health and Family Welfare Deptt. to prevent blindness and to conserve sight. Blindness is one of the most severe of human scourages. It is now possible to control and dramatically reduce major blinding diseases. Noel West has rightly suggested the need of eye relief camps. because our permanent eye hospitals are over-flowing and we would otherwise miss much of the rural population. It has been found that eye specialists work in isolation from other health workers engaged in eye care functions.

They should rather engage themselves in organising training programmes for these workers so that they can deliver proper eye care to the rural population or those who cannot afford specialists attention.

It is essential to improve awareness among health care workers at all levels about the need for preventive measures and importance of early identification.

Programme Priorities during Ninth Plan

- To improve the quality of cataract surgery, clear the backlog of cataract cases.
- To improve quality of care by skill upgradation of eye care personnel.
- To improve service delivery through NGO and Public Sector collaboration.
- Increase coverage of eye care delivery among under-privilege population.[28]

Targets for the period 1997-2002

- 17.5 million cataract operations.
- 100,000 corneal implants.[29]

6. Health Education of the Masses

Right from the start of the programme: In 1963, the main emphasis has been on mass education of the public. This has been done quite effectively through visits to each and every home in the remotest villages by basic health workers, both in the first stage of the specialized Trachoma Control Programme and after its integration with general health services. Village schools have been an essential port of call in the daily round of the health worker. Being the most vulnerable and at the same time the most impressionable age-group, children of 6 to 12 years are visited at school where the co-operation of teachers in enlisted for both treatment and health education. The health worker examines infected eyes and applies ointment. The teachers are supplied with more ointment to continue the treatment till the next visit. Visits are made usually once a month, since the health worker's "beat" includes from 20 to 30 villages and a total population of about 10,000.

When calling at private homes, health workers apply ointment if necessary and distribute tubes free of charge to the villagers after careful explanations. Health education talks are enlivened by the use of charts, flannel-graphs, photographs and posters.

In urban areas, the programme works mainly through school teachers. They are trained in the detection of suspected cases of trachoma and in the application of antibiotic ointment. They also educate the children in matters of personal hygiene. The health worker helps the school health programme by regular visits and by supplying drugs.

The use of antibiotic eye ointments is now being very effectively promoted at family planning centres. In a subtle way, this has in turn helped the family planning programme as more and more mothers flock to village centres. It is in the villages that the incidence of trachoma and associated infections is highest.[30]

CONCLUSIONS

There is already much improvement. People are definitely more conscious now about their personal hygiene and general health than they were, say, then year ago. The Indian villager now seeks medical assistance much sooner than before. Although a time limit for the successful control of the disease cannot be set, our work is being actively supported by the population. This is a healthy sign. We still face some resistance from the population, but it is gradually disappearing. Old customs and traditions are breaking down with improving economic and educational standards in the country. Our activities have created an increased consciousness in the people of the need to seek medical care at the onset of the disease.

Notes and References

1. Final Report of The Task Force on Health and Family Welfare, Govt. of Karnakata, April 2001, p. 75.
2. Ministry of Health and Family Welfare, GOI, Annual Report, 2006-07, p. 87.
3. *Ibid.*, pp. 88-89.
4. Phyllida Brown, "A disease that is alive and kicking" in *World Health*, July-Aug. 1993, p. 5.

5. India, *op. cit.*, pp. 1721-73.
6. *World Health*, July-Aug., 1993, p. 12.
7. *Ibid.*, p. 3.
8. *World Health*, January, 1982, p. 16.
9. *Ibid.*, p. 11.
10. *World Health*, January 1982, p. 13.
11. *Ibid.* p. 3.
12. John Parter Keith McAdam and Richard Frachem, "The Challenge is International", in *World Health*, July-Aug. 1993, p. 12.
13. Karl Huus, Tenget it Nine Die, in *World Health*, July-Aug., 1993, p. 29.
14. *World Health*, March-Apirl 1998, p. 15.
15. Ninth Five Year Plan, *op. cit.*, p. 169.
16. Ministry of Health and Family Welfare, GOI, Annual Report 2006-2007, p. 90.
17. Final Report of The Task Force on Health and Family Welfare, Govt. of Karnakata, Apri, 2001, pp. 79-80.
18. Bjorn Thylefors, "Foresight Presents Blindness", in *World Health*, May 1987, p. 3.
19. Ministry of Health and Family Welfare, GOI, Annual Report, 2006-07, p. 96.
20. Annual Report, Ministry of Health and Family Welfare, 1998-99, p. 160.
21. Ministry of Health and Family Welfare, GOI, Annual Report 2006-2007, p. 96.
22. Pararajasegaram, Partners in Eye Health in *World Health*, May 1987, p. 78.
23. *Ibid.* pp. 6-7.
24. Moses C. Chirambo, "Ophthalmic medical Assistants", in *World Health*, May 1987, p. 9.
25. Richard Homeier, "Low Cost Spectacles", in *World Health*, May 1987, p. 19.
26. Alferd Sommer, Blincling Malnutrition, in *World Health*, May 1987, p. 20.
27. Edourd M. De Mae Yer, A Three Pronged Programme, in *World Health*, May 1987, p. 22.
28. Ninth Plan, *op. cit.*, p. 175.
29. Ministry of Health and Family Welfare, GOI, Annual Report, 2006-007, p. 95.
30. A.S. Kochar, "India is Tackling Trachoma" in *World Health*, June 1970, p. 15.

5

CHAPTER

National Leprosy Eradication Programme

Skin infections are an important public health problem in our country. Most of the skin diseases can be attributed to bad personal hygiene of the persons. One of the reasons for this is, apart from ignorance, lack of adequate water for washing and bathing, particularly in the rural areas and urban slums. Though skin infections *per se* may not be life threatening, these are important, since some of the skin infections can lead to infection of vital organs. Leprosy is a chronic communicable disease characterized by lesions of the skin and involvement of nerves.

INTRODUCTION

Dr. T. Parthasarthy, Joint Director (Leprosy) Karnataka Government very clearly states that Leprosy is a public health problem and also social problem. National Leprosy Eradication Programme (NLEP) was conceived of as a control programme and launched in 1954-55. Its main thrust was early detection, sustained and regular treatment of all patients with 'Dapsone' tablets. This had some time limitations like; treatment was to be taken for a long leading to irregular treatment, which led to development of drug resistance and deformities.

Leprosy, a chronic bacterial disease with long incubation period between 9 months to 20 years after infection can affect all age groups. The signs/symptoms may vary between PB to MB depending upon the degree of patient's immunity to M. Leprae, the causative agent. Nevertheless, 95% of the people in our community are immune to leprosy. Since the leprosy bacilli affect the peripheral nerves and if not properly cared the patients loose sensation by and large in their hands, feet and eyes and injuries to these insensitive parts may lead to disfigurement, which is main consequences of disease that generates fear and stigma. The early detection

CHART 5.1

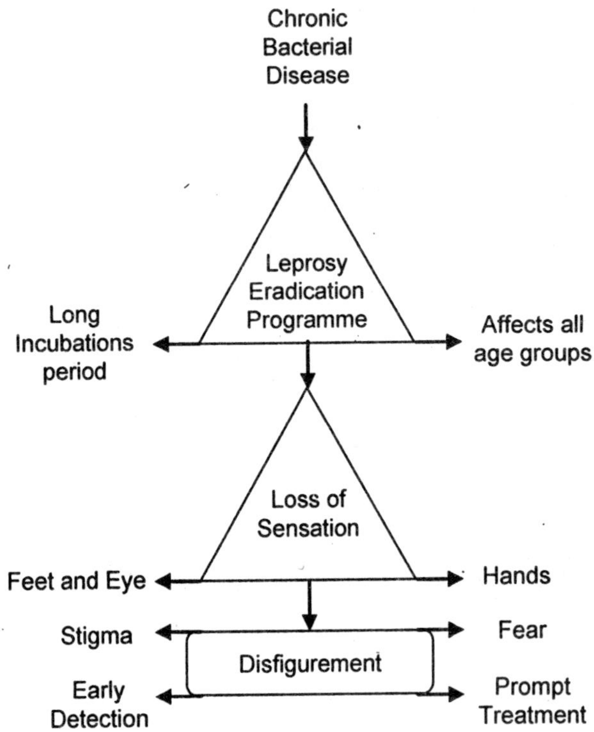

and prompt treatment of leprosy with prescribed MDT not only cures leprosy but also interrupts its transmission to others.

The World Health Assembly in 1991 took a major initiative towards global elimination of leprosy, an age old public health problem with devastating effects on its suffers. The WHO's leadership, strong commitment of endemic countries and active support of NGO's/VOs as well as donor agencies have jointly helped in reducing the global situation of leprosy by about 90% and the elimination level achieved in more than 100 countries. Currently only a dozen countries have leprosy as a major problem and India contributes about 60% of global leprosy burden as leprosy had been widely prevalent in this vast country for centuries.[1]

Leprosy continues to remain a serious public health problem in the developing countries, particularly if one considers that the populations at risk of contracting the disease are very large, and that more than one-third of all leprosy patients face the threat of permanent and progressive physical and social disability. It should be emphasized here that the problem of leprosy is far more serious than what is represented by the numbers alone, particularly in terms of the intense human suffering involved resulting from the physical deformities and the related social problems.

Leprosy is a chronic bacterial disease caused by Mycobacterium leprosy. It affects the skin, peripheral nerves and the upper airway. The main clinical presentations are the tuberculoid and lepromatous forms. Though the distribution is worldwide, the chief endemic areas are in South and South-East Asia, tropical Africa, and some areas of Latin America. Man is the only reservoir of significance.

The exact mode of transmission has not been established but household and prolonged contact appear to be important. Environmental factors such as overgrowing and poor hygiene facilitate the spread of the disease. The incubation period ranges between 9 months and 20 years. Leprosy is rarely seen in children below three years of age. At present, there is no effective vaccine against this disease. Unlike some other diseases, such as tuberculosis, there does not appear to be a connection between leprosy and HIV infection.

Geneses, Growth and Development

Leprosy is scourge of mankind. It is a major public health problem in all the developing countries. It is widely prevalent in India and 58% of global recorded leprosy patient load is in India. The disease primarily affects skin mucous membrane and peripheral nerves. The public health importance of leprosy lies in the capacity of the disease to produce deformities as well as psychological and social disabilities.[2]

LEPROSY SITUATION IN INDIA

With efficient implementation of well planned efforts since 1953-54, India has very substantially controlled leprosy. The goal of leprosy elimination at National level (i.e. PR of <1 case/10,000 population) as set by National Health Policy 2002 has been achieved in the month of December 2005 when the PR was 0.95/10,000 population.

Major Initiatives taken

Modified Leprosy Elimination Campaign (MLEC) with the package of teaching/training, intensified Information Education Communication (IEC) case detection and prompt MDT were put together and implemented in the entire country to facilitate efforts towards leprosy elimination. 5 such MLEC were conducted during 1997-98 to 2003-05 which helped in bringing out 9.9 lakh new cases for treatment over a short period of time and also in increasing leprosy awareness amongst the masses.

Special Action Project for Elimination of Leprosy (SAPEL) for Rural and Leprosy Elimination Campaign (LEC) for Urban areas were carried out to cover population residing in difficult and inaccessible rural/tribal areas as well as slums in urban areas, respectively which were not generally covered by regular programme activities.

During the year 2004-05 and 2005-06, focus of attention under National Leprosy Eradication Programme was shifted from endemic states to high priority districts and blocks based on Prevalence Rate where PR>5/10,000 in 20005 and PR>3/10,000 in 2005-06 was taken as cut-off point. Special activities in the form of Focused Leprosy Elimination Plan (FLEP) were carried out in identified district and blocks in 2005-06.

Urban Leprosy Control Programme has been implemented since 2005 under which assistance is being provided by Govt. of India to urban areas having population size of more than 1 lakh. For the purpose of providing graded assistance, the urban areas are grouped in four categories, i.e. Township-I, Medium Cities-I, Medium Cities-II, Mega Cities.[3]

Infrastructure

In endemic rural areas, the Leprosy Control Units (LCU) provides Survey leprosy services; Survey, education and treatment (SET) have been attached to Primary Health Centres (PHC) or hospital existing in low endemic areas to provide services to leprosy patients. At present, the existing infrastructure is as under:

Unit	
Leprosy Control Unit or Modified Leprosy Control Unit (LCU/MLCU)	778
Urban Leprosy Centre (ULC)	907
Survey, Education and Treatment Centre (SET)	5744
Temporary Hospitalization Ward (THW)	290
Reconstructive Surgery Unit (RSU)	75
Sample Survey Assessment Unit (SSAU)	40
Mobile Leprosy Treatment Unit	350

Objectives of the Programme

National Leprosy Control Programme had been in operation since 1955. Initially it started as centrally aided scheme with primary focus on rural areas of high and moderate endemicity. It was converted into 100% centrally sponsored scheme since 1969. The main objective that time was to control leprosy through domiciliary Dapsone Monotherapy. In view of scientific advancement and availability of highly effective treatment of leprosy, the programme was redesignated as a National Leprosy Eradication Programme in 1983 with an aim to achieve arrest of the disease activity in all the known leprosy cases in the country by the year 2000 AD. After the World Health Assembly Resolution in the year 1991, the objective of the programme was defined to achieve the elimination of leprosy by the end of century in the country thereby reducing the case load to 1 or less 10,000 population.

SPECIAL EFFORTS FOR LEPROSY CASE DETECTION AND PROMPT MDT

Modified

Leprosy Elimination Campaign (MLEC) with the package of teaching/training, intensified IEC case detection and prompt MDT were put together and implemented in the entire country to facilitate efforts towards leprosy elimination. While involving the General Health Care Staff, District Technical Support Team (DTSTs) and Community volunteers, three such nationwide campaigns have been carried out by all States/UTs between (i) February 97-September 98, (ii) January-March 2000 and (iii) October 01-February 02; during which 4.63 lakh, 2.13 lakh and 1.65 lakh leprosy cases were detected and treated with MDT, respectively. The 4th MLEC during the year 2000-03 will be undertaken from September 2002 in the country for which the specific strategy will vary according to the endemicity of different states and blocks in the districts, viz:

Category 1: 8 Endemic States

Bihar, Uttar Pradesh (new state of Uttaranchal), West Bengal, Jharkhand, Chhattisgarh, Madhya Pradesh and Orissa where mix of IEC and reorientation training, active search and Voluntary Reporting of Cases (VRC) will be undertaken. In these states VRC will be organized in all urban areas and in those rural block population where PR is less than 5/10,000 the population. In all rural areas with PP>5/10,000 the active search through house to house visit by a team of health workers and trained volunteers will be carried out.

Category 2: 14 Moderate/Low Endemic States

Andhra Pradesh, Arunchal Pradesh, Goa, Gujarat, Karnataka, Maharashtra, Tamil Nadu, Chandigarh, Daman and Diu, Dadra and Nagar Haveli, Pondicherry, Andman and Nicobar Island, Delhi and Lakshadweep where extensive IEC with training to engaged staff and Passive case detection through VRCs will be adopted.

Category 3: 13 Very low Endemic States

Haryana Punjab, Himachal Pradesh, Nagaland, Sikkim, Tripura, Meghalaya, Mizoram, Jammu and Kashmir, Assam, Manipur, Rajasthan and Kerala where extensive IEC and passive detection of cases in all the health centers will be undertaken.

SPECIAL ACTION PROJECT FOR ELIMINATION OF LEPROSY (SAPEL) FOR RURAL AND LEPROSY ELIMINATION CAMPAIGNS (LEC) FOR URBAN AREAS

Besides regular surveillance activities, the SAPELs and LECs have been designed for early detection and prompt MDT of leprosy cases along with proper IEC in the difficult and inaccessible rural/tribal areas as well as slums in urban areas, respectively. A total of 1440 SAPEL/LEC projects have been decentralized along with guidelines to States/UTs for implementation during the period 2001-03 (3 years).

WORLD BANK SUPPORTED PROJECT ON NLEP

NLEP is 100% centrally sponsored scheme. The 1st Phase of the World Bank supported Project from 1993-94 was completed on 31.3.2000 with further 6 months extension to complete the preparation of proposal for 2nd phase project. This project involved a cost of Rs. 550 crores of which World Bank loan/assistance/reimbursement was 292 crores. During this phase, against a target of 2 million cases 3.8 million leprosy cases were newly detected and on the whole 4.4 million leprosy cases were cured with MDT. The prevalence rate reduced from 24/10,000 population in 1992 before starting 1st phase project to 3.7/10,000 by March 2001 and the disability grade-II and above reduced to 2.7% from 7% whereas the MDT coverage of registered cases increased from 62% to 99.5%.

The 2nd phase of World Bank Project on NLEP started for a period of 3 years from 2001-02 involving project cost of Rs. 249.8 crore including World Bank assistance/loan of Rs. 166.35 crore and WHO to provide MDT drugs free of cost worth Rs. 48.00 crore. This phase is being implemented with the objectives towards:

- Decentralization of NLEP responsibilities to States/UTs through State/District Leprosy Societies,
- Accomplish integration of leprosy services with General Health Care System (GHS), and
- Achieve elimination of leprosy at National level by the end of the Project.

This 2nd phase of NLEP also aims to detect 11.0 lakh new leprosy cases and cure 11.5 lakh leprosy cases with MDT while reducing the disability rate to 2% among new leprosy cases,

This project thus envisages the following strategy towards Leprosy Elimination in India:

- Decentralization of NLEP to States and Districts,
- Integration of leprosy services with General Health Care System,
- Leprosy Training of GHS functionaries,
- Surveillance for early diagnosis and prompt MDT, through routine and social efforts,
- Intensified IEC using Local and Mass Media approaches,
- Prevention of disability and care,
- Monitoring and Evaluation on regular (Monthly/Quarterly/Annually) basis as well as with special efforts such as

independent Evaluation, Leprosy Elimination Monitoring (LEM), Annual Survey(s) and Validation of Elimination, etc.

Well planned activities are efficiently implemented in close association of various NLEP partners viz. State and UT/Governments, World Bank, WHO, ILEP, DANLEP, NGOs and Community, Pvt. Medical Practitioners and various concerned Government Ministries/Departments such as Information and Broadcasting, Social Justice and Empowerment, Education, Railways, Defence/paramilitary, labour and industries, etc.

Major Initiatives taken during 2nd Phase NLEP

(a) The 2nd phase of NLEP launched on 7th-8th June 2001, when all the States/UTs Health Secretaries, DHS and State Leprosy Officers (SLOs) were sensitized and state specific orientation of senior health officials from the state and district level e.g., CMHOs, DLOs and NGOs were carried out.

(b) State Leprosy Societies (SLS) have been formed in all the states/ UTs except in 8 small states/UTs where the HQ district leprosy society will function as SLS for the State/UT. In the country all the districts are covered through 576 District Leprosy Societies (DLS).

(c) Release of NLEP Fund as Grant-in-Aid to all the State Leprosy Societies and adequate quantity of anti-leprosy drugs (MDT) supply to States/UTs have been maintained. funds are also provided to the State governments as Cash Assistance for maintenance of cost of vertical units created during the particular plan period and also through District leprosy Societies for meeting the cost of other treatment activities.

(d) A nation-wide IEC through mass media (TV, AIR, News Papers) is being undertaken through M/s LINTAS (SOMAC) at cost of Rs. 11.32 crores. In addition State/District Leprosy Societies are made responsible to plan, implement, monitor and supervise rural/local IEC upto periphery.

(e) Integration of leprosy services with general health care system has been operationalised with daily availability of diagnosis and MDT of leprosy patients upto PHCs/Sub-Centers and process of merging the existing vertical NLEP staff with General Health Care system initiated which is required to be accomplished by the end of the project in the country.

(f) Based on the recommendations of national workshop held during May 02 the guidelines on simplified information system under NLEP have been issued to all the States/UTs for their implementation by September 2002.

(g) A national workshop of all concerned experts and NLEP partners, including NGOs, during July 02 extended the recommendations on "redefined roles and responsibilities of NGOs/VOs in context of leprosy elimination and integration with General Health Care System" and the same have been communicated to all the States/UTs, NLEP partners and others concerned for necessary actions at their ends.

(h) All the States/UTs through their respective leprosy societies have been equipped and empowered with all requisite guidelines, manpower and capacity building, equipments and various procurements, etc. for achieving the national objectives of leprosy elimination by the year 2004. Almost all the general health care and IEC functionaries have been oriented/trained on leprosy. Various community educational as well as advocacy activities are in full swing through out the country.[4]

Let us take a Case study of Karnataka As stated by Dr. T. Parthasarty, Joint Director, Leprosy:

Multi-Drug Treatment (MDT) for leprosy was conceived in 1981. In 1986 MDT Services were introduced in Karnakata in a phased manner to cover all the districts by 1992-93. Leprosy services has been integrated into General Health Care system in Karnataka in its G.O. No. HFW 324: CGE: 2000 Bangalore dated 15/4/2002 as per Government of India guidelines letter No. Z 14020/4/99/Lep (CCD) dated 16/12/1999. 893 Leprosy vertical staff have been absorbed into General Health Services and 813 vacant posts have been abolished. Only 25% of the vertical staff are remaining as nuclear staff at taluka level in endemic areas, at district level and at state level for monitoring of the National Leprosy Eradication Programme (NLEP) activities. With intense information, Education and Communication (IEC) activities, awareness has been and is being created for encouraging voluntary reporting to nearest Health Centres, Leprosy services are made available daily, as diagnosis is made easy merely on clinical grounds and MDT treatment, is done for any other simple disease. The unreachable/forgotten areas where pockets of hidden cases are suspected, are brought into mainstream by undertaking SAPEL/LEC projects. The Districts Technical Supporting Team are supporting in endemic districts; NLEP State coordinator (WHO) and DTST State Coordinator are assisting at State Level in planning, monitoring and implementation of NLEP.

Remarkable achievements have been made after the introduction of MDT Services regarding Prevalence of Leprosy Cases and in Prevention of Deformities. So far, 4,59,855 Leprosy Cases have been cured with MDT from 1986 and 21,810 villages are free from leprosy out of 27,066 villages in state as on 31/3/2003. The cases on hands as on 31/1/204 are 8292 cases.

The Epidemiological Trends are as follows:

The goal of NLEP is to bring down the Prevalence Rate to <1 Case per 10,000 population by the end of 2004 and in Karnataka this has already been achieved in 10 districts viz. Chitradurga, Tumkur, Chickmagaur,

Sl. No.	Particulars	31/3/1986	31/3/1993	31/3/2003	31/1/2004
1.	PR/10,000	40	69	1.9	1.57
2.	MB Proportion	16%	15%	35%	44%
3.	PB Proportion	84%	85%	65%	56%
4.	Female Rate	-	-	-	37%
5.	NCDR	7.66	5.88	4.04	1.7
6.	Child Rate	19.5%	29%	21%	15.5%
7.	Deformity Rate	17%	2.49%	1%	0.81%
8.	No. of new cases Detected and Treated	24026	26449	13070	9229
9.	No. of RFT Done	8759	39529	15340	10690
	PR	No. of Dists.	No. of Dists.	No. of Dists.	No. of Dists.
	> 10	20	17	—	—
	5-9	—	3	1	—
	2-4	—	—	11	8
	1-2	—	—	7	9
	<1	—	—	8	10
Total		20	20	27	27

Dakshina Kannada, Banglaore (U), Bangalore (R), Mysore, Mandya, Hassan and Kodagu as on 31/1/2004

The rest, i.e. in 17 districts the Prevalence rate is still between 1 to 4 with the dedicated General Hospital Care Staff and District Monitoring Nucleus staff strengthened by Dist. Staff, it is hoped to achieve the goal of NLEP in entire Karnataka by the end of 2004.

MDT Services

- Diagnosis of Leprosy and Classification is made easy by the number of anesthetic patches over the skin and peripheral nerve affections.
- The Drugs are supplied by WHO through Government of India free of cost.
- There is no shortage of supply of MDT drugs.
- Stocking of Drugs are to be maintained from sub-centre right upto Major Hospitals depending on the case load as per norms (3 months Buffer Stock).
- Validation of new cases detected (within 1 month for PB and 3 months for MB); cleaning of registers to avoid false reporting.

- The Reporting System is made very simple by Simplified Information System (SIS) Good records keeping.
- Fixed Duration Treatment (FDIT) PB 6/6 MB 12/12.

Welfare and Rehabilitation Measures for Cured Leprosy Patients:

- MCR Foot Wear, Goggles to protect the eyes, Woollen Blankets, Splints and Crutches have been provided to the needy Leprosy Patients as a Welfare Supportive Measure.
- Reconstructive surgery for those who need Surgical Corrections for the Deformities, by Orthopedic Surgeons, Eye Surgeons, and Plastic Surgeons. NGO Hospitals providing Reconstructive Surgeries are:
  (a) Swami Vivekananda Institute of Rural Health Centre, Pavagada, Tumkur.
  (b) St. Father Muller's Hospital, Kankanady, Mangalore.
  (c) Hubli's Hospital for the Handicapped, Hubli.
  (d) Belguim Leprosy, Hospital, Hindalga, Belguam.
  (e) Baptist Hospital, Bangalore.
- Government of Karnataka has reserved 5% Jobs for Group 'D' posts for those who have Grade II Deformities.
- Loans and Pensionary benefits for those who are physically handicapped.
- Housing Scheme for houseless under Ashrya Yojana, Slum Clearance Board, etc.
- NGOs are providing Training in Leather and Printing Technology as a Rehabilitation Measures (Self-Employment).[5]

SUGGESTIONS

1. Strengthen Health Care Services

In planning the strategy for the introduction of multi-drug therapy, it must be appreciated that the new challenge, resulting from the increased complexity of the treatment technology, will involve fundamental reconsideration of the various activities relating to leprosy control involving restructuring of the services to ensure high levels of case finding and case holding, strengthening of the laboratory services, retraining of staff, closer collaboration between the primary health care system and the leprosy control services, and full community participation.

2. Rehabilitation

WHO stated: "By rehabilitation is meant the physical and mental restoration, as far as possible of all treated patients to normal activity, so that they may be able to resume their place in the home, society and industry. To achieve this, treatment of physical disability is obviously necessary, but it must be accompanied by the education of the patient, his family and the public, so that not only can be take his normal place, but society will also be willing to accept him and assist in his complete rehabilitation."

To quote Dr. G.K. Shivamurthy, District Leprosy Officer, Mangalore "Footprints on Sands on Time" about Rehabilitation Leprosy still being considered a disease with social stigma, just imagine the plight of leprosy patients a couple of years ago when they were subjected to social humiliation. There were good number of patients who meekly accepted this and merely led a life of social deprivation and detachment voluntarily.

But very rarely we do come across a rare personality like Sri K.V. Shetty who till about a decade ago was a leprosy patient, but today the main spring of a rehabilitation effort for other victims of the disease. He had come across a series of obstacles in his existence. He was deserted by his own relatives and laid off by the employers of his own district; state and Maharashtra state private sector units. His deformities betrayed him on several occasions. In spite of his capacities he was put to severe distress. He also experienced several brakes in getting operation for his bilateral claw hands. But his determination and a stony will to live in dignity made him self-reliant in getting himself cured of the disease and also successfully getting operated for his deformities. Now he is able to hold his pen and write legibly after 20 years. There is now no boundary for his overwhelming joy of success. He now experiences a new breath of life.

Then started Sri Shetty's new thinking on rehabilitation of his fellow victims. His motto was to make them live with dignity. He raised funds from philanthropists and private organisations for construction and development of his brainchild "Bright India Rehabilitation Center" at Maddadka, Belthangady. Now he is rehabilitating several patients by training them in horticulture and farming. He has made provisions to provide food and shelter of the destitute. His thirst for learning has made him to author two books on leprosy, namely, "UNTOLD TRUTH ABOUT LEPROSY" AND "PROVOKING THOUGHTS ON LEPROSY."

Mr. Shetty is married to a healthy woman and is blessed with two beautiful and intelligent children. His contribution towards the cause of leprosy rehabilitation has been recognized and awarded by government of Karnataka, District Leprosy society as well as Maharashtra Government by nominating him as member of study team on leprosy. His services to leprosy patients continue uninterruptedly. He has managed to tour entire part of South Canara, Udupi, Kodagu and Chikkamagalur district. He took crusade against leprosy by propagating IPC with school children. He has proved his metal and rose from the edge of the doom.

3. Involvement of Primary Health Care

- To give orientation in leprosy to already employed MPWs. To give orientation in leprosy to community health workers.
- To include a module on leprosy during the training of MPWs.

- To train community health workers in leprosy.
- To supply adequate health education material and train them to use it properly.
- Adequate training must be provided to all PHC doctors and medical graduates.

4. Community Education

This could be greatly facilitated by the community health workers and Multipurpose workers. It is easy for them to identify the various channels of communication in the society. There should be non-formal education regarding teaching and learning process for PHC team. These information's are helpful for social science research. A systematic approach by the medical and social scientist to communicate to the periphery will help the PHC in turn to be effective to bring in the desired change in the community.[6]

5. Removal of False beliefs from the Community

Leprosy earned its sinister reputation because of its potential to disable and disfigure human beings. The dread of the deformities it causes only served to burden the sufferers with a further handicap: that of social ostracism.

The ostracism that leprosy patients face is likely to be overcome only slowly, as communities realize that former leprosy patients living among them have been totally cured, cannot transmit the disease to others, and must be encouraged to overcome their residual impairments and to in-integrate themselves into the community.[7]

6. Involvement of NGO's for Leprosys Elimination

Non-Governmental organisations (NGOs) have been involved for the cause of leprosy elimination For many decades and their contributions have made a positive impact in reducing the prevalence of leprosy. More than 290 NGOs are working in the field of leprosy throughout the country of which 30 NGOs are getting grant-in-aid from Govt. of India under SET scheme. Another 35 NGOs have been given recognition for conducting reconstructive surgeries (RCS) and are given reimbursement for undertaking major RCS operations on disabled leprosy patients @ Rs. 2500 per surgery and for supply of a pair of MCR Chappal @ Rs. 160 per pair and MRC insole @ Rs. 40 per sheet to the needy patients. GOI guidelines laying down the pattern of assistance to the NGOs have been developed which are followed for functioning and release of grant-in-aid to these organisations. As mentioned earlier, the involvement of NGOs/VOs, both, from field of leprosy and other health areas are being encouraged to play key roles on various leprosy elimination-related activities in the country.

The NGOs serve in remote, inaccessible, uncovered, urban slums, industrial/labour population and other marginalized population groups. The various activities undertaken by the NGOs are, IEC, Prevention of

Impairments and Deformities, Case follow-up and MDT delivery. From current financial year (2006-07), Grant-in-aid is being disbursed to NGO by the State Leprosy Society directly.

7. Financial and Personal Support and Psychological Assurances

Aside from the purely medical aspects of the drive against leprosy, there is the human and social side. While the cure is certain for every person with leprosy who comes forward for MDT, many still face ostracism from their own communities, even from their own families. The social suffering lingers on and together with the totally unjustifiable loss of human rights, adds a heavy psychological burden to in the physical damage that they have undergone. So it is essential for everyone concerned in public health to spread the word that leprosy is curable, that it is extremely hard to "catch", and that sufferers need not and must not be shunned. Unless this message reaches every patient in every village, and unless they come forward for the drugs—which should be available at every clinic and primary health care centres in the leprosy—endemic countries—the disease will still lurk in isolated and dangerous pockets.

It is important to avoid triumphalism and the tendency to count our chickens before they are hatched. But provided the impetus is maintained and provided there is no shortfall in the human and financial resources required we should be able to put paid to this age old disease and ensure a leprosy-free world in the 21st century.[8]

There is a need to put all these suggestions into practice. We do mere paper planning than execution. Jupinderjeet Singh reporting from Patiala (*Newsline, Indian Express,* January 31, 2000) on the basis of the study of Dr. Khushdeva Singh Leprosy Colony, suggests the need of putting in practices the promises we make. "Anti-leprosy Day was observed here today. Every year scores of functions promising schemes for the uplift of the lepers and their acceptance in the "healthy" society are organised. But most of the time such plans are forgotten by the end of the day.

And the lepers continue to be shooed away by the general public. And have to earn their bread and butter through the humiliating act of begging. This is what has happened with the inmates of Padamshri Dr. Khushdeva Singh Leprosy Colony Tafazalpura here in the suburbs of the city. The renowned doctor, famous for his work in the field of tuberculosis and leprosy, had single-handedly roped in few like-minded individuals in 1956 to set-up this colony experiment, first of its kind in the country, had objectives of regular treatment of lepers, saving their children from contracting the dreadful disease and enable the patients to live gracefully through self-earning and grants.

All these targets are on the verge of coming to a naught as the colony inmates have again resorted to begging, courtesy the failure of the once sponsored self-help business of candle making and poultry farming, the non-supply of pensionary grants as well as the apathetic attitude of the administration towards daily needs e.g. a doctor, medicines and water and power supply to the lepers."[9]

During the Ninth Plan the strategy for NLEP were:

- Strengthening laboratory services in PHC/CHC, establishing surveillance system for monitoring time trends in prevalence of the disease throughout the country.
- Accelerating the pace of activities, intensifying case detection and MDT coverage in high prevalence states and areas that are difficult to access.
- Maintaining activities in the previously highly endemic areas.
- Preparing for and initiating horizontal integration of the leprosy programme into the primary health care system.
- Greater emphasis on disability prevention and management through: (a) transfer of knowledge and technology to affected persons, families, community, (b) strengthening local treatment facilities for ulcers/leprosy-related deformities, (c) supply of aids and appliances to prevent further impairment, (d) developing trained manpower resources and improving facilities for corrective surgery for deformities.
- Implementation of Modified Leprosy Elimination campaign and bringing mass public awareness, training of general health care staff and detection of hidden cases. Ensuring rehabilitation of cured patients.
- Repeal of discriminatory provision under marriage act where leprosy is one of the grounds of divorce.

The target for the Ninth Plan is to reduce prevalence of leprosy to 1/ 10,000 by 2002 A.D.

8. Monitoring and Evaluation of NLEP

NLEP is equipped with an inbuilt information system for concurrent monitoring and feedback for timely corrective measures at various levels of programme implementation. In addition, the independent evaluation(s) of NLEP are undertaken and last such evaluation was conducted while involving NIHFW, New Delhi and NIE (CMR), Chennai in March-April 2000, with the following main observations:

- 99.7% of leprosy patients were found to be receiving MDT.
- A declining trend in prevalence rate was seen in all the states.
- Quality MDT services, accuracy in diagnosis and classification, fixed duration MDT/Treatment, regularity of treatment were being provided in most of the states.
- The drug position was found to be satisfactory in all the states/ UTs.
- Awareness of community about leprosy was found to be higher in urban areas.

Leprosy Elimination Monitoring (LEM)

The LEM is required to assess the performance of Leprosy Services and envisages to collect key information on the issues like integration, quality of leprosy services like diagnosing and treatment (MDT), Drug Supply Management and IEC, etc. the LEM exercise was carried out with WHO assistance through the National Institute of Health and Family Welfare (NIHFW), New Delhi during June 2002 in the 12 priority endemic states and the same will be repeated every year for next 3 years. During the current year another such survey is being carried out through an independent agency, "The Leprosy Mission", New Delhi in the seven high endemic States of Bihar, U.P., M.P., Orissa, West Bengal, Chhattisgarh and Jharkhand with the funds of World Bank supported 2nd National Leprosy Elimination Project.

Validation of Leprosy Elimination

Twelve States/UTs have so far reached the Goal of Elimination, i.e. Prevalence Rate, less than 1/10,000 population. There is no standard method to assess low levels of leprosy prevalence in a population for certifying achievements of elimination level. The WHO Technical Advisory Group had suggested a Pilot Testing of Validation of Elimination of Leprosy by Lot Quality Assurance Sampling Technique. Govt. of India is undertaking this study in the 2 states of India viz. Himachal Pradesh and Meghalaya, through the Central Leprosy Teaching and Research Institute (CLTRI), Chengalpattu.

CONCLUSION

Early diagnosis and prompt initiation of treatment are now considered important in the control of leprosy. Active search for cases of leprosy in endemic areas is recommended. Survelliance of household and close contact will help in detecting a large number of cases of leprosy. Health education emphasizing the availability of effective treatment and that with prompt treatment the infection can be contained is essential. There are a lot of misconceptions that leprosy is hereditary, due to impure blood, the disease always leads to deformities, etc. There is unjustified social stimga. The community should be encouraged to seek medical assistance in all the cases of suspected hypopigmented skin patches.

- Microorganisms like bacteria, fungus are the main causative agent for skin infections (boils, ringworm, impetigo, etc.) Scabies is however, caused by an insect—itch mite.
- Skin infections effect all individual but they are more common in children (except leprosy—in adults only).
- Low standard of living, unhygenic personal habits are the main causes of skin infections.
- Direct contact with the patient in most cases helps in the spread of infections.

- Proper cleanliness of the body helps prevent the occurrence of skin infections.
- Drugs and skin ointments are used to treat skin infections.
- Health Department should create Self-confidence and positive thinking among leprosy patients.
- Health Departments need to pay personal attention with sympathy and love.
- Health Department should try for their rehabilitation.
- People should be told to be sympathetic to them.
- Health education about the disease, medicine may be provided.
- Good examples as mentioned earlier may be hammered again and again.

FUTURE STRATEGY

After elimination of leprosy at National level, the country has still many areas in State, District and Block level that need extra focus. The programme will continue with following strategy:

- Maintaining the gains achieved in each of the States/UTs in which elimination has already achieved by providing existing MDT services through integrated General Health Care system.
- Achieving elimination of Leprosy in remaining States, Districts and Blocks by providing quality MDT services with Focused attention on Endemic Districts, Endemic Blocks, Endemic Urban localities, Districts with high disability rate and States with high child proportion
- Capacity Building of all categories of staff by Induction and reorientation training.
- Increase emphasis on Disability Prevention and Medical Rehabilitation (DPMR) for prevention of development of disabilities in newly detected leprosy patients and to provide medical rehabilitation services to existing deformity cases.
- Increasing awareness about Leprosy among masses and Inter-Personal Communication (IPC) to remove social stigma.[10]

In 1983-84, National Institute of Communicable Diseases (NICD), was made the nodal agency by the Ministry of Health and Family Welfare, Government of India, for planning, coordination, guidance and evaluation of Guinea Worm Eradication Programme (GWEP). At the beginning of the Programme, i.e. in 1984, about 40,000 GW cases were reported in 12,840 guinea worm endemic villages across 89 districts of seven endemic states, viz., Andhra Pradesh, Gujarat, Karnataka, Madhya Pradesh, Maharashtra and Rajasthan. The State of Tamil Nadu remained free from GW disease since 1982. The last case from Maharashtra occurred in 1992 and in 1994 in Karnataka and Madhya Pradesh. Andhra Pradesh and Gujarat reported their last cases in 1990. The last guinea worm case was reported in July 1996 in Jodhpur district of Rajasthan. World Health Organisation certified India as guinea worm disease free country in February 2000. However, WHO recommended routine surveillance and IEC to be continued till global eradication of the disease, which are being undertaken in all formerly guinea worm disease endemic states. An amount of Rs. 0.332 crore was released to different states as "Grants-in-Aid" during 2005-06.

Notes and References

1. Annual Report, Ministry of Health and Family Welfare, GOI, 2002, p. 33.
2. *Ibid.*, pp. 153-55.
3. Annual Report, Ministry of Health and Family Welfare, GOI, 2006-07, pp. 85-86.
4. Annual Report, Ministry of Health and Family Welfare, GOI, 2002, pp. 34-36.
5. Karnataka State Leprosy Society, Department of Health and Family Planning Welfare Services, Bangalore, Vol. I, No. 1, March 2004.
6. Dr. (Mrs.) E. Thangaraj, "Leprosy in Primary Health Care" in *Health Administrator*, Vol. 6, No. I, July, 1988, p. 65.
7. Denis Doumerie, The Legacy of Leprosy, in *World Health*, Sept.-Oct. 1995, p. 28.
8. WHO: *World Health*, March-April, 1998, p. 19.
9. Newsline, *Indian Express*, January 31, 2000.
10. Annual Report, Ministry of Health and Family Welfare, 2002-03, p. 87.

6

CHAPTER

HIV/AIDS

A Serious Increasing Disaster

India, the second most populous country in the world with more than 100 crore people (half of whom are adults in the sexually active age group), is the home of 16% of world population. However, the country accounts for only 2.4% of the world area. These statistics tell us how the country is crowded. Apart from these, the low literacy rate (63%) and less urbanization (more than 70% of the total population is living in rural areas) necessitates specialized programmes for making people aware of any kind of situation, particularly about various health aspects such as control and spread of infectious diseases, precautionary measurements, availability of vaccines, etc. the same is true with respect to AIDS also. India, the home of more than 4.6 million AIDS cases, earned the distinction of having the largest number of AIDS cases among South Asian countries and second place in the world (The first place goes to South Africa). According to UN estimates, there were 2.7 million AIDS deaths in India between 1980 and 2000. CIA's National Intelligence Council predicted 2025 million AIDS cases in India by 2010, more than any other country in the world. The spread of HIV within the country is mainly via heterosexual contacts and injection drug users (IDUs). The first case of HIV infection in India was diagnosed among commercial sex workers in Chennai in 1986. At present, almost all the states and Union Territories of the country are infected with AIDS, with Tamilnadu at the top with more than 24,000 cases. Only Arunachal Pradesh, Dadra and Nagar Haveli and Lakshadweep do not have any reported AIDS victims. (See Chart 6.1)

Although, in India, AIDS is concentrated among high risk populations such as commercial sex workers, IDUs and truck drivers, the surveillance data suggests that the epidemic is moving beyond these groups and in some regions into the general public.[1]

GOI, UNICEF Master Plan of operations, 2003-07 states that there

CHART 6.1

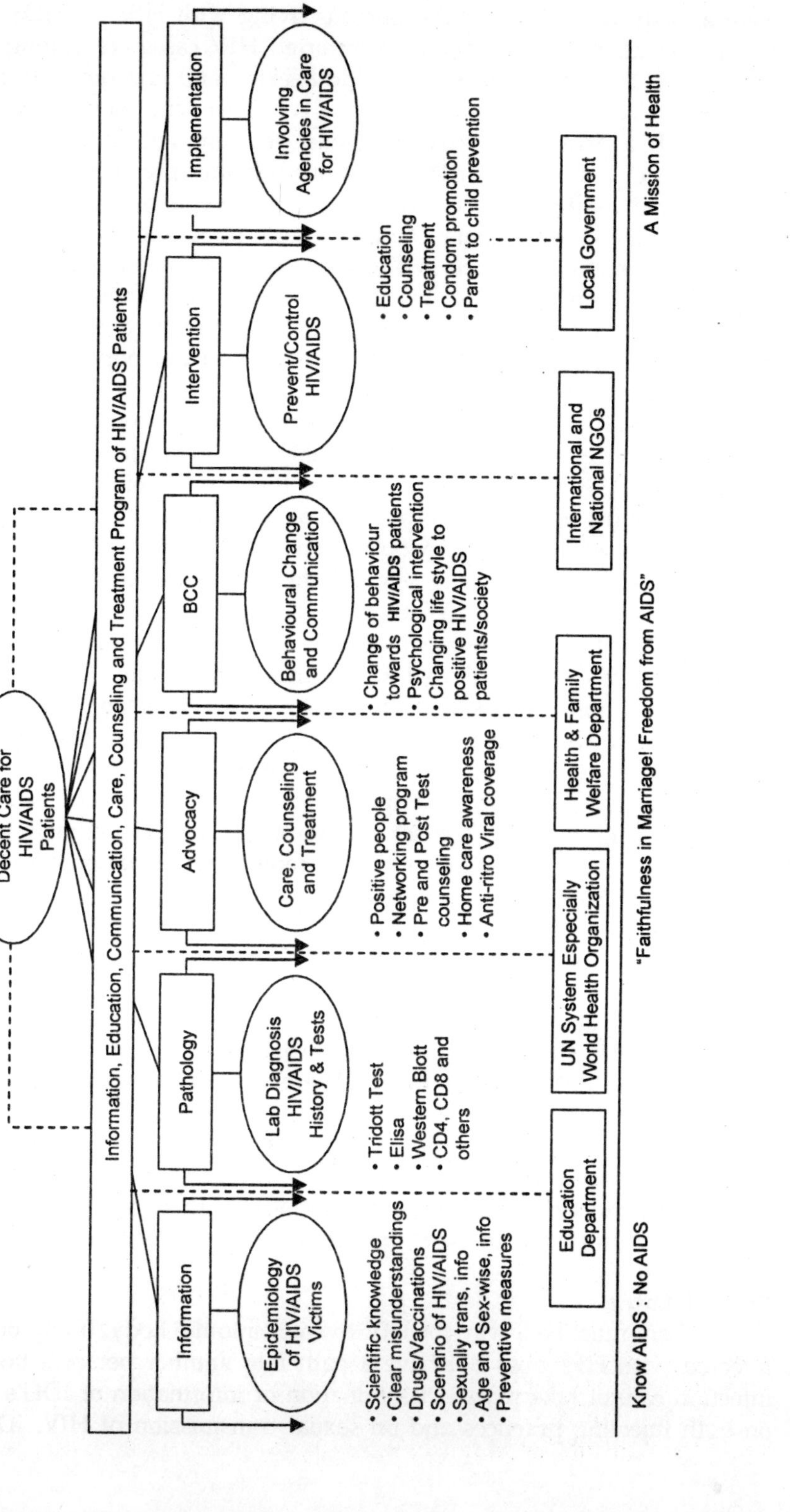
A Model for Decent Care for HIV/AIDS Patients
Information, Education, Communication, Care, Counseling and Treatment Program of HIV/AIDS Patients
Information
Pathology
Advocacy
BCC
Intervention
Implementation
Epidemiology of HIV/AIDS Victims
Lab Diagnosis HIV/AIDS History & Tests
Care, Counseling and Treatment
Behavioural Change and Communication
Prevent/Control HIV/AIDS
Involving Agencies in Care for HIV/AIDS
• Scientific knowledge
• Clear misunderstandings
• Drugs/Vaccinations
• Scenario of HIV/AIDS
• Sexually trans, info
• Age and Sex-wise, info
• Preventive measures
• Tridott Test
• Elisa
• Western Blott
• CD4, CD8 and others
• Positive people
• Networking program
• Pre and Post Test counseling
• Home care awareness
• Anti-ritro Viral coverage
• Change of behaviour towards HIV/AIDS patients
• Psychological intervention
• Changing life style to positive HIV/AIDS patients/society
• Education
• Counseling
• Treatment
• Condom promotion
• Parent to child prevention
Education Department
UN System Especially World Health Organization
Health & Family Welfare Department
International and National NGOs
Local Government
Know AIDS : No AIDS
"Faithfulness in Marriage! Freedom from AIDS"
A Mission of Health

were an estimated 3.97 million persons living with HIV or AIDS in 2001. Ninety per cent of the cumulative reported HIV cases are among persons aged 15-49, the age group that is child-bearing and economically the most productive. The national prevalence rate is 0.7 per cent, though there are six states with a prevalence exceeding one per cent which together have a population of 291.7 million. There are much higher prevalence rates among certain groups with high-risk behaviour, but the epidemic is now primarily driven by heterosexual contact in the general population. Indeed, the great majority of pregnant women found to be HIV-positive in teaching hospitals in high-prevalence states in 2000-01 had no known risk factor. Transmission is also facilitated by sexually transmitted infections, which have been found to affect 3-4 per cent of some rural populations.

Mother-to-child transmission is responsible for approximately one per cent of all HIV infections. It is estimated that about 100,000 HIV-positive women deliver every year, and that 30,000 infants acquire HIV as a result. At the end of 1999, it was estimated that there were 160,000 children aged 0-14 years living with AIDS (4 per cent of total cases). Half of all new HIV infections are among young people aged 15-29 years.

The Government has recognized the seriousness of the situation and responded to the epidemic. Working under the aegis of the National AIDS Control Board, the National AIDS Control Organisation (NACO) administers the National AIDS Control Programme (NACP-II). The Government has launched a five year strategic plan, using various approaches and strategies including the Prevention of Mother-to-Child Transmission (PMTCT), HIV/AIDS education, information and communication, advocacy and mobilization of officials, and surveillance and monitoring. NACP-II has set two key goals for 2004, namely to reduce the spread of HIV infection and to strengthen the national capacity to respond to HIV/AIDS on a long-term basis.

MEANING

AIDS-Acquired Immuno-Deficiency Syndrome is caused by a virus known as HIV (Immuno-Deficiency-Virus). It is the most talked about disease in the entire world today. There are two requirements for HIV infection to take place.

Minimum Infective Dose

There must be a sufficient quantity of HIV to allow infection to occur. If the concentration is too low, the possibility of infection does not exist.

Port of Entry

There must be a way for HIV to enter into the body. If any body fluid infected with HIV does not have a path into another person's body, then infection cannot take place. Dissemination of information of IDU's must be on both injecting practices and on sexual transmission of HIV. IDU's face the same risks and problems of sexual transmission, as do other sectors of the community. The sharing of injecting equipment increases the risk of contracting and transmitting HIV, resulting in the virus being passed onto sexual partners through unprotected sexual intercourse.[2]

The predominant mode of transmission of both HIV and other STD agents is sexual, although other routes of transmission for both include blood, blood products, donated organs, and from infected mother of her child (vertical transmission). Many of the measures for preventing sexual transmission of HIV and other STD agents are the same. There is a strong association between the occurrence of HIV infection and the presence of certain STD's making early diagnosis and effective treatment of such STDs an important strategy for the prevention of HIV transmission. STD clinic services are important access point for the people at high risk of contracting both AIDS and other STDs not only for diagnosis and treatment but also for education and counselling. HIV can be transmitted from mother to child. It is important that information on transmission includes details about all the routes of transmission. Often people may be aware of one route of transmission but not of another. IDUs in particular, need to be informed about the risks of infecting their partners through sex and or unsafe injecting practices and the subsequent risk of infecting a child.

A healthy immune system serves as the body's first line of defence for diseases. Scientific research conclusively documents that illicit drug use, including heroin, alcohol, amphetamines and marijuana, weakens and suppresses the immune system, impairs human judgment regarding safe sexual behaviour, and facilitates sexually transmitted diseases.

Alcohol and drugs also influence the progress of HIV in the post-transmission period. The numerous health problems caused by alcohol and drug abuse added to the lowered immunity status of the HIV positive individual, hastens the process of development of HIV into full-blown AIDs. So, it becomes important to recognize the link between alcohol, drugs and HIV prevention and intervention.

Alcohol and HIV

- Heavy alcohol/cannabis use can reduce the number of white blood cells which are responsible for fighting infection leading to reduced immunity level.
- Those clinically diagnosed as alcoholics appear to be more prone to bacterial infections and certain forms of cancer.
- The individual's vulnerability to being infected with HIV increases if exposed to the virus.
- In those already infected with HIV, alcohol can speed up the course of the disease.

How does alcohol consumption increase the risk of being infected with HIV through sex?

- Alcohol reduces inhibition and leads a person into high risk sexual activity. One who hesitates to make sexual overtures to a new partner or visit a sex worker may do so with less hesitation under the influence of alcohol.
- Alcohol acts as a depressant, affects perception and motor coordination which interferes with the sexual act. In his desperation to experience satisfaction he may attempt other forms of sexual activity like anal sex. Poor coordination could further discourage condom use as he may find it difficult to use.
- Alcohol impairs the ability to process negative consequences of an action. There is a tendency to overlook risks. Even one who uses condoms routinely may not do so under the influence of alcohol. He may pressurize or force the other to have sex when the other is unwilling.
- Heavy use of alcohol over a period of time impairs sexual performance. After giving up alcohol, a person craves for a sexual relationship but is doubtful whether he will be able to perform. In order to avoid failure in front of spouse, he may visit sex workers to reassure himself of his virility.

Partners of substance abusers are equally susceptible to HIV and a number of factors affect women's ability to protect themselves from HIV/AIDS..

- Lower literacy levels.
- Limited mobility.
- Limited access to information.
- Limited access to appropriate services for sexually transmitted diseases and substance use disorders of their partners.

Psycho-social, cultural and legal barriers to women's decision-making powers and independence.

After a positive test result, post-test counselling should

- ensure that the person understands what a positive HIV test result means,
- discuss how he feels about being infected,
- provide support to help the person deal with these feelings,
- discuss his plans for the immediate future,
- establish a relationship with the person as a basis for future counselling,
- schedule appointments for medical evaluation and follow-up counselling, and
- counsel partner if possible.[3]

It mainly spreads through sexual intercourse, blood contacts and from mother to child. No specific control or treatment measures are yet known. Not only survival beyond three years is unlikely but those with the disease are to go through acute physical, mental and social anguish, trauma and pam.

Who is Particularly at Risk?

- Injecting drug users and their partners
- CSWs and their clients
- Men who have sex with men
- STD clients
- Migrant workers
- Long distance truck drivers
- Women of child-bearing age

How can HIV Infection be Prevented? Health Education Measures?

- If you know you are uninfected and are sexually active, have sex only with one mutually faithful partner who is also known to be uninfected.
- In all other situations a condom should always be used during sex.
- Women with HIV should seek advice before getting pregnant because they may pass HIV to their babies.
- When you need a blood transfusion, insist on having blood that has been tested for HIV. It is safer when your relatives donate blood for you.
- When you cannot avoid skin-piercing instruments such as blades, needles and syringes insist on having sterilized instruments.
- Do not share needles and syringes in any situation.
- Cover cuts and wounds with waterproof plasters. If you do not have plasters, use a piece of clean cloth to cover the wounds.
- Women should be extra careful as they are more at risk of getting infected with HIV because they have.
- Greater chances of catching the infection during sexual intercourse.
- Greater chances of needing a blood transfusion because of bleeding associated with HIV infected pregnancy and child-birth.[4]

Progression of Infection

- Infections and acute sero-conversion illness,
- Asymptomatic infection (latency period),
- Early symptomatic illness, and

- The "full blown" AIDS stage, i.e. opportunistic infections, opportunistic tumors and other AIDS defined conditions.

Window Period

When a person is infected with HIV, it usually takes about 3 to 6 months for the antibodies to show in a blood test. This period is commonly referred to as the window period. When a blood test detects the presence of antibodies, the person tested is referred to as 'sero-positive' or 'antibody-positive test'. During the window period, an infected person can unknowingly infect others.

Later some of these Symptoms may Appear

- Dry cough or shortness of breath Diarrhoea,
- Fitigue, Fever,
- Furry white spots in the mouth (thrush),
- Significant weight loss,
- Skin rashes, swollen lymph glands,
- Lack of resistance to infection,
- Loss of appetite,
- Memory or movement difficulties,
- Night sweats, and
- Red or purplish spots on the body.[5]

PREVENTING HIV INFECTION

Even in the absence of an effective vaccine against AIDS, we know that it is possible to prevent the spread of HIV infection through individual behaviour. Information and education about personal habits are therefore essential to the Global AIDS Strategy.

These information and education measures, designed to assist people to modify or to refrain from behaviours that carry a risk of HIV infection, stress the following messages:

- Sexual intercourse is the most common route of HIV transmission. The sexual spread of HIV can be avoided by remaining with a faithful, uninfected partner or by not having sexual intercourse at all. Otherwise, people should restrict their number of sexual partners as far as possible, and should always use a condom—properly—whenever having sexual intercourse with someone who might possibly be infected with HIV; HIV can be transmitted through infected blood. As far as possible, blood for transfusion should be tested for infection with HIV, and discarded if it is found to be contaminated. Needles and other skin piercing instruments should be sterilized after each use. They should not be shared with other people; if they are, they must first be properly sterilized.

- An infected mother can pass HIV infection to her foetus or infant. Women infected with HIV should therefore consider avoiding pregnancy.

Information and education are essential to AIDs prevention programmes; but alone, they are not sufficient. Counselling and other forms of health and social services must be provided in order to motivate and encourage people to avoid the behaviours that carry a risk of HIV transmission, and to provide those who are infected with HIV, as well as their families and friends, with practical assistance and psycho-social support.

Finally, to be successful, AIDS prevention and control measures must be introduced and implemented in a social environment that is conducive to risk reduction. This means social norms and policies which respect and uphold the rights and dignity of people infected with HIV including people with AIDS.

Measures such as isolation, quarantine, and other forms of discrimination on the grounds of a person's infection status are harmful. They cause unnecessary additional suffering to people infected with HIV; and they also threaten public health more generally: thus, discriminatory policies can have the effect of discouraging people at risk of HIV infection from seeking advice and information on risk reduction, including HIV testing, and this in turn can lead to an increase in the spread of infection.[6]

Steps in Post-Test Counselling (Role Play)

The 41st World Health Assembly, which met in May 1988 in Geneva, expressed the conviction that respect for the human rights and the dignity of HIV-infected people and people with AIDS is vital to the success of AIDS control programmes. It therefore adopted a resolution on the avoidance of discrimination in relation to HIV-infected people and people with AIDS, and this now forms an integral part of the WHO Global AIDS Strategy.

Steps in Post-test Counselling for (Positive Result)

- Re-establish rapport and review pre-test notes.
- Find out what the waiting period was. Reveal test result gently.
- Client's understanding of test result checked.
- Facilitating ventilation of feelings and coping with those feelings.
- Explain the difference between HIV and AIDS.
- Ascertain support system—family, friends and relatives and medical.
- Arrange for referral services if required.
- Arrange for screening tests—blood test and chest X-ray.
- Emphasis on a "positive outlook to life", medication, yoga, good diet and adequate rest. Advice them to seek medical help for early treatment of minor ailments.

- Encourage client to bring spouse/partner and children for counselling.
- Arrange follow-up visits, ongoing supportive counselling.

Components of HIV/AIDS Counselling

WHO defines HIV counselling as a:

Dialogue between the client and the care provider aimed at enabling the client to cope with stress and to take personal decisions relating to HIV. Counselling includes evaluation of personal risks of HIV transmission and the facilitation of preventive behaviours.

HIV counselling is recommended for:

- Persons already HIV infected and their families.
- Persons wanting to be tested for presence of HIV.
- People seeking help because of past or present behaviours.
- Persons not seeking help, but who are practicing 'risky' behaviours.

Counselling in relation to HIV infection and health education of the public is the primary way of (1) reducing resistance to behavioural change, (2) helping people adjust to the need to change behaviour; (3) assisting individuals, families, and communities to use social, medical, spiritual and economic support systems; and (4) reinforcing healthy behaviours which may already exist. (An orientation to HIV/AIDS Counselling, WHO). Education is an important tool for counselling. Therefore, health education and counselling complement each other.[7]

India had launched the National AIDS Control Programme (NACP) in 1987 aimed at containing the spread of HIV in order to reduce the future morbidity and mortality. In the year 1992 a comprehensive Phase-I AIDS Control Programme was initiated with the assistance of World Bank for a period of 5 years (1992-97), but was extended upto March 1999. The Phase II of the National AIDS Control Programme (NACP-II) with the assistance of World Bank and two bilateral agencies, namely United States Agency for International Development (USAID) and Department for International Development (DFID) was initiated with effect from 1st April 1999 for a period of 5 years (1999-2004). The national AIDs Control Programme, Phase-II has two key objectives, namely: (i) to reduce the spread of HIV infection; and (ii) to strengthen the capacity of Central/State Governments to respond to HIV/AIDS on a long-term basis. Operationally, the Phase-II programme would seek to achieve the following benchmarks by the end of year 2004.

TEN POINTS ON AIDS FOR WORLD AIDS DAY

1. AIDS is a New World-wide Problem

Over 150,000 cases of AIDS have been reported from more than 145 countries around the world. All communities can be affected by AIDS because the human immunodeficiency virus, HIV, that can cause AIDS can cross all boundaries, geographical and social. Worldwide, an estimated 5 to 10 million people are already infected with HIV.

2. We Know How HIV Spreads

Fortunately, HIV can only be spread in three ways:

- Sexual intercourse,
- Blood, and
- From infected mother-to-infant.

3. To Know How HIV Spreads is to Know How to Prevent Infection

HIV can be spread by sexual intercourse—from man to woman, from woman to man and from man to man. HIV can also be spread through blood in two major ways: by receiving a transfusion of contaminated blood; or if needles or other skin-piercing instruments are used more than once without being properly cleaned and sterilized after each use. Finally, HIV can spread from infected mothers to their infants, either before, during, or after birth.

4. The Sexual Spread of HIV can be Prevented

The most effective means of preventing the sexual spread of HIV is by remaining with a faithful, uninfected partner or not having sexual intercourse at all. Otherwise, a person should reduce their number of sexual partners as much as possible. People should avoid sexual intercourse with prostitutes or other people who have many sexual partners. Whenever having sexual intercourse with someone who might possibly be infected with HIV, a condom should be used—properly—from start to finish.

5. Infection through Blood can be Stopped in a Variety of Ways

Fortunately, blood for transfusion can be tested for infection with HIV and discarded if contaminated. Needles and other skin-piercing instruments can be sterilized after each use. Drug users can—and should—stop injecting drugs; if they continue, they should use only sterile needles and not share them with anyone.

6. It is Important to Know How HIV is NOT Spread

HIV is NOT spread by causal contact at work or school, shaking hands, touching or hugging. It is NOT spread through food or water, by sharing cups or glasses, by sneezing or coughing, by insects, in swimming pools or on toilets. Knowing how HIV is NOT spread helps people understand that there is no danger of becoming infected from causal contact.

7. AIDs Affects us All

There is no reason to fear people who are HIV-infected or have AIDS. They should not be discriminated against. They need our support to help them with the physical and emotional difficulties they face.

8. Information and Education are Vital

Some day, medical research may give us a drug to cure AIDs or a vaccine to prevent AIDS. Untill then, we must rely on changes in personal behaviour to prevent the spread of HIV. Information and education are therefore vital in the fight against AIDS.

9. A Global Mobilization for a Global Threat

National AIDS programmes already exist in nearly all countries of the world. These programmes inform and educate people about AIDS, how to avoid becoming infected and how to protect others. National AIDS programmes are linked through the Global Progrmme on AIDS of the World Health Organisation, which directs and coordinates the Global AIDS Strategy. Because AIDS is a global problem, it can only be stopped in one country if it is stopped in all countries.

10. Together, we can stop AIDS[8]

You can contribute to stopping AIDS, by making sure that you understand the facts about AIDS and helping others to do the same. The risk of AIDs is not about who you are or where you are. It is about what you do. We now have the opportunity to talk about AIDS, to learn, to teach and to speak out. Join the worldwide effort to stop AIDS.

Since most of the HIV cases are found in developing countries like South Africa and India, more emphasis should be given on research to find out new antiretroviral molecules, vaccines and more affordable treatments. It is also important to stress the dissemination of information on preventive care. It is essential to give health education to high-risk groups on preventive methods. Screening of blood donors and proper sterilization of surgical instruments, needles must be ensured. The prevalence of the disease in many parts of the country is on increase, which indicates the thrust of preventive strategies to reach every corner of the country. The social isolation of infected persons, especially children, has to be brought down by awareness programmes. United States and western European countries successfully reduced the incidence of disease by preventive measures and highly active antiretroviral therapy.

Even after 20 years of intense research, we have been unable to find a curative drug or vaccine against HIV. However, the biology of the virus and pathology of disease process are well documented. Rapidly mutating virus and development of drug resistance during long-term treatment is a challenge to researchers. Innovative new approaches like designer molecules and recent advances in genetic research may help to find a cure in the future.

A CASE STUDY OF KARNATAKA

The National AIDS Control Programme is being implemented in the State as per the Guidelines of National AIDS Control Organisation, Ministry of Health and Family Welfare, GOI. This is a 100% centrally sponsored scheme. The activities under National AIDS Control Programme are being implemented through Karnataka State AIDS Prevention Society.

Objectives of Phase-II AIDS Control Project

1. To reduce the spread of HIV infection in Karnataka state.
2. To strengthen Karnataka States capacity to respond to HIV/AIDS on long-term basis.

Project Interventions

(a) To keep HIV prevalence rate below 3% of adult population in Karnataka.
(b) To reduce blood borne transmission of HIV to less than 1%.
(c) To attain awareness level of not less than 90% among the youth and others in the reproductive age group.
(d) To achieve condom use of not less than 90% among high risk behaviour groups.

Programme Components

Sl. No.	*Component Nos.*	*Description*
1.	Component-I	Targetted Intervention STD/RTI services including condom promotion
2.	Component-II	IEC, Blood Safety, and VTC
3.	Component-III	Institutional Strengthening
4.	Component-IV	Low Cost Care and Capacity Building
5.	Component-V	Intersectoral Collaboration including AIDS Education in Schools

HIV/AIDS Control Programme

The morbidity attributable to sexually transmitted disease has continued to increase through this century, relative to that caused by other infectious diseases. Sexually Transmitted Disease now rank among the 5 most important causes of loss of years of healthy productive life in developing countries. Many Sexually Transmitted Diseases (including HIV/AIDS) are often encountered as syndromes.

Sentinel Surveillance data in Karnataka 2002 reveals that almost 11-22% of STD patients are infected with HIV. HIV prevalence is high in the rural areas and among women. Therefore, it is pertinent to immediately expand the services of STD across the state, especially in the rural areas. Karnataka being one among the high prevalence states, the Sentinal Surveillance over the years indicated that there is a continuous rise in the incidence of HIV infection in the State. At present 34 STD centres are existing in the state, and they have been strengthened by way of supply of Drugs and Chemicals.

(a) Information, Education and Communication

To create awareness on HIV/AIDS in the Community, Information, Education and Communication activities are being implemented. All India Radio, Doordarshan and leading daily news papers are also utilized for conveying the messages to the community. TV spots on HIV/AIDS with the involvement of religious leaders and cine artists are being advertised through Doordarshan. Video and Audio cassette are being used by District Health and Family Welfare Officers, Information and Publicity Department and Field Publicity Department, Government of India in their publicity activities. In addition to this, Folk Media programmes such as Thogalu Gombe Aata. Yakshagana are also taken up especially in the rural areas and high prevalence districts. Tin plates with messages on Condom promotion have been displayed behind driver's seat of SKRTC buses. Folders, Booklets, Brochurs are printed and supplied to all the districts and NGOs.

(b) Observance of World AIDS Day on 1st December 2002

World AIDS Day was observed with the involvement of college students, NCC and NSS students. The Hon'ble Health Minister inaugurated the Jatha and also the State level function. Folders on Stigma and Discrimination "Live and Let Live" were printed and supplied to all the districts and NGOs. A combined message on Hon'ble Health Minister, Chief Minister and Medical Education Minister were advertised through regional news papers. TV spots involving cine artists were produced and telecasted through Doordarshan.

(c) Launching of Legislators Forum on HIV/AIDS

The State Level Legislators Forum on HIV/AIDS was launched by the Hon'ble Chief Minister of Karnataka on 3rd May 2002. Mr. Peter Poyat Executive Director, UNAIDS and Asstt. Secretary General UNO and Dr. David Miller, Country Advisor to UNADIS, and Hon'ble Speaker, Karnataka Legislative Assembly and Hon'ble Karnataka Legislative Council, Hon'ble Ministers, Members of Parliaments (Lok Sabha and Rajya Sabha), MLAs and MLCs were present.

Voluntary Counselling and Testing Centres

There are 29 VCTS functioning in Karnataka. The six old VCTCs are attached to Microbiology Department of Medical Colleges. The new 23

VCTCs in District Hospitals started functioning from 15-08-2002. They provide Pre-Test, Post-Test Counselling and HIV Testing for Diagnosis and Surveillance purposes.

Blood Safety

Under Blood Safety Programme it is ensured that the safe Blood is Transfused to a patient. Now all the Blood Banks come under the purview of Drugs and Cosmetics Act of India. All the Blood Banks require License from Drugs Controller. The Drugs Controller, Government of Karnataka and Drug Inspector of KSAPS will supervise and monitor all the Blood Banks in the state for statutory stipulations.[12]

All the Blood Banks are ensuring that before transfusion of blood to the recipient the mandatory tests for HIV, VDRL, Hepatitis-B, Hepatitis-C and Malaria are done. Under Blood Safety programme 52 Blood Banks were modernized (34 Government Blood Banks, 9 Voluntary Blood Banks run by NGOs and 9 ZBTC's) and strengthened with the NACO assistance by way of providing drugs and chemicals, consumables and supporting staff.

Two Blood Component Separation Centres are functioning, i.e. Blood Bank, NINHANS and Kidwai Memorial Institute of Oncology, Bangalore.

CD4/CD8 Count Facility

At present the facility for CD4/CD8 count is available in one, centre that is NIMHANS at Bangalore.

NGO Support

Targetted Interventions for Vulnerable Populations

Targeted Interventions through NGOs is a very crucial component of NACP-II. Under this Programme the State AIDS Society has been successful in reaching out to vulnerable populations who are otherwise not reachable through the government system.

NGOs are being supported financially and technically to reach and intervene with these vulnerable populations. The main aim of the programme is to reduce vulnerability and promote safer behaviour by promoting condom usage, with populations who are most vulnerable to the epidemic of HIV/AIDS due to various socio-economic and occupational reasons.[12]

The existing 20 targeted interventions funded by KSAPS include 4 Migrant workers' projects, 3 Commercial sex workers projects, 9 Truckers' project, 1 project each with street children, MSM and Trans-sexuals, Telephone counselling and people living with HIV/AIDS.

Care and Support is a priority area for Karnataka. Providing care and support to people living with HIV/AIDS helps the care providers to break the myths and misconceptions about HIV in the community and increase acceptability of PLWHA. This component aims at providing timely and quality treatment of opportunistic infection and sexually transmitted diseases.[13]

Population Service International (PSI)[9]

Operational Lighthouse (OPL) in its study, "The Balbir Pasha Story: An Innovative Approach to Reducing AIDS/HIV prevalence through targeted Mass Media Communications from Nov. 2002 to Feb. 2003 suggests the following lessons to make the AIDS/Control Affective:

Targeting

Allocate scarce resources to activities (from communications to counselling) that promise highest impact among those likely to contract and transmit the HIV/AIDS virus.

Integration

In an integrated approach, mass media, mid-media and inter-personal communications are designed to inform, motivate and create demand for services and products, which include phone help-lines, STI and VCT services and condoms.

Information

Changing behaviour is an iterative process, demanding an ever-expanding base of knowledge across a wide range of topics, including beliefs and habits, socio-cultural characteristics affecting gender and empowerment, patterns of migration and sexual behaviour. Over time, steady production, analysis and use of qualitative information feeds into continuous programme improvement.

Better Handling of Criticism

Key stakeholders in a city must be taken into confidence prior to reintroducing 'Balbir' into Mumbai, in order to build up an 'ally base' that can help protect the full execution of the campaign messages. It is important not to have these individuals to dictate the course of the campaign, but, rather to help mediate criticism from those who may react negatively on the basis of misinformation, misunderstanding, etc. of the campaign's objectives.

Greater Consideration of Public Sentiments

It is important to take into consideration the sentiments of individuals that may be exposed to campaign messages, and control the hype that media campaigns can create by determining appropriate compromises that will ultimately benefit the cause of HIV/AIDS communication.

Replication

Reception of 'Balbir Pasha' mass media campaign in other communities depends on prevalent attitudes in that community regarding HIV/AIDS. Campaigns must be 'tailor-fitted' to account for regional variations.

NGO Guidebook, Department of Family Welfare, Ministry of Health and Family Welfare, GOI observes that Reproductive Tract Infections (RTI) including Sexually Transmitted Infections (STI) are being recognized as a major problem. This has been brought into the reproductive health agenda. Many RTIs are sexually transmitted. The emergence of HIV and identification of STIs as a facilitating factors of designing appropriate programmes to address unmet needs for RTIs/STIs. Young people are at a greater risk of contracting sexually transmitted diseases including HIV/AIDS, due to early onset of sexual activity, reluctance/ignorance to use preventive methods and frequency of partner change.

The common causes of RTI among women include infections due to inadequate medical procedures such as unsafe abortions, unclean deliveries, and other diagnostics and therapeutic procedures, infections associated with inadequate personal, sexual and menstrual hygiene practices and sexually transmitted infections. Men also experience RTI in the form of uretheritis and genital infections. Though both men and women get infected, the prevalence and the consequences are much more severe for women.

Women hesitate to discuss the issue of RTI since it is related to sexual activity. Untreated RTI/STI create complications resulting from spread of infection to other parts of reproductive tract or other organs of the body. Major complications include, infertility, entopic Pregnancy, and cervical cancer resulting in mortality or psychological problems for women. Some infection may cause fetal wastage, preterm delivery, low birth weight babies or infecting the newborn during the delivery.

Treatment of women for STD and RTIs without the cooperation of men is an area of concern in the management of RTIs and STDs. Self-reporting of gynaecological problems is low. This is because it is associated with a sense of embarrassment and shame. This affects chances of being diagnosed and treated. Extra marital sexual behaviour of male partners contributes to the problem. Lack of negotiating ability of women in the practice of unsafe sex by partners also contributes to the problem. Treatment options available to the women are limited by a number of factors. These include a symptomatic nature of these diseases in women, their access to services, non-availability of female doctors, cultural resistance to internal examinations, and lack of availability of non-stigmatizing treatment in public sector. Patients find it easier to use the services offered by unqualified quacks though the quality of service is poor. There is need to increase the availability of quality services to people to meet their unmet needs for the management of RTI.[10]

In *The Tribune* Editorial AIDS Bomb: Defuse it the Karnataka way rightly observes:

Karnataka's plan to make AIDS test mandatory for couples before getting married is a step in the right direction. The whole country will be watching with interest how the state goes about the task of implementing it. Much will depend on the legislation it contemplates. To be effective, the onus of certifying that a prospective couple had undergone the test and they know each other's result should rest on the celebrant of the marriage like the priest or the designated official. Whatever be the manner in which the proposed law is implemented, the need for such a step cannot be overemphasised. AIDS is no longer a taboo word in India, where 5 million people are reportedly carrying the virus. Available data on the disease suggests that the AIDS bomb is ticking away and it can explode into a pandemic.

Unlike Africa where women are disproportionately afflicted with AIDS, in India men outnumber women as carriers of the disease. In most cases, wives contract the disease from their husbands, and they realise it only when their spouses die. Many men do not reveal their HIV status when they get married and by the time their wives know about it, they too would have contracted it. The proposed law will tackle this problem. But, to be effective, the state should provide AIDS testing facilities at the village level at affordable rates, if not altogether free. At present, the facility is available only at. the district level and that, too, at a cost which is beyond the means of the poor.

In view of the large size of the population, the lack of awareness and the subordinate role women play in society, the possibility of AIDS becoming an epidemic cannot be ruled out.

Unfortunately, there are sections of public opinion that mistakenly believe that AIDS is more of a scare than a reality. The random test conducted on some pilgrims to a shrine in Punjab revealed that some of them were indeed HIV+ and their percentage was above the national average. Yet, if Brazil, a developing country comparable to India, can successfully fight the disease, unlike, for example, Zimbabwe and Botswana where one-third of the adult population is HIV+, there is no reason why India should lag behind. Let other states take their cue from Karnataka and carry forward the fight against AIDS.

DECENT CARE FOR HIV/AIDS PATIENTS

Introduction

Acquired Immune Deficiency Syndrome (AIDS) was first reported in the United States of America in 1981. Today, the Human Immunodeficiency Virus (HIV), which causes AIDS, is present in virtually all countries of the world. In the South-East Asia Region, AIDS was first reported in Thailand in 1984. The rapid spread of HIV, however, began during the late 1980s in many countries of the South-East Asia region. Apart from people with high-risk behaviour, such as homosexuals, female sex workers and injecting drug users, HIV infection rates have begun to increase in the general population as well. Heterosexual intercourse is the major route of transmission in the region. People with thalassaemia who require frequent blood transfusions are also at risk. The Global Program on AIDS (GPA), established by WHO in 1987, was succeeded by UNAIDS, a joint program of various UN agencies (WHO, UNICEF, UNDP, UNESCO, UNFPA and the World Bank) in January 1996 to fight against this deadly disease.

Preface

HIV/AIDS has emerged as a formidable challenge to public health over the last decade. HIV prevalence in India among adults is estimated at 0.9% to 1.4% in 2004; 25% of whom are women. The spread of HIV infection is not uniform across all states. Six states of Indian Union (Andhra Pradesh, Karnataka, Maharashtra, Manipur, Nagaland, Tamilnadu) have been categorized as high prevalence states. Key factors fuelling spread of HIV infection have been identified as labour migration from economically backward pockets to more developed regions, low literacy levels, particularly among marginalized and vulnerable sections of society, gender disparity, prevalence of reproductive tract infections and sexually transmitted diseases among both men and women. The following measures have been adopted in India to deal with HIV/AIDS:

- The National AIDS Control Organisation was set-up in 1992.
- Phase II of the National AIDS Control program launched in 1999 has a specific focus on strengthening the capacity of the Central/State governments to respond to HIV/AIDS on a long-term basis.
- The National AIDS Control and Prevention Policy 2002 makes special mention about the protection of rights of HIV positive women in making decisions regarding pregnancy and childbirth.
- There has been a change in approach from seeing transmission mechanism as mother-to-child to seeing it as parent-to-child. The Government commits itself to providing prophylaxis for prevention of parent to child transmission and the requisite counselling to all infected mothers based on informed consent.
- Safe blood transfusion is assured at district level.
- As per agreed guidelines of WHO and GOI, by 2005, 3 million persons with HIV were covered by anti-retroviral (ARV) drugs. From April 1, 2004 free ARV drugs are being made available to mothers having HIV.
- The Family Health Awareness Campaign is an effort to address the management of Sexually Transmitted Infections (STIs) and HIV/AIDS by generating awareness among the vulnerable groups, residents of rural and urban slums, particularly vulnerable women.

The key lesson to be learnt is that the world is now just a large neighbourhood. A threat from HIV/AIDS to one corner is an attack on all of us. Whether in developed or developing countries, we all have a common destiny, and a common enemy, which must be defeated by a common strategy to realize our goal of harnessing nature to our advantage and ensuring continued development.

Observed Statement of the Problems

One of the crucial factors about HIV/AIDS is that it is different from most other diseases and consequently requires a radically different and a broader response, one which goes beyond the health sector. The various factors which make it different from other diseases are:

1. HIV occurs through specific risk behaviours that are within the realm of private life, i.e. extra-marital sexual intercourse, which is intimate and private and not open to public debate.
2. HIV selectively affects two groups—the young adults and the very poor, eighty to ninety per cent of those affected are young adults, at the prime of their productive and reproductive lives.
3. HIV/AIDS retains a long period of invisibility. The danger is that during this period, most are unaware that they are infected and they continue to spread the disease.
4. The prognosis for HIV/AIDS is bleak. Currently there is no vaccine and no medical cure. Treatment options are very expensive HIV/AIDS essentially an incurable and fatal disease as at present.
5. HIV/AIDS aggravates existing health problems like tuberculosis, hepatitis, enteric fever, etc.
6. HIV/AIDS destabilizes society because of the fear, blame and stigma attached to it. It threatens basic human rights and invades the right to privacy and human dignity.
7. The scale of the epidemic is vast and almost every country is involved as compared to other infectious diseases.
8. Its less visible consequences, constitute an urgent and massive threat to development, i.e. deteriorating child survival, reduced life expectancy, increasing number of orphans, and loss of the most productive section of the population.

Thus unlike other diseases, HIV/AIDS has serious implications for the individual, family and the community. The hardships faced by the AIDS patients are innumerable—Social isolation, lack of diagnostic and treatment facilities, lack of counselling and rehabilitation centers, harassment from family members and the police, scarce medical care, sense of shame and treatment as a criminal, etc. are some of the painful situations faced by the AIDS patients in their daily lives.

The 41st World Health Assembly which met in May 1988 in Geneva felt that safeguarding the dignity of HIV/AIDS infected people is vital to the success of any AIDS Control program.

Decent Care

At present, HIV/AIDS affected people carry a serious social stigma. Their life is miserable and a discussion with most of them in confidence in some parts of India, i.e. Chandigarh, Punjab and Haryana reveals that such people prefer to die rather than lead a life of shame, guilt, insult as well as mal-treatment.

Even interactions with family members indicate that they are considered a blot on the fair name of the family. Indian people being superstitious and dogmatic, have no sympathy for HIV/AIDS patients who indulge in sexual activities through extra-marital relations and violate the codes of good behaviour of the society. It is a matter of great concern that even medical and health professionals do not provide sympathy, love and affection. The HIV/AIDS patients feel frustrated due to internal as well as external environment leading to suicidal tendencies. Rampant poverty accentuates risky practices like using used syringes, unsafe blood transmission, etc.

There is a need for a care system which is active and holistic led by a professional team at a time, when the patients stop responding to curative treatment and life expectancy is relatively short. The goal of palliative care is to provide physical, psychological, social, spiritual support and care for patients in the last phases of the diseases so that they can live as fully and comfortably as possible and maintain their dignity till their death and in death.

Decent Care for HIV/AIDS in India: Some Suggestions

1. The staff engaged in Indian Health infrastructure consisting of 1,37,311 sub-centers (each serving a population of 5000), 22842 Primary Health Centers (each serving a population of 30000), 3043 Community Health Centers (each serving a population of one lakh), Sub-Divisional Hospitals, District Hospitals, Super Specialty Hospitals, need to be trained, sensitized and re-oriented in the science and art of decent health care for HIV/AIDS patients, family and community.
2. Sex-Education must be introduced for children, adults, and the whole community so that people can understand the causes of HIV/AIDS and take preventive measures. Suzanne Cherney in an article, "AIDS: A Glance Back, a Look Forward" in *World Health,* March-April, 1995 states, "Global Program on AIDS (GPA) thus invests a great deal of time in explaining why preventive methods such as school AIDS education are effective and not harmful. It argues for the empowerment of women, millions of whom are unable to negotiate safe sex or leave a relationship that puts them at risk. GPA advocates against coercive measures such as mandatory HIV testing which not only flout human rights but threaten to make the epidemic worse by driving people away from prevention and care program.

3. John Bland in his article, "Issues of Life and Death", in *World Health,* Nov. 1982, states that "Small hospitals may be started for the incurable sick where the reality of death can be faced in a loving and caring environment to help the patient to live to the limit of his/her potential in physical strength, in mental and emotional capacity and the social relationship."
4. As with all sexually transmitted diseases from time immemorial, there is one sure fine way of avoiding HIV/AIDS, though abstinence, prevention and early detection.
5. Making people aware of their rights and responsibilities to help them to determine their own health priorities and to take part in solving their own health problems, is a step so essential in the process of empowerment of the people for prevention of HIV/AIDS.
6. The prevention and control of HIV Infection must be closely integrated with existing services for women, mothers and children.
7. HIV/AIDS programs cannot be conducted by health sector alone. It demands coordinated action by governmental and voluntary organisations and local authorities.
8. Teachers and students can help the victims of HIV/AIDS through health education to lessen their grief and take proper measures to motivate them to lead a decent life. Higher education, in this way can act as a bridge between the community and government.
9. Health professionals need not isolate themselves in health institutions for diagnosis of HIV/AIDS positive cases but should initiate public campaigns to remove the false impressions about MW/AIDS only when the public at large would be educated, the HIV/AIDS patients will be able to lead a decent life.
10. Since the problem of HIV/AIDS is going to be bigger and bigger especially in developing countries, there is a need to carry out research on priority basis firstly to find a permanent solution to the problem and secondly to discover new medicines, as an interim measure.
11. Health professionals, family members, NGOs, Self-Help Groups (SHG), Social Activists and the leaders of the community should provide counselling to HIV/AIDS affected patients repeatedly as they become psychologically, emotionally, morally very weak.
12. Media especially through Wall Posters, Pamphlets, Information Booklets, Wall Slogans, Cultural Programs, etc. can help the prevention of Spread of HIV/AIDS by advocating abstinence from unsafe sex.
13. HIV/AIDS positive cases can be kept busy in some small-scale industries so that they consider themselves to be productive rather than a burden on family and society.

We can help the victims of AIDS by:

- Making them comfortable and protecting them from problems that can make them feel worse.
- Helping them to be as independent as possible.
- Assisting them in coping with, the continuing physical and financial losses, they experience.
- Helping them and their families prepare for death. This may include making a Will, tending to relationships in the family or the community, and arranging for the transfer of responsibilities.
- Keeping them within the community and family groups for as long as possible through a caring approach.
- Involving Religious leaders who have great influence on the community. The Union Territory (UT) Chandigarh (India) AIDS Control Society is trying to involve religious leaders to educate on HIV/AIDS, the stigma attached with it, high risk behaviours and safe practices. The results of such innovative practices may be replicated in other places also to provide enduring care for HIV/AIDS.
- Provide physical contact to MW/AIDS patients by touching, holding hands and hugging to make them feel wanted and live with dignity.
- Reaching out to the vulnerable and the poor.

It is high time that comprehensive strategies for HIV prevention, treatment and decent care be universalized for ushering in an AIDS free Generation.

CONCLUSION

There is a need to tackle this disease through sustained efforts otherwise this disease can take huge tolls.

During the Ninth Plan the focus is on:

(1) more effective implementation of the programme for ensuring safety of blood/blood products;
(2) increasing the number of HIV testing network;
(3) augmenting STD, HIV/AIDS care facilities;
(4) improving hospital infection control and waste management so as to reduce accidental HIV infection;
(5) enhancing efforts to improve HIV/AIDS awareness, counselling and care; and
(6) strengthening sentinel surveillance.[11]

We recognise that the AIDS situation is likely to become even more serious during the next few years. In the face of this global emergency, we cannot give AIDS a "grace period", and the opportunity for prevention must not be lost. We have a collective and historical responsibility to take action now against a world-wide epidemic whose ultimate scope and dimensions we cannot yet predict. The awareness of our collective strength heightens our sense of responsibility. What has so far; amazingly, been accomplished during the past seven years is a credit to many throughout the world.

The global challenge which lies ahead will truly demand the best of us all.[12]

Race against Time

Professor Luc Montagnier, Chief of the Viral Oncology Unit, Pasteur Institute, Paris, observes that AIDS is becoming beyond doubt a major health problem for some developed and developing countries. Because there are no medical solutions available, it has also raised serious social problems. Researchers have therefore a heavy responsibility and, as one among the first to be involved in unraveling the viral origin of this epidemic, I am acutely aware of this responsibility.

The aims of AIDS research are, of course, to find efficient treatment to cure AIDS patients or to eradicate HIV infection in seropositive persons, and to find a vaccine. But if there are already some hopes of progress in these fields, I feel strongly that more fundamental research is still needed before we arrive at the right solution. Viruses of the type to which the causative agent of AIDS belongs are old, almost perfect biological objects for survival. The more we study them, the more we are surprised by many ways in which they act. Fighting against such viruses calls for hard and skilled work, and perhaps the deployment of new concepts as well. International collaboration in this field is also absolutely necessary. No doubt, we will win the race against this new epidemic, but body as yet can predict when and how.[13]

Notes and References

1. Dr. M.V.S.S.T. Subbarao, "Aiids and the Silent Killer", Science in India, *The National Science Magazine*, Vol. 7, No. 8, August 2004, pp. 17-18.
2. UNICEF, Master Plan of Operations, 2003-7, p. 43.
3. United States Office on Drugs and Crime, Regional Office for South Asia and Ministry of Social Justice and Empowerment, Govt. of India, Drug Use and HIV/AID Prevention and Management, New Delhi, 2004, p. 10.
4. Drug use and HIV/AID, Prevention and Management, *op. cit.*, pp. 11-13.
5. *World Health*, WHO and the Global AID Strategy, Oct. 1989, pp. 4-5.
6. Drugs and HIV/AIDS Prevention and Management, *op. cit.*, pp. 17-18.
7. Annual Report, 2002-03, Ministry of Health and Family Welfare, pp. 49-54.
8. *World Health*, AID, A World Wide Effort will Stop it, Oct. 1989, p. 27.
9. Annual Report, 2002-03, Govt. of Karnataka, pp. 8-11.
10. Ministry of Health and Family Welfare, NGO, Guidelines, p. 41.
11. Ninth Five Year Plan, para 3.4.17.
12. *World Health*, March 1988, p. 8.
13. *World Health*, March 1988, p. 12.

7

CHAPTER

Mental Health and Mental Retardation

Mental Health Care, unlike many other areas of health, does not generally demand costly technology. Rather, it requires the sensitive deployment of personnel who have been properly trained in the use of relatively inexpensive drugs and psychological support skills on an outpatient basis. What is needed, above all, is for all concerned to work closely together to address the multi-faceted challenges of mental health.

—*Dr. Vijay Chandra*

NEED

The component of Primary Health Care has promotion of Mental Health as one of the eight specified areas. The battle for healthy minds and healthy behaviour has to be fought at the front line of our struggle for Health for All: in the community, in the family, in the school and in the factory—that is to say, at the level of primary health care. Victories won at that front line will strengthen our conviction that psychosocial distress, alcohol and drug abuse, and health damaging behaviour don't need to be the price paid for socio-economic development.

Success in this field will also help to relegate to the past the tainted image of mental health as an euphemism for lifelong impairment, social stigma an custodial dependency.

Though mental health problems have been in existence since times immemorial, but in the modern civilization, it has its serious effects on the health of the people. Urbanization, over-population, competition, stresses and strains of modern life are adding to the mental problems. Mental disability has not achieved the attention it deserves.

CHART I

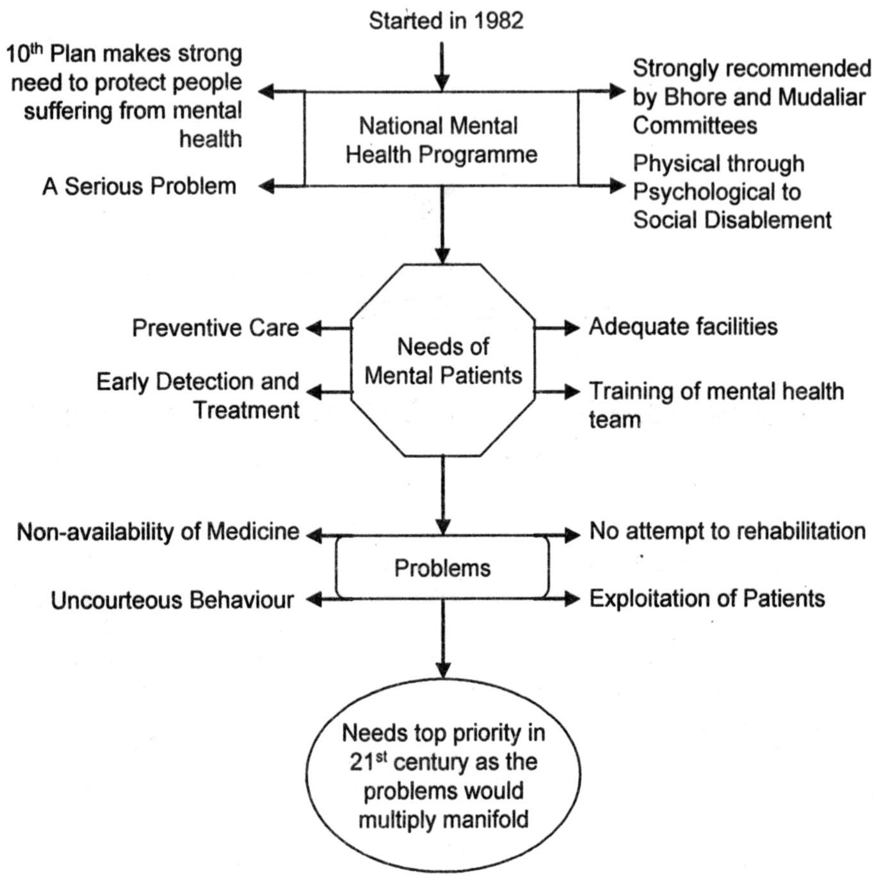

Scope and Importance of Mental Health

Govindaswamy has rightly said: "The field of mental health in India has THREE objectives. One of these has to do with mentally ill persons. For them the objectives is the restoration of health. A second has to do with these propel who are mentally healthy but who may become ill if they are not protected from conditions that are conducive to mental illness which however are not the same fore every individual. The third objective has to do with the promotion of mental health with normal persons, quite apart from any question of disease or infirmity. This is positive mental health. It consists in the protection and development of all levels of human society to secure, affectionate and satisfying human relationships and in the reduction of hostile tensions in the community.[1]

J.S. Naki in his Article "Mental Disability" rightly stresses this disability is a complex concept. It ranges from physical, through psychological, to social disablement. Its manifestations differ widely in visibility and hence in the concern they evoke. Such physical disabilities as blindness and deafness, being most visible, have easily attracted the active interest not only on health professionals and charitable organisations, but also of many governments. Disability resulting from mental disorder, on the other hand, has attracted insufficient attention from the public even while it generates greater anxiety, disgust and repulsion than physical disability. Yet it can often be equally devastating, and afflicts not only the disabled but also many of those around them, especially members of their family.[2]

Even World Health Organisation has realized the need of raising awareness about mental health. The promotion of mental health and the prevention of mental disorders both require that people should be aware of what mental health means. Many of the basic concepts involved are quite simple, but are not necessarily seen by people as relating directly to their own lives.

The physical and mental health of an individual are inter-related and no health programme can be considered complete without adequate provision for the treatment of mental ill-health and for the promotion of positive mental health. Positive mental health is characterized by discriminative self-restraint associated with consideration for others. A man in such positive health uses effectively his intelligence and talents to obtain the maximum satisfaction from life, with the minimum of discomfort to others. He will not allow himself to be overwhelmed by the stresses and strains inseparable from ordinary existence. He not only profits from experience but, under favourable circumstances, can transcend such experience. It should be the aim of every health programme to include measures meant to assist the individual to achieve mental stability and poise and develop into a useful citizen.[3]

According to the American Psychological Association (APA), division-12, the field is involved with:

> ...research, teaching and services relevant to the application of principles, methods and procedures for understanding, predicting and alleviating intellectual, emotional, biological, psychological, social and behavioural maladjustment, disability and discomfort applied to a wide range of client populations.[4]

The Indian Association of Clinical Psychologists (IACP) preferred to define clinical psychology as:

> ...an applied branch of psychology which, drawing heavily from the biological medical and social sciences, aims to study systematically all kinds of pathological deviations of human behaviour and experience from the normal pattern with a view to develop and apply adequate diagnostic, therapeutic, rehabilitative and preventive (including legal) techniques and measures.[5]

Mental and behavioural disorders account for 12% of the global burden of disease. It is estimated that nearly 450 million people suffer from a mental or behavioural disorder in the world. Nearly 10% of total population suffers from these disorders. In 1990, it was estimated that 10% Disability Adjusted Life Year (DALYs) across all age groups were due to depressive disorders, suicides and alcohol-related problems. A selective examination in 15-44 years and in gender specific terms indicates that depressive disorders, alcohol abuse, suicides, schizophrenia, bipolar disorders and panic disorders rank high among causes. Depression ranks third among men and second among women. Yet, mental health budgets of most countries are less than 1% of their total health expenditure. Further, 40% of the countries have no mental health policy and 30% have no mental health programme.[6]

A major cause for this scenario in India is lack of epidemiological data and absence of policy driven epidemiological data and research driven mental healthcare policies. It is estimated that India alone has about 1000 million people in need of mental health services.[7]

A recent study by NIMHANS submitted to the Commission on Macro Economics and Health estimated that nearly 100 million or about 10% of our population are in need of specific mental and neurological care. Several epidemiological studies in India, and some recent reviews by the Ministry of Health and Family Welfare, Government of India, have clearly established that nearly 10 million people suffer from serious mental disorders, 60 million people have moderate and minor mental disorders and about 30 million people have neurological disorders.[8]

National Health Policy 2002 stipulates, "A network of decentralized mental health services for ameliorating the more common categories of disorders is envisaged. The programme outline for such a disease would involve the diagnosis of common disorders, and the prescription of common therapeutic drugs, by general duty medical staff. In regard to mental health institutions for in-door treatment of patients, the Policy envisages the upgrading of the physical infrastructure of such institutions at Central Government expense so as to secure the human rights of this vulnerable segment of society."

The Promotion of Positive Mental Health: Bhore Committee Recommended

The pursuit of positive mental health requires the harmonious development of man's physical, emotional and intellectual equipment. Measures designed to create and maintain an environment conductive to healthful living and to control the specific causes responsible for all forms of physical and mental ill-health are essential for promoting such development. The comprehensive programme of health reconstruction which we have recommended in this report, will if implemented, constitutes in itself no small contribution to the development of positive mental health in the community. Apart from provision for the prevention and cure of specific forms of ill-health, physical and mental, many of our proposals, e.g. those dealing with health and physical education, the social aspects of our programmes for mothers and children, for the school going population and for industrial workers, the removal of slums and the creation of parks and other facilities for promoting community life should also help to raise the level of mental health in the community.

The development of an integrated personality, which will help the individual to adjust himself to the stress and strain of life, is essential if sound mental health is to be achieved and maintained. The mental health programme, if properly organized, should be able to assist in the endeavour to secure the unhampered development of human personality. Psychologists agreed that the child requires a domestic environment which assures it a sense of security "based upon affection, consistency, fairness, regularity and serenity" if its mental development is to proceed on sound lines. At a later age the child's mental development is also influenced to a large extent by the teacher. An educational campaign for imparting to parents and teachers knowledge regarding the ways in which they can help the normal mental growth of the children for whom they are responsible is an essential part of a mental health programme. Such education will supplement the provision that the mental health service will make through child guidance clinics, to correct unsatisfactory mental or emotional states in children which, if left uncared for, lead to the development of "an aggressive anti-social attitude that is socially destructive or to a regressive attitude which is destructive to the personality."

The mental health programme should also include within it scope educational propaganda for the adult. Opportunities for self-expression through work and recreational facilities are of great importance for the maintenance of a man's mental health. He should therefore be encouraged to create for himself as wide a field of cultural activity as is compatible with his main occupation. The development of hobbies helps to keep alive an active interest in life. A cultivation of the love of nature enables the individual to escape from the cramping limitations of his daily round of duties and to obtain, from the changing panorama of nature, refreshment which invigorates him without leaving behind any adverse after-effects. The arts also provide a varied field for self-expression outside a person's normal range of duties.

Economic insecurity probably plays a part in preventing the attainment of full mental health in the case of many adults. The view is widely held that unemployment promotes the incidence of psycho-neurotic conditions and some evidence has been advanced in support of this view. The wider aspects of the social security problem are clearly beyond the scope of our investigation. We may, however, draw attention to the fact that the provision of adequate medical care, preventive and curative for the individual, without regard to his ability to pay for it, is becoming recognized in all progressive countries as part of the National Social Security Programme. We have advocated in this report the adoption in India of this objective of a full and free medical service to all.

The Central Council of Health adopted the following resolutions for the promotion of Mental Health Services (held on 18-20 August 1982).

Mental health must form an integral part of the total health programme and as such should be included in all national policies and programmes in the field of Health, Education and Social Welfare. Realizing the importance of mental health in the course curricula for various levels of health professionals, suitable action should be taken in consultation with appropriate authorities to strengthen the Mental Health Education components. While appreciating the efforts of the Central Government in pursuing legislative action on Mental Health Bill, the joint Conference expressed its earnestness to see that the bill takes a legal shape at the earliest."

Mudaliar Committee Report 1961 recommended that:

There is, therefore, urgent need for the setting up of preventive mental health services, for the expansion and improvement of curative services, for the institution of training facilities, for meeting these needs and for research and survey programmes. The administrative organisation at the Centre and in the States survey programmes. The administrative organisation at the Centre and in the states would need to be geared upto meet these needs. In the preventive field there should be:

- Provision for mental health services at pre-primary, primary and secondary schools by the employment of not only psychiatrists and psychiatric social workers, but also by the employment of school counselors among the teachers who have undergone intensive training and who would be able to deal with children with emotional difficulties and other problems.
- Marital and pre-marital guidance in the social field.
- Child guidance and psychiatric clinics in all teaching and other major and district hospitals.

The following curative psychiatric services for adults need to be provided to a far greater extent than at present:

(i) In-patients and out-patient departments at lay hospitals.

(ii) Independent psychiatric out-patient clinics or mental health clinics.

(iii) Institutions for mental defectives.

Training

Training of psychiatric and mental health personnel. Orientation in mental hygiene for various professional groups in the field of family welfare and child welfare such as pediatricians, school teachers, nurses, social administrators, etc. All medical and public health personnel should be given orientation in the subject of mental health. There is a need of a plan for starting schemes of training and psychiatric services on a pilot scale with the assistance of voluntary organisations and/or existing colleges and mental institutions.

Research

Research to increase the knowledge of the multiple causes of mental diseases and disorders, research in the factors which promote positive mental health, studies of personal and educational problems of children, the studies of the genesis of unhealthy parent/child relationships, research in association with the practitioners of indigenous systems of medicine in the treatment of mental illness with a view to benefit from the rich and ancient heritage of Ayurvedic and Unani systems of treatment, study of the possibilities of integrating psychiatric teaching within the medical curriculum, study of the role of malnutrition in the aetiology of psychiatric disorders, survey of the incidence of suicides and factors in relation to psychiatric aspects of crimes, need to be undertaken.

There is an acute shortage of personnel trained in mental health. Psychiatrists, clinical psychologists and psychiatric nurses need to be trained in large number. We are glad to note the increased demand on the training facilities in the All India Institute of Mental Health, Banglore. Such facilities need to be multiplied. The Ranchi Mental Hospital should be developed into a full-fledged training institution and ultimately each region if not each state should become self-sufficient in the training of mental health personnel.

FACILITIES OF MENTAL HEALTHCARE

Each district hospital should have a psychiatric clinic in the course of the next 10 years. Five to ten beds at the district level may be earmarked for psychiatric cases. Mental hospitals should be developed on a regional basis, the optimum strength being about 750. The majority of the mental hospitals are at present extremely overcrowded and understaffed. It is only in some places that there is an evidence of their transition from custodial to curative institutions. We have laid stress elsewhere on the importance of developing preventive psychiatric services, but even so the existing institutional facilities for the treatment of mental illness fall so short of the needs that within the next 10 years the number of mental hospital beds should at least be doubled.

Tenth Five Year Plan suggested the following points:

1. Redesigning the DMHP, around a nodal institution, which in most instances will be zonal medical college.
2. Strengthening the medical colleges with a view to develop psychiatric manpower, improve psychiatric treatment facilities

at the secondary level, and to promote the development of general hospital psychiatry in order to reduce and eventually eliminate to a large extent the need for large mental hospitals with a huge proportion of long-stay patients.

3. Streamlining and modernization of mental hospitals to transform them from the present mainly custodial mode to tertiary care centers of excellence with a dynamic social orientation for providing leadership to research and development (R&D) in the field of community mental health.
4. Strengthening of central and state mental health authorities in order that they may effectively fulfil their role of monitoring ongoing mental health programmes, determining priorities at the central/state level and promoting intersectoral collaboration and linkages with other national programmes.
5. Research and training aimed at building up an extensive database of epidemiological information related to mental disorders and their course/outcome, therapeutic needs of the community, development of better and more cost-effective intervention models, promotion of intersectoral research and providing the necessary inputs/conceptual framework for health and policy planning. Focused Information, Education and Communication (IEC) activities, formulated with the active collaboration of professional agencies, such as the Indian Institute of Mass Communication and directed towards enhancing public awareness and eradicating the stigma/ discrimination related to mental illness, will form an important component of this policy objective.

GENESIS AND GROWTH OF MENTAL HEALTH PROGRAMME[9]

The National Mental Health Programme was started in 1982. Severe mental disorders that include schizophrenia, bipolar disorder, organic psychosis and major depression affect nearly 20 per 1000 population. This population needs continuous treatment and regular follow-up attention. Close to ten million severely mentally ill are in our country without adequate treatment by this estimate. More than half remain never-treated. Lack of knowledge on the treatment availability and potential benefits of seeking treatment are important causes for the above. With a large population in our country and very few psychiatrists being available for every 3 lacs population. The psychiatrist/population ratio in rural areas that account for 70% of country's population, could well be under one for every million.

To address this huge burden NMHP was started in 1982 with the following objectives:

- To ensure availability and accessibility of minimum mental health care for all in the near foreseeable future, particularly to the most vulnerable sections of the population.
- To encourage mental health knowledge and skills in general health care and social development.
- To promote community participation in mental health service development and to stimulate self-help in the community.

A model for delivery of community-based mental health care at the level of district was evolved and field-tested in Bellary district of Karnataka by NIMHANS between 1986-1995.[9]

The District Mental Health Programme was launched in 1996-97 in four districts, one each in Andhra Pradesh, Assam, Rajasthan and Tamil Nadu. The programme has been extended to seven more districts, one each in Himachal Pradesh, Uttar Pradesh, Haryana, Punjab, Madhya Pradesh, Maharashtra and Arunachal Pradesh in 1997-98. The programme envisages a community-based approach to the problem, which includes: (i) training of the mental health team at the identified nodal institution within the state, (ii) increase awareness in the case of necessity about mental health problems, (iii) provide services for early election and treatment of mental illness in the community itself with both OPD and indoor treatment and follow-up of discharged cases, and (iv) provide data and experience at the level of community in the state and center for future planning, improvement in service and research. The training to the trainers at the state level is provided by the National Institution of Mental Health and Neuro Sciences, Bangalore.

This model was adapted as the District Mental Health Programme (DMHP) and it was implemented in 27 Districts across 22 states/UTs in the IXth plan beginning in the year 1996.

NMHP during the Xth Plan

An evaluation of the NMHP was undertaken in 2003 and the programme was restrategised to incorporate the following changes and it became from single pronged to a multi-pronged programme for effective reach and impact on mental illness.

Main strategies of NMHP during the 10th plan-period was as follows:

- Expansion of DMHP to 100 districts all over the country.
- Strengthening and Modernization of Mental Hospitals.
- Up gradation of Psychiatry wings in the General Hospitals/ Medical Colleges.
- IEC Activities.
- Research and Training in Mental Health for improving service delivery.

Re-strategised National Mental Health Programme—10th Five Year Plan

- NMHP with a total outlay of Rs. 139 crore for 10th Five Year Plan was launched in the year 2003.
- National Human Rights Commission conducted a review of the functioning of all state run mental health institutions and psychiatric wards in general and medical college hospitals.
- Hon'ble Supreme Court of India has been monitoring the condition of mental health institutions and accordingly passing directions to the State Governments and Central Government to improve the status of these institutions and health care facilities for the mentally ill patients.
- District Mental Health Programme.

It now covers 94 districts in 29 States/Union Territories all over the country. In addition, Proposal for covering 22 more districts under DMHP, upgradation of 6 more Medical Colleges and strengthening and modernization of one Mental Institute have been approved during the year 2006-07. Its main objective is to provide basic mental health services to the community and to integrate these with other health services. The programme envisages a community-based approach to the problem, which includes:

- Training of mental health team at the identified nodal institutions.
- Increase awareness about Mental Health problems.
- Provide service for early detection and treatment of mental illnesses in the community (OPD/Indoor and follow up)
- Provide valuable data and experience at the level of community, at the state and center for future planning and improvement in service and research.

Problems

Mental Health facilities are in bad shape in the India. Based upon observation, study and analysis, we mention the following problems faced by psychiatric patients:

1. Poor facilities resulting into acute problems. The environment of mental hospitals is so disgusting that the patients become more sick rather than recover. There are not adequate facilities in terms of accommodation, personnel, medicine, dietary services, etc.
2. Exploitation of patients, especially women, for sexual purposes-patients are exploited by personal working there. Besides, family members also do not bother much about them.
3. Uncourteous behaviour of health staff.
4. No attempt at Rehabilitation.

5. Political and administrative interference to keep patients in hospitals for extra purposes like misusing property rights.
6. No dedication among health personnel essential for such services.
7. Non-availability of medicine.
8. No adequate arrangements for food, etc.

Suggestion

1. Emphasis on Prevention rather than Providing Secondary and Tertiary Care of Hospitals.

Secondary and tertiary care have engaged the attention of psychiatrists, but not the primary care. At present, health systems rarely contribute their full potential to the prevention of mental health. There are two main reasons for this. Firstly, the prevailing concept of health relates to physical well-being. Mental health rates too low in the scale of priorities to justify large investments in prevention action. Secondly, there is a relative scarcity of mental health technologies in the filed of primary prevention which are cost-effective and acceptable, and can be readily introduced by the health systems. Prevention as a humane alternative to custodial care of the mentally ill was advocated long ago by leading representatives of European psychiatry.

A good point of departure for disentangling this complicated issue is an awareness that the mental well-being of the patient is an asset of tremendous importance to limit the negative effects of any illness. Any investment aimed at securing the mental well-being of the sick must thus be "cost-effective", apart from being a human act, even of the benefits are too intangible to be expressed in terms of statistics. If health systems could become more receptive to this kind of reasoning, the integration of mental health care would be greatly facilitated. And we would be a step nearer towards fulfiling the recommendations of the 1978 Alma-Ata Conference.[10] Same view is expresses by Norman Sartorius.

It is becoming increasingly clear that many mental and neurological disorders can be effectively prevented. There are exciting opportunities to prevent psycho-social problems such as self-injury caused by excessive risk taking behaviour, alcohol and drug abuse and attempted suicide. In addition, the occurrence, course and outcome of many of the so-called physical diseases could be significantly influenced by change in behaviour of people. Both promotion of mental health and the efforts to help those with disorders and impairments are of essential importance.[11]

2. Emphasis on Rehabilitations to Promote Permanent Treatment

It is should be the effort of psychiatrists to rehabilitate the mentally ill so that they can become an asset to them and the society.

"Rehabilitation", as one of the more recent developments in mental health care, has the potential to be either one more method of professional definition and domination or, alternatively, to become a joint enterprise in which professionals and users combine to transform the social roles of services recipients. If the latter approach is to prevail, it is essential that user groups be brought into the process of designing, implementing and evaluating programmes and services to ensure that they permit users to enter the worlds of work and community living in ways that respect individual choice and human dignity.

If, on the other hand, rehabilitation is to remain a strictly professional field in which old ways of thinking prevail, it will become just one more element of mental health care from which users will develop ways of extricating themselves.[12]

3. Integration with Primary Health Care

The promotion of community mental health, the prevention of specific mental health problems and the identification, management and effective follow-up of psychiatric patients are among the key areas of health care where a primary health care approach can have a direct impact on the health status of any population. There is also no doubt that a community-oriented primary health care approach, with the active involvement of the patient's family and other members of the community, is the most effective way of rehabilitating a psychiatric patient.

This is mainly because many of the current mental health problems in the developing world are intimately related to psychosocial and inter-personal factors which can only be effectively solved or dealt with in a collaborative manner involving the patient, his family, and several community workers from different sectors.

The traditional dichotomy between body and mind has created an artificial gulf between physical health and mental health, to the point where many health workers forget that most of their day-to-day health activities also have a good deal of promotional and preventive effects on community mental health, and may result in a dramatic reduction of mental health problems in a particular community. This point is only too often forgotten.

The mental health programmes deal with the promotion of mental health and of psychosocial development. They are concerned with many psychological aspects of provision of care and of socio-economic development. But they also deal with the prevention and control of specific mental disorders, which present a major public health problem.[13]

4. Involving NGO's in Mental Health Programmes

There is general agreement that the NGOs, international, national and local, engaged in promotional and preventive health programmes play a vital role in the development effort exercised in this domain by governments and by inter-governmental agencies such as WHO.

There is an even greater inherent potential in the impact, which they could have on progress in mental health development. What is needed is still more effective coordination of action between them and the concerned national government. WHO has an essential role to play in this process.

Mental health programmes the world over, but especially in developing countries, would have everything to gain of collaborative WHO-NGO groups on mental health, under WHO leadership, would engage at both global and regional levels-in joint planning, programming and even joint fund-raising, preferably within the framework of primary health care.[14]

The greatest common strength, which the voluntary movement seems to share, lies in the NGOs' human resources-a reservoir of people highly motivated, with initiative, vision and great devotion to their mission.

5. *Equipping the Schools to Provide Congenial Environment and Promote Socialization*

School experience constitutes a major social influence on behaviour. It is not just a matter of learning to read, write and do sums; schools constitute social groups of children working and playing together, supervised by adults who serve as models for their behaviour. Whether or not schools aim to do more than teach, they will have social effects. The challenging is to ensure that the effects are positive, rather than negative.

Schools cannot be expected to compensate for the ills in the rest of society. Nevertheless, they can be a force for the good, with benefits that are especially marked for the disadvantaged. The overall psychological impact of the school is relatively modest compared with that of the family. But in terms of prevention, schools have a major advantage in that they can affect many children, while at the same time society has the power to ensure that the schools do indeed provide good environments in which to live and to learn. That is no small advantage, but its potential for preventing mental ill-health has not yet been fully realized.[15]

6. *Encouraging Indigenous Practices of Relaxation and Removal of Stresses and Tensions.*

People who regularly practice meditation or relaxation techniques produce measurable bodily changes, including slower heart rate, decline in blood pressure and slower metabolism, as well as increased feelings of calmness and well-being. Physical exercise, like a vigorous walk or sport activity is also a healthy way to relieve tension.[16]

7. *Availability of Drugs and their Administration*

The WHO Expert Committee's report on essential drugs (1979) recommended five or six drugs which could be sufficient for the treatment of most mental health problems and epilepsy. Most PHC workers at different levels can be trained to assess, identify, administer, and evaluate effects of at least two or three of these drugs, indeed a report of the WHO Regional Expert Panel of Mental Health in Africa has recommended that even the most peripheral community health worker (or village health worker) should have chlorpromazine and phenobarbitone available to him or her.[17]

Recent Developments

Modern Democratic Psychiatry

An association in Basle, Switzerland, founded to encourage psychiatric patients to assume responsibility for themselves, has become a model of self-help and voluntary cooperation.

The main aims of the group are:

1. to reserve inpatient stays for shot-term interventions in acute crises;
2. to encourage outpatient facilities outside hospitals for aftercare (counselling, accommodation, work, leisure, meeting points);
3. to promote self-responsibility and the right to dialogue;
4. to use the patient's own resources and promote self-help;
5. to extend patients 'rights';
6. to break down hierarchical grading so that the patient is no longer the lowest link in the chain;
7. to find pathways leading out of isolation and back into society; and
8. to involve relative in work with patients.[18]

During the Eighth Plan, NIMHANS developed a district mental health care model in Bellary district with the following aims:

(1) to provide sustainable basic mental health services to the community and to integrate these services with health services;
(2) early detection and prompt treatment of patients;
(3) to provide domiciliary mental health care and to reduce patient load in mental hospital;
(4) community education to reduce the stigma attached to mental illness; and
(5) to treat and rehabilitate patients with mental problems within their family setting.

During the Ninth Plan period the experience gained in implementing mental health care both in Central and State Sector is being utilized to provide sustainable mental health services at primary and secondary care levels and to build up community support for domiciliary care. IEC on mental health, especially prevention of stress-related disorders through promotion of healthy lifestyle and operational research studies for effective implementation of preventive, promotive and curative programmes in mental health through existing health infrastructure, are receiving due attention.

The approach to the treatment of mental disorders is based upon the following strategies:

- Integrating mental health with primary health care through the National Mental Health Programme.
- Provision of tertiary care institutions for treatment of mental disorders.
- Eradicating stigmatization of mentally ill patients and protecting their rights through regulatory institutions like the Central Mental Health Authority and State Mental Health Authority.

Mental health should form an integral part of the total health programme and as such should be included in all national health policies and programmes. It is now recognized that it is possible to prevent a number of mental, neurological and psychological problems of public health importance. There is a need to provide more resources for mental health and emphasize preventive and rehabilitative mental health.

The National Human Rights Commission (NHRC) has done well to direct the state governments once again to ensure that mentally ill persons are not kept in jail under any circumstances.

NMHP Issues and Challenges

- Strengthening of DMHP and enhance its visibility at grass root level.
- Filling up manpower gap in the field of psychiatry in general and DMHP in particular.
- Harnessing NGO's help in the Community-based care of mentally ill.
- Focusing on preventive and promotive components of Mental Health in addition to treatment of serious mental ailments.
- Strengthening the IEC activities particularly in the School Health Programme.
- Training of general practitioners in Mental Health Programme.
- Need to develop the urban Mental Health Programme.
- Development of standardized training manuals for doctors and health care workers.

Identified thrust areas based on experience gained during 10th Five Year Plan

- To expand DMHP in an enlarged and more effective form.
- Strengthening/modernization of remaining mental hospitals in order to modify from largely custodial role to therapeutic role.
- Upgrading Departments of psychiatry in Medical Colleges and enhancing the psychiatric content of the medical curriculum at the UG/PG level.
- Information, Education and Communication activities for creating awareness and reducing stigma.

- Research and Training in Mental Health.
- School Mental Health Programme.

Involvement of NGO's and Public Private Partnership in Community based care of mentally ill patients to fill the service gap in mental health delivery.

Mental Health and Substance Abuse

For many years, the Regional Office has advocated community-based mental health services for meeting the mental health needs of the community. This strategy received a boost in the Health Minister's meeting held in Dhaka, Bangladesh in August 2006, which called upon WHO to assist Member-countries in strengthening community mental health services as a part of health system development. This strategy emphasizes the integration of mental health care into the existing primary health care system. It also recommends focusing on the most common and disabling neuropsychiatric disorders in the community (epilepsy and psychosis affecting 1% and 1.5-2% of the population, respectively). Most Member countries of the Region organized extensive training programmes for basic health workers to overcome the shortage of qualified mental health manpower so that essential services could reach the community. WHO developed training tools and manuals for community-based health workers, to identify and manage the most common and disabling neuropsychiatric conditions in the community.

All Member-countries have initiated various activities, such as school mental health promotion, community-based mental health promotion with the use of traditional yoga and mediation in selected districts. A regional review was undertaken in December 2006 with particular emphasis on mental health promotion for adolescents.[19]

Acharya Mahaprajna as told to Lalit Garg in *Times of India,* dated 18-4-2008 has suggested the following to improve mental health.

Mental health promotes physical health. The reverse is also true. The mind and the body are two mutually connected entities. However, the mind's influence on the body is deeper than that of the body on the mind. Mental health is connected with the feeling of equality. Without this feeling the mind cannot be healthy. The principle of equality is also the principle of mental health.

The first principle of mental health is: Know thyself. One who does not know his own strength and weakness cannot be mentally healthy. We do not know our strength because we are weak and we feel a sense of being wretched. We become excited when somebody misbehaves with us because we do not know our weakness. In such cases we overlook ourselves and try to find fault with others.

The second principle of mental health is the willingness to admit one's responsibility for whatever has been done. We are not prepared to visualise the consequences of our actions and that is why our mind has no peace. It is unhealthy to avoid responsibility for our actions. It can lead to mental illness. One needs courage to admit his faults. A weak mind does not have this courage.

One should take responsibility for the good as well as bad consequences of one's actions. It is the weak who find fault with others. They want to save their own skin. We generally like to be praised for our good actions but are not prepared to be blamed for the bad consequences of our actions.

Devotion to truth is the third principle of mental health. Truth is experience of the law governing the universe. Death is a universal law. It has no exception. All the prophets and great men of the world met death. Nobody is immortal. Everyone who is born must die one day. Death is, therefore, a truth. In the same way karma (action) and tela (time) are also truths. One who admits the operation of the laws, which govern nature, is a mentally healthy man.

Tolerance is the fourth principle of mental health. An intolerant man is always miserable. Moreover, the behaviour of an intolerant man is always unpredictable. If an intolerant man is meditating and if the fan is stopped, his mind will be upset and his meditation will break.

He who commands tolerance is indifferent to losses and gains. Wealth and riches are not lasting. Heat and cold, comfort and pain and convenience and inconvenience do not affect the tolerant man. They affect those who do not possess the requisite strength to face them. Those who have been born and brought up in the midst of difficulties and privations ultimately develop in themselves the spirit of tolerance.

The fifth principle of mental health is that we should present ourselves as we are. We should not put up appearances. Generally people are snobs in their social life and when people see them in their true colours they are put in a quandary Secretiveness creates ill feelings.

Those who put up appearances not only deceive others, they deceive themselves also. They create difficulties for all. We try to create false impressions on the minds of others in order to hide our own real state. You cannot hide reality for a long time. Only he whose mind is weak tries to hide facts. On the other hand he whose mind is strong and sound will always present himself as he is.

CONCLUSION

In order to be able to absorb the resources allocated for mental health care and to spend the money effectively and efficiently, we need a large pool of trained human resources. There are today only about 3500 psychiatrists, 700-800 psychologists and a like number of social workers. This is hardly adequate in a country of over a billion people. The urgent need is to augment the human resources within the shortest possible time.

How do we augment the human resources? Capacity has to be built in a systematic and scientific way. New mechanisms must be identified for overcoming the critical shortage in human resources. Government will look forward to another major contribution from NIMHANS for the development of innovative projects to augment the human resources gap in the area of mental health care.

RECOMMENDATIONS

- Train the medical officers and others at the Primary Health Centres to recognize mental health problems early, manage them effectively or refer them wherever necessary.
- Have District Mental Health Programmes in all districts on the model of Bellary District Programme.
- Ensure availability of essential drugs for the management of mental disorders.
- Have counselling centers with qualified and trained personnel.
- All districts hospitals to have mental health units with qualified psychiatrists and other trained staff and facilities for outpatient and inpatient care of the mentally ill persons.
- All medical colleges to have qualified psychiatrists and facilities for teaching medical students and for outpatient and inpatient care of mentally ill persons.
- Upgrade the Dharwad Mental Hospital, converting it into a center of active treatment in a humane way.
- Encourage community-based rehabilitation of persons with mental disorders, who have recovered from acute illness.
- Encourage community-based rehabilitation of persons with mental retardation, integrating them into the society.[20]

National Institute of Mental Health and Neuro Sciences (NIMHANS), Bangalore[21]

National Institute of Mental Health and Neuro Sciences (NIMHANS) is a premier research and training center in the area of mental health and neuro sciences. The Institute was established in 1974, as an autonomous institution under Ministry of health and Family Welfare, Government of India, funded by Central Government and State Government. Multidisciplinary and integrated approach is the main stay of this institute. Based on the work done at NIMHANS since its inception, the University Grants Commission declared this as a Deemed University from 1994. Health care, Manpower development and Research are the three main activities.

The functioning of the Institutions is under the direction of the NIMHANS Society, with the Union Minister of Health and Family Welfare as President and the Minister for Health and Family Welfare, Government of Karnataka as Vice-President. The principal organ of management is the Board of Management. The other statutory bodies are Finance Committee,

Academic Council, Planning and Monitoring Board, Selection Committee, Board of Studies, Grievance Redressal Committee, Ethics Committee, Building and Works Committee, Rehabilitation Committee and Hospital Management Committee.

Department

(1) Biophysics, (2) Biostatistics, (3) Clinical Psychology, (4) Epidemiology, (5) Human Genetics, (6) Mental Education, (7) Neuromicrobiology, (8) Neuroanaesthesia, (9) Neurochemistry, (10) Neurology, (11) Neur-opathology, (12) Neurophysiology, (13) Neuro Imaging and Interventional Radiology, (14) Neurosurgery, (15) Neurovirology, (16) Nursing, (17) Psy-chiatry, (18) Psychiatric and Neurological Rehabilitation, (19) Psychiatric and Social Work, (20) Psychopharmacology, (21) Speech Pathology and Audiology, and (22) Ayurvedic Research Unit.

Central Facilities

(1) Library and Information Centre, (2) Biomedical Engineering, (3) Central Animal Research Facility, (4) Photography and Documentation Centre, (5) Engineering, and (6) Publication.

New Facilities

(a) Liquid Medical Oxygen system to cater to the oxygen demands of the hospital was inaugurated on 19 January 2006.
(b) Gamma Knife for treating small sized lesions of brain without surgery was installed on 1 march 2006 at the Gamma Knife Centre.
(c) Stealth Station for Image Guided Surgery.
(d) The state-of-art Microscope Pentero by Carl-Zeiss.
(e) The department of Biophysics had developed Electrophysiological recording and laser scanning confocal microscopy facilities.

The Department of Psychiatry: (i) Initiated a yoga therapy service for schizophrenia and alcoholism, (ii) initiated MRI analysis facility funded by the Fogarty ICOHRTA grant, (iii) started Perinatal Psychiatry Service for Pre-pregnancy counselling for: (a) Women with psychiatric problems, (b) Pregnant women with psychiatric problems, (b) Pregnant women with psychiatric problems, (c) Post-abortion mental health problems, and (d) Postpartum women till the first year after childbirth.

The Department of Neurophysiology acquired state-of-the art cellular imaging facility. This includes laser confocal microscope with softwares for qualitative and quantitative imaging of neurons in invivo and in vitro preparations. This facility allows quantifying cell density, dendritic arborization, spines, and 3D reconstruction and imaging of individual neurons.

The Department of Mental Health and Social Psychology developed standardized Batteries for Neuropsychological testing viz. (i) WMS III India norms, and (ii) NIMHANS Neuropsychological Battery for Intractable epilepsy.

The Department of Neurovirology developed: (i) New tests for Ante mortem diagnosis of rabies by detection of antigen and immune complexes in CSF, (ii) HIV viral load by Real Time PCR, (iii) Molecular epidemiology.

Development of New Technologies/Transfer of Technologies/Patents

The Department of Psychiatry Developed: (i) Interactive CD for Doctors-Interactive Computer-based Learning Modules for primary care physicians and 6 Episode film on life skills education to be telecast using the EDUSAT. This has been done as part of NIMHANS-DERT collaboration, and (ii) A manual for "Caregiver Training in Dementia in South India" as a part of Fogarty International Project. The manual was evolved after carrying out the needs assessment in family caregivers of persons with dementia and adapting an earlier manual used by the US collaborators. This manual has now been filed-tested and at present the programme is being trailed in a randomized control study to look at the efficacy and applicability in the South Indian population.

The Tobacco Cessation Centre which is the coordinating center for 18 WHO/Ministry of Health and Family Welfare sponsored TCCs in the country has developed the TUPAQ (Tobacco use and problem assessment questionnaire), an internet-based assessment and follow-up questionnaire for tobacco use.

The department of Mental Health and Social Psychology developed the syllabus for the post-graduate Certificate course in Forensic Psychology.

The Department of Neurovirology developed: (i) Hybridoma Technology for production of monoclonal antibodies to rabies proteins, (ii) Real Time PCR for estimation of HIV viral loads in plasma and CSF, (iii) Real Time PCR for the antemortem diagnosis of Rabies, (iv) Molecular Epidemiology of Rabies and HIV-viruses (deposition of Viral gene sequences to the Gen Bank), and (v) Cloning and expression of Rabies virus protein using Baculovirus expression system.

The Department of Speech Pathology and Audiology developed: (i) Introduction of Gap-in-Noise (GIN) Test for detecting temporal dysfunction, and (ii) PAN Registry (iii) Swallowing therapy.

Hospital Services

NIMHANS is the apex secondary and tertiary care hospital in the country in the fields of psychiatry, neurology and neurosurgery, for inpatient and outpatient care and subsequent neuro-rehabilitation of the affected to enter back into society as useful citizens. The institute renders services to the patients from all over the country as well as neighbouring developing countries. During the year 2005-06, 3,36,784 patients have been treated.

The institute has an 805 bedded hospital. Out of this, 650 beds are for psychiatry and 155 for Neuyrology and Neurosurgery. There are general wards, paying wards and ICUs. NIMHANS Outpatient services are available on all days. The emergency and causality services are available round the clock with modern facilities of CT Scan, Angiogram, latest MRI and Digital Subtraction Angiography's (DSA).

Teaching and Training

District Mental Health Programme (DMHP)

The Department of Psychiatry has been actively involved in the training and monitoring of the DMHP. As part of the programme a number of training workshops were conducted at Shimoga, Karwar, Gulbarga and Chamarajnagar. Two hundred and eighty-nine doctors and 66 health workers were trained. A 2-day workshop for programme officers for implementation of DMHP was organized. Twenty programme officers working in various districts attended 6 programmes.

Monitoring visits of Deaddiction Centres and Review meeting

As part of the mandate set by the Department of Health and Family Welfare and the Government of India the Deaddiction Centres staff conducted a review visit to monitor the state and functioning of the Deaddiction Centres initiated by the Union Government.

Continuing Medical Education

The Department of Neurology organized a CME program for postgraduate students in Medicine sponsored by Karnataka Medical Education Research Trust, Banaglore on 18 October 2005.

Another CME program in Neurology was held at NIMHANS on 18th March 2006

Manpower Development

100 Students joined for different kinds of Post-graduate Degree/ Diploma and Certificate Courses for the academic year 16/06/2006 to 15/ 11/2006.

Training and Visiting of Students

The total number of students from Government/Private Institutions have visited NIMHANS from all over the Country during the period 16/06/ 2006 to 15/11/2006 are: 1117. Students passed-out in July 2006 and August 2006 exams.[21]

Central Institute of Psychiatry (CIP), Ranchi

Central Institute of Psychiatry is a premier Institute in the field of Mental Health in India. It offers clinical services to mentally ill, trains manpower in the field of Mental Health and carries out various research programmes. Clinical services are provided both at the level of outpatient and inpatient. Apart from Adult Psychiatry, services are available for Child and Adolescence Psychiatry, Addiction Psychiatry, Community Psychiatry and Neuropsychiatry. A number of special clinics are run to render services in areas of Epilepsy, Headache, Dermatology, Mood Disorder, Chronic Schizophrenia, De-addiction, etc. Community Psychiatry are a various programme and runs seven outreach services, which includes Child and School Mental Health.

Patient OPD Attendance, Admission and Discharge

In the year during January 2006-November 2006 the total number of OPD cases were 57,484 (including Psychiatric Cases (Adult and Child), Staff OPD, Clinical Psychiatry, Extension Clinics, Skin Clinics, Cardiology Lab (Staff), Psychiatric New Cases were 8986, Psychiatric old cases were 26398; 2963 patients were admitted, 2941 discharged and only (3) deaths occurred during the period. Average stay of patient was 55 days and bed occupancy 418 beds. During January 2006-November 2006, Special Clinic have also been opened such as chronic Schizophrenia Clinic, Skin and Sex Clinic, Neurology Clinic, Sleep Clinic, Movement Clinic, Epilepsy Clinic, Memory Clinic, Headache Clinic, De-addiction Clinic, Child Guidance Clinic, Mood Clinic, etc.

During January 2006-Nov., 2006, 817 patients suffering from the problem of Alcohol Drug addiction were seen in the OPD of Centre for Addiction Psychiatry. During the same period, 469 (New-1302, Follow-up-3387) patients visited for treatment at OPD of Centre for Child and Adolescent Psychiatry.

Courses and Training Programme

This Institute runs the following courses; MD (Psychiatry), DPM (Psychiatry), M.Phil and Ph.D. (Clinical Psychology, M.Phil (Psychiatric Social Work) and Diploma in Psychiatric Nursing (DPN). Nursing Department arranged 5 Continuing Nursing education/Training Programmes which were attended by 168 participants, Seminar-23 (1075 participants), Case Conference-26 (1134 participants), Journal Club-19 (760 participants), Programme 2 (25 participants). The Institute has acquired during January-November 2006, campus server, colour Doppler and 16 slices CT Scan.[22]

Disability and Mental Health

Coping with challenges of living in a rapidly developing society and increasing exposure to a violent world has led to a perceptible increase in mental stress. Provision of mental health care is thus vital. From the children of farmers who commit suicide to victims of violence, calamities and sexual abuse, all need counselling support. Yet this has been a much-neglected areas in our country. Even today there is a stigma attached to mental illness, which prevents many from reaching out. The 11th Plan will recognize the importance of mental health care and will concentrate on providing counselling, medical services and establishing help lines for all—especially people affected by calamities, riots and violence. Adequate budgetary provisions will be made available for this purpose.[23]

Mental Retardation

Mental retardation is a common condition. In surveys in the general population in India among people of all ages. it has been found that around 2% have mental retardation. In other words, in a village of 1,000 people one can expect to find around 20 people with mental retardation. But if one estimates the problem only in children. (under 18 years of age) there will be about 3% of cases with mental retardation among all children under 18 years of age in the same village. Regarding learning disability, a study by UNICEF in Sri Lanka revealed that 12% of primary school children had learning disability. Another report from Sri Lanka estimated that 15% of school going children suffered from some form of disability. A study in children (aged 2-9 years) from Bangladesh found that around 7% had some form of disability. Mental retardation. the second most common form of disability was seen in around 2% of children. Severe mental retardation in Bangladeshi children (2-9 years old) was estimated to be around 6 per 1,000 in keeping with the reports from other countries. In 1999. the Planning Division. Department of Mental Health of Thailand conducted ari epidemiological study on mental health problems countrywide and found that the rate of occurrence of mental retardation was 1.3%.

Mild mental retardation is much more common than severe mental retardation accounting for 65 to 75% of all cases with mental retardation. Looked at in another way in a village of 1,000 people. of the 20 who will have mental retardation. about 15 will have mild mental retardation and about five will have more severe forms.

It has been found that mental retardation. especially mild mental retardation. is more common in rural areas. and in low-income groups. Reasons like poor access to health facilities under-stimulation. and under-nutrition could account for this observation.

Why does mental retardation occur ? As noted earlier, anything that damages and interferes with the growth and maturation of the brain can lead to mental retardation. There can be hundreds of such causes. This might happen before, during or after the birth of the child. While a few examples are explained below, a more detailed list of causes is given in Table 7.1.

Iodine Deficiency Disorder (cretinism)

Iodine is essential for the normal development of unborn babies. Lack of adequate availability of iodine from the mother restricts the growth of the brain of the foetus and leads to a condition called hypothyroidism. Babies

TABLE 7.1

Causes of Mental Retardation

Category	*Type*	*Examples*
Prenatal (Causes before birth	Chromosomal disorders	Downs syndrome* Fragile X syndrome, Prader Wili Syndrome, Klinefelters syndrome
	Single gene disorders	Inborn errors of metabolism: such as galactosemia*, phenylketonuria*, mucopolysaccaridoses Hypothyroidism*, Tay-Sachs diseases Neuro-Cutaneous: Syndromes such as tuberous sclerosis, and neurobibromatosis Brain malformations such as genetic microcephaly, hydrocephalus and myelo-meningocele* Other dysmorphic syndromes, such as Laurence Moon Biedl syndrome.
	Other conditions of genetic origin	Rubistein Tabi syndrome De Lange syndrome
	Adverse maternal/environmental influences	Deficiencies* such as iodine deficiency and folic acid deficiency. Severe malnutrition* in pregnancy Using substances* such as alcohol (maternal alcohol syndrome), nicotine, and cocaine during early pregnancy Maternal infections:

		such as rubella*, syphillis* toxoplasmosis, cytometalovirus and HIV Others such as excessive exposure to radiation* and Rh incompatibility
Perinatal (around the time of birth)	Third trimester (late pregnancy)	Complications of pregnancy* Diseases* in mother such as heart and kidney disease and diabetes Placental dysfunction
	Labour (during delivery)	Severe prematurity, very low birth weight, birth asphysxia Difficult and/or complicated delivery* Birth Trauma*
	Neonatal (first four weeks of life)	Septicemia, severe jaundice*, hypoglycemia
Postnatal (in infancy and childhood)		Brain infections such as tuberculosis—Japanese encephalitis, and bacterial meningitis Head injury* Chronic lead exposure* Severe and prolonged malnutrition* Gross understimulation*

with this problem have mental retardation, hearing impairment and dwarfism. In addition, they may have lethargy, coarseness of facial features, rough and dry skin, feeding problems, constipation. cold extremities, and neck swelling because of enlargement of the thyroid gland. A severe form of this condition, in which all the features mentioned are very pronounced is called cretinism. Iodine occurs naturally in food. But in some places, the soil and the food are deficient in iodine. In such places naturally a pregnant woman's intake of iodine is less and therefore their infants would also be deficient in iodine and manifest hypothyroidism. Iodine deficiency is prevalent in large areas in some Member Countries of SEARO.

Difficult/Complicated Delivery

Till they are born, babies receive their supply of food and oxygen from the mother. Immediately after birth, babies begin to breathe on their own. Normally, this transition occurs smoothly. When, for any reason, the delivery becomes difficult, prolonged, or complicated, oxygen supply to the baby is diminished. As the brain is very sensitive to oxygen deprivation. this can result in brain damage. This is called birth asphyxia. Such babies may have problems in development such as mental retardation or cerebral palsy.

Brain Infection (Brain Fever)

An important cause of mental retardation after birth is brain infections caused by bacteria or viruses. In this condition, children who are otherwise normal, suddenly develop fever, headache, vomiting, convulsions and loss of consciousness. If this infection is severe, there may be irreversible brain damage leading to mental retardation. Such children, when they recover from acute illness, are noticed to have lost many skills which they had learnt earlier. Young children are more at risk for brain fever in regions where Japanese encephalitis and tuberculosis are common.

Nutrition and Mental Development

A balanced diet rich in calories, protein, vitamins and minerals is required for pregnant women and young children for normal brain development. Lack of adequate diet can have direct and indirect effect on brain development and thereby increase the risk of subnormal development.

Studies have shown that birth weight is an important indicator of the future health of the baby. A baby with low birth weight is more likely to have problems in mental development. The height and weight of would-be mothers and the extent of weight grain in pregnancy are important factors determining birth weight.

Common Health Problems Associated with Mental Retardation

Many children and adults with mental retardation are otherwise physically and mentally healthy, except that they have lower intelligence. Several others, however, frequently have other problems. The common health problems associated with mental retardation are as follows:

Behaviour Problems

Symptoms like restlessness (continuously moving around; unable to sit in one place), poor concentration, impulsiveness, temper tantrums, irritability and crying are common. Other disturbing behaviour, like aggression, self-injurious behaviour (such as head banging) and repetitive rocking may also be seen. When such behaviour is severe and persistent, it can become a major source of stress for families. Therefore, attention should be paid to reduce such behaviour while providing treatment and care.

Convulsions

About 25% of people with mental retardation get convulsions. Many types of convulsions can occur involving the whole body, or only one half of the body, or sudden single jerks leading to a fall. Convulsions, although alarming to watch, can be easily controlled with proper medication.

Sensory impairments

Difficulties in seeing and hearing are present in about 5-10% of persons with mental retardation. Sometimes these problems can be resolved by using hearing aids or glasses, or undergoing surgery for cataract. As noted earlier, other developmental disabilities, such as cerebral palsy, speech problems and autism, can occur along with mental retardation. Persons with many disabilities, or multiple disabilities, pose a big challenge in terms of providing care.

Individual and family approaches

Mental retardation is generally a life-long condition and it cannot be 'cured' with medical treatment. Given this fact, what can be done and what should be the aims and objectives in providing care for these individuals? The following considerations should be kept in mind to guide actions.

Scientific evidence

Scientific research has shown that by providing the right kind of support and services. It is possible to ensure that those with mental retardation can live healthy and relatively independent lives. These services comprise many areas such as health care, early intervention, education, vocational training, and so on. Studies have also shown that considerable ill health. physical or behavioural, in people with mental retardation is caused by lack of appropriate care and is hence preventable.

Humanistic need

As citizens of a civilized society, it is the right of people with mental retardation to lead their lives with respect and dignity. It is possible to achieve this goal by bringing about positive changes in societal awareness. attitudes and beliefs about this condition.

Family perspective

Very often, the problem of mental retardation is inseparable from the problems faced by the families. It is clear that organized services are definitely needed for families to adapt well and face the situation with confidence and the least amount of stress.

To achieve these aims. professionals from many fields families. governmental and non-governmental organisations. and society as a whole have to work together. The following principles should help in guiding and directing the development of appropriate services:

Normalization

This concept. which originated in the Scandinavian countries. has had a powerful influence. In simple terms, normalization means ensuring that the same environmental conditions of everyday life are available to people with mental retardation as they are for anybody else. It also means providing them with facilities to enable development of their full potential.

Integration

Individuals with mental retardation should become an integral part of society; they should not be isolated, segregated or discriminated against in any fashion.

Home-based Care with Parents as Partners Research has shown that the best place for children with mental retardation to grow in is their own families where they can be nurtured with appropriate stimulation. Therefore, services should be organized so that the families are supported, strengthened and empowered to look after their affected member. Families have different needs at different stages in the life cycle of its members (such as childhood, adolescence, and adulthood); this should be recognized and attempts made to fulfil these needs. It should also be recognized that families are not just recipients of services but care-providers as well. In other words, they are partners in care.

Community-based Approaches

Very often, services tend to be concentrated in well-to-do urban localities. To overcome this lop-sided approach, a community orientation is necessary, so that services are available to large sections of society in their own vicinity. No programme is likely to succeed without community involvement and participation.

Services for Individuals with Mental Retardation

Medical and Psychological (clinical) Services

The first requirement is for appropriate facilities for a good medical/ health evaluation and accurate diagnosis. Doctors should be in a position to recognize and manage treatable disorders such as hypothyroidism. Associated problems such as convulsions, sensory impairments and behaviour problems, can be corrected or controlled with proper medical attention. It is desirable to have facilities for psychological assessment of strengths and weaknesses in the child which can form the basis for future training. Adequate parental counselling in the initial stages is essential. Doctors, nurses psychologists and social workers can make a big difference to parents by correctly explaining the condition and the options for treatment as well as by clarifying their doubts.

Parental counselling also involves providing emotional support and guidance and strengthening morale. Once the parents get a grasp of the condition they need to learn appropriate ways of rearing and training the child. Parents continue to need such assistance guidance, and support as the child grows up especially during adolescence early adulthood and during periods of crisis. There are many claims that some drugs and herbal preparations can improve intelligence. But no drugs or any other treatment can completely cure mental retardation. It is important to ensure that parents do not spend a lot of their valuable money and time in pursuing treatments that are of doubtful or no value.

National Institute for the Mentally Handicapped (NIMH) a national asset in India. NIMH was established as an apex body in the field of mental retardation by the Government of India in 1984 at Secunderabad in Andhra Pradesh. The main objectives were to develop human resources, models of care and rehabilitation, and to undertake research, documentation, and information in the field of mental retardation. Since its inception, NIMH has grown by leaps and bounds, with many achievements to its credit and a visible impact on the national scene. Its major contributions have been manpower development, numerous and very popular publications on early stimulation, education, training, and rehabilitation. The Institute has been able to develop innovative models of family and community-based care that have undergone research evaluation, and has functioned as a clearing house of information at the national level. Recently, it has been instrumental in promoting and supporting the parental self-help group movement in India. Other notable activities include an annual national seminar on mental retardation, an annual meet of parent organisations, Special Olympics, awareness campaigns and a national meet of special employees. The Institute has many regional centres all over India, mainly to run training courses for manpower development.

Primary prevention refers to a set of approaches that .reduce or eliminate the risk of mental retardation in the community. As mentioned earlier, these concern promoting the health status of the community as a whole and affording specific protection against certain conditions. Knowledge of the causes of mental retardation can help to reduce cases by at least 25% by practising primary prevention. There are many methods of primary prevention. Some of these are simple, whereas others are more complicated.

Simple methods

These apply to large segments of the population and basically mean implementation of certain practical and effective interventions at the community level. A large number of these practices concern maternal and child health care. Some of the important steps are:

- Improving the nutritional status of the community as a whole, especially the girl child in order to reduce the risk factors for mental retardation such as low birth weight, and prematurity in the offspring of these children in future;

- Universal iodization of salt to prevent iodine deficiency disorders which are endemic in some parts of SEAR Member-countries;
- Administration of folic acid tablets to reduce the occurrence of neural tube defects;
- Nutritional supplementation during pregnancy, focusing on intake of calories and iron;
- Universal immunization of children with BCG, polio, OPT, and MMR to prevent many disorders having the propensity to damage the brain and thereby causing mental retardation. Rubella immunization (part of MMR) can totally eradicate the occurrence of maternal rubella syndrome;
- Avoiding pregnancy before 21 years and after the age of 35 years as complications of pregnancy and labour are more common before 21 years. The risk of Downs syndrome and other chromosomal disorders increases as the maternal age at pregnancy crosses 35 years;
- Spacing pregnancies to help the mother to nutritionally replenish herself before the next pregnancy;
- Avoiding exposure to harmful chemicals and substances including alcohol, nicotine and cocaine during pregnancy.
- Especially early pregnancy. Failed abortions are caused by chemicals often administered by quacks, using harmful medicines. All pregnant women should inform their doctors about their pregnancy status;
- Detection and care for high-risk pregnancies;
- Screening pregnant women for infections such as syphilis and promptly treating it;
- Preventing Rh iso-immunization, a situation that can arise when the mother has Rh negative blood group. The damage to the foetus can be prevented by administration of a medicine called Anti-D immunoglobulin immediately after the first delivery;
- Prompt treatment for severe diarrhoea and brain infections during childhood to reduce the chance and extent of brain damage;
- Providing an enriching and stimulating environment for children from infancy to ensure proper intellectual development;
- Chronic low-grade exposure to lead can impair brain development; steps should be taken to reduce the sources of environmental pollutants (such as using unleaded petrol), and
- Health education about the nature causes and prevention of mental retardation especially during the formative years can lead to healthy practices during pregnancy and child-rearing.

Levels of Prevention

Level	Approach	Interventions
Primary Prevention (preventing the occurrence retardation	Main promotion	Health education, especially for adolescent girls Improvement of nutritional status in community Optimum health care facilities Improvement in pre, peri and postnatal care
	Specific protection	Universal iodization of salt Rubells immunization for women before pregnancy Folic acid administration in early pregnancy Genetic counselling Prenatal screening for congential malformation and genetic disorders Detection and care for high-risk pregnancies Prevention of damage because of Rh incapability Universal immunization for children
Secondary Prevention (halting disease progression)	Early diagnosis and treatment	Neonatal screening for treatable disorders Intervention with 'at risk' babies Early detection and intervention of developmental delay
Tertiary prevention (preventing complications and maximization of functions)	Disability limitation and rehabilitation	Stimulation, training and education, and vocational opportunities Mainstreaming/integration Support for families Parental self-help groups

Note: Primary prevention strategies remain the optimum solutions in SEAR Member-countries. Not only are these effective, there is no 'cure' for most cases of mental retardation, and knowledge and facilities for secondary and tertiary prevention are limited.

Based on WHO Document on Mental Retardation.

NOTES AND REFERENCES

1. Final Report of the Task Force on Health and Family Welfare, Government of Karnataka, April 2001, pp. 160-61.
2. J.S. Neki, "Mental Disability", in *World Health,* Aug-Sept., 1985, p. 18.
3. GOI, Bhore Committee; Health Survey and Development Committee, Vol. II, Simla, Govt. of India Press, 1946.
4. Resnick, J.H., Finally, a definition of clinical psychology: A message from the President, Division 12. The Clinical Psychologist 1991; 44:3-11.
5. IACP, IACP Constitution: Amended 1995, Jaipur: IACP Secretariat, 1985.
6. World Health Organisation, World Health Report, 2001, Mental Health; New Understanding, New hope. Geneva: WHO, 2001.
7. Chanbdrashekar, C.R., Isacc, M.K., Development of psychiatric epidemiology in India, *NIMHANS Journal,* 1999; 17(4): 297-306.
8. P. Chidambram, Human Resources Gap in Mental Health Care, *University News,* 43(36), September 05-11, 2005, p. 16.
9. Annual Report, 2006-07, Ministry of Health and Family Welfare, NRHM, GOI, pp. 139-42.
10. Atanas Maleev, Prevention Through the Health System, in *World Health,* Aug.-Sept. 1985, pp. 24-25.
11. Norman Sartorius, Protecting the Mind, The Role of Prevention in Mental Health, in *World Health,* Aug.-Sept., 1985, p. 4.
12. *World Health,* Sept.-Oct., 1995, pp. 16-17.
13. V.B. Vankiri, Healthy Minds Healthy Bodies, in *World Health,* Dec., 1982, p. 11.
14. Stanisias Flache, Education and Mental Health, The Role of Schools, in *World Health,* Aug.-Sept., 1985, p. 27.
15. Michael Rutter, Education and Mental Health, The Role of Schools, in *World Health,* Aug.-Sept., 1985, p. 29.
16. *World Health,* Aug.-Sept., 1985, p. 12.
17. V.B. Vankiri, Healthy Minds Healthy Bodies, *World Health,* Dec., 1982, p. 12.
18. Margot Wicki Schwarzschild, Democratic Psychiatry, in *World Health,* May-June, 1992, p. 18.
19. The Work of WHO, Report of the Regional Director, 1st July 2006-30-June 2007, Non-communicable diseases and mental health, pp. 21-22.
20. Govt. of Karnataka, Karnataka Towards Equity, Outlay and Integrity in Health: Rural Report on Health and Family Welfare, 2001, Bangalore, p. 169.
21. Annual Report, 2006-07, Ministry of Health and Family Welfare, GOI, NRHM, pp. 247-49.
22. *Ibid.,* p. 216.
23. Planning Commission, GOI, 17th November 2006, Towards Faster and More Inclusive Growth, An Approach to the 11th Five Year Plan, p. 72.

8

CHAPTER

Cancer Control Programme

Knowledge available today allows us to predict that—given the right measures, sufficient resources and continued goal-directed research—upto one-third of existing cancers can be prevented, upto one-third can be cured, and most incurable cancer patients can be spared pain.[1]

WHAT IS CANCER

The human body consists of different organs tissues which are made up of very small structure called cells Although cells of different body tissues may have distinctly different functions, they all reproduce by dividing. Normally this process of dividing is well controlled so that new cells are formed to replace those that have died and the tissues of the body are kept in their proper proportions. However, sometimes this cell division becomes uncontrolled and an abnormal growth occurs. These abnormal growths may be either benign or malignant. A benign growth is usually confined and does not spread to other parts of the body When completely removed there is no chance that the growth will continue. A malignant growth cancer, spreads in an uncontrolled fashion; Invading the surrounding tissue, and often travels through the blood or lymph system to other parts of the body, forming separate growths, or metastases

Cancer can arise in any organ or tissue of the body. It is not one disease, but rather is a collection of more than 100 diseases. These separate diseases arise because the cancer may evolve from various types of cells, such as cells of the skin, bone, or blood, and the cancer may originate in various sites such as a lung or breast.

Some cancers grow very slowly, and destroy neighbouring tissue by local invasion. Others are very aggressive and metastatize rapidly. Cancer occurs roughly equally in both sexes, and develops most often in persons

CHART 8.1

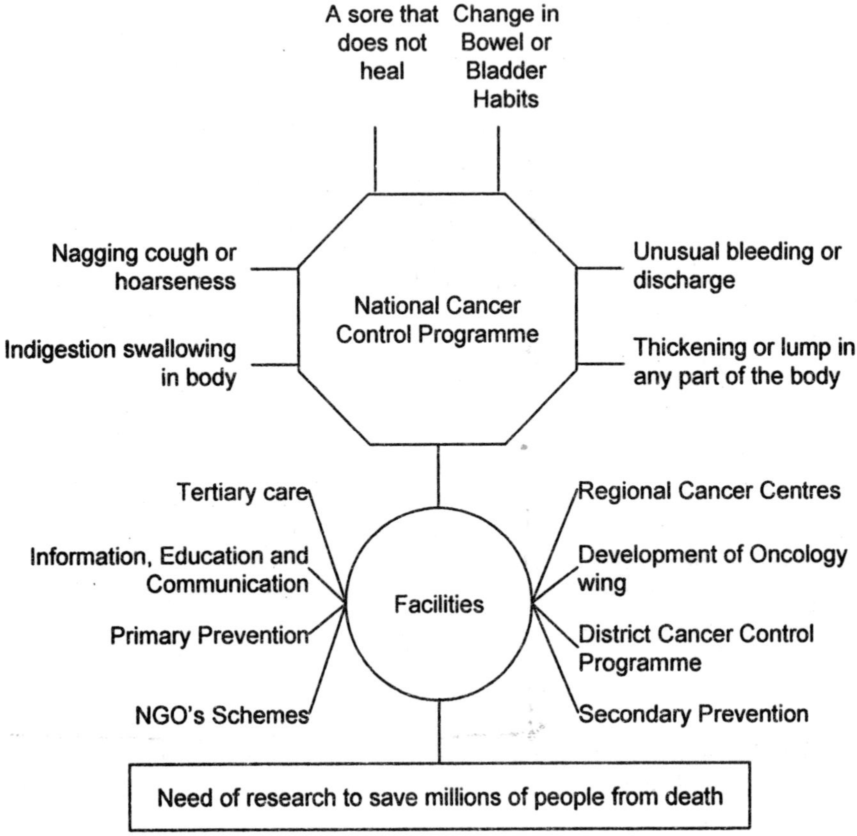

who are middle-aged or older. We know the cause of some cancers and can prevent their occurrence. For other cancers we have 10 reliable information about the cause. It is quite clear however, that a patient with cancer cannot transmit the disease to a healthy individual.

Therapies that work well in some cancers do not work at all in others. The problems have proved to be a great deal more formidable than most scientists anticipated 10 or 20 years ago. Progress is being made today in understanding this disease and developing therapies to treat it, although at times this progress seems agonizingly slow. However, the public need not wait for the scientific community to develop cures for the various types of cancer. Effective action can be taken today by the community to prevent some of these cancers from occurring.[2]

The cancer-causing factors that have so far been identified account for a large proportion of the existing cancers. But there is no doubt which is the dominant factor: it is tobacco.

Recent estimates suggest that 30 percent of cancers in the USA were caused by smoking Cancer may be avoidable. The fight to reduce smoking as a means of ending most forms of lung cancer, and many other diseases, may prove to be one of the most significant health victories of the century. Unlike the magnificent conquest of smallpox, it will result from a change in human behaviour. Smoking as a habit produced an epidemic of serious diseases. Ending the habit can point the way to protecting health through decisions made by individuals and communities. It can prove to be a clear example of individual responsibility.[3]

Two myths

Two myths have to be killed. One is that all cancer is unavoidable, and the other that cancer is only a disease of industrialized countries.

Cancer is, to some extent, avoidable. Environmental factors which cause cancer include not only man-made chemicals but also such factors as tobacco, diet and a large number of natural carcinogens. For the same ethnic groups, there are differences in cancer incidence relating to geographically different living areas. Populations who migrate have a change in incidence of some cancers and changes over a period of time correlate with the introduction of cancer-causing factors such as smoking. When a known cancer-causing factor is eliminated, certain cancer incidences go down, as has been shown for lung and bladder cancer.

All of these findings demonstrate that some cancers can be avoided. Although much is known about causation, not enough is known about how to change human behaviour or lifestyles associated with cancer, nor about the real value of screening for cancer. Goal-directed research is badly needed.

Epidemiological surveys show that many tumours, such as cancer of the skin, oral mucosa, oesophagus, liver and cervix, are more frequent in developing countries. Once an individual has survived the first five years of childhood, cancer is one of the three major causes of death both in developed and developing countries. We don't have to wait for industrialization for cancer to appear in developing countries. It is already there and, as the proportion of the aged population increases in these countries, the cancer problem must be expected to increase as well. Counter-measures should be planned now.[4]

Symptoms[5]

Seven Warning Signals of Cancer are:

- Change in bowel or bladder habits.
- A sore that does not heal.
- Unusual bleeding or discharge.
- Thickening or lump in breast or elsewhere.
- Indigestion or difficulty in swallowing.
- Obvious change in wart or mole.
- Nagging cough or hoarseness.

Known Causes of Cancers

Agent or Circumstances	*Site of Cancer*
Aflatoxian	Liver
Alcohololic drinks	Mouth, pharynx, larynx, oesophagus, liver
Alkylating agents:	
Cyclophosphamide	Bladder
Melphalan	Marrow
Aromatic amines:	
4-Aminodiphenyl	Bladder
Benzidine	Bladder
2-Naphthylamine	Bladder
Arsenic (certain compounds only)	Skin, lung
Asbestors	Lung, pleura, peritoneum
Benzene	Marrow
Bis (chloromethyl) ether	Lung
Busulphan	Marrow
Cadmium (certain compounds only	Prostate
Chewing (betel, tobacco, lime)	Mouth
Chromium (certain compounds only)	Lung
Chlornaphazine	Bladder
Chlorophenol/phenoxy acids	Sarcoma, lymphoma
Furniture manufacture (hardwood)	Nasal sinuses
Immunosuppressive drugs	Reticuloendothelial system
Ionizing radiations	Marrow and probably all other sites
Isopropyl alcohol manufacture	Nasal Sinuses
Leather goods manufacture	Nasal sinuses
Mustard gas	Larynx, lung
Nickel (certain compounds only)	Nasal sinuses, lung
Estrogens:	
Unopposed	Endometrium
Transplacental (DES)	Vagina
Overnutrition (causing obesity)	Endometrium gallbladder
Phenacetin	Kidney (pelvis)
Polycyclic hydrocarbons	Skin, scrotum, lung

Reproductive history:	
Late age at first pregnancy	Breast
Zero or low parity	Ovary
Parasites:	
Schistosoma hae... atobium	Bladder
Chlonorchis sinenesis	Liver (cholangioma)
Sexual promiscuiety	Cervix utteri
Steroids:	
Anabolic (oxymetholone)	Liver
Contraceptives	Liver (hamartoma)
Tobacco smoking	Mouth, pharynx, larynx, lung, oesophagus, bladder
UV light	Skin, lip
Vinyl chloride	Liver angiosarcoma
Virus (hepatitis B)	Liver (Hepatoma

(Adapted from R. Doll and R. Petro, *Journal of the US National Cancer Institute,* June 1981).

Relative Importance of known cancer causing factors:

Factors	*Percentage of all cancer deaths*	
	Best estimate	*Range of acceptable estimates*
Tabacco	30	25-40
Alcohol	3	2-4
Diet	35	10-70
Food additives	< 1	-5.2
Reproductive and sexual behaviour	7	1-13
Occupation	4	2-8
Pollution	2	< 1-5
Industrial Products	< 1	< 1-2
Medicines and medical procedures	1	0.5-3
Geophysical factors	3	2-4
Infections	10 ?	1-?

Source: Ibid.

Why you should quit smoking

Risks of smoking	*Benefits of quitting*	*Low-tar, low-nicotine*	*Risks of smoking*	*Benefits of quitting*	*Low-tar, low-nicotine*
Shortened life expectancy Risk propotional to amount smoked. A 25 year old person who smokes two packs a day can expect to live 8.3 years less than a non-smoking contemporary	After 10 to 15 years ex-smokers risk approaches that of those who never smoked	Reduced risk of death from certain diseases suggests increased life expectancy	**Cancer of Pancreas** Risk of fatal cancer is 2-5 times higher than for non-smokers	Since risk seems related to dos, stopping smoking should reduce it	No identified benefit
			Coronary Heart Diseases Smoking a major factor, causing 120,000 heart deaths each year	Risk decreases sharply after one year. After 10 years risk is the same as for those who never smoked	With low T/N brands, men have 12 per cent lower risk, women 19 than smokers of high T/N brands
Lung Cancer Cigarettes are major cause in both men and women. Overall, smokers' risk is 10 times greater than non-smokers	After 10-15 years risk approaches that of those who never smoked	Filter tips reduce risk, but the risk is still 5 times that of non-smokers, Low T/N brands reduce risk to men by 20 percent to women by 40 percent	**Bronchitis and Emphysema** Smokers face 4 to 25 times greater risk of death; lung damage even in young smokers	Within weeks cough sputum disappears, lung function may improve, slower deterioration	No identified benefit
Larynx Cancer Smoking increases risk by 2.9 to 17.7 times that of non-smokers	Gradual reduction in risk, reaching normal after 10 years	No identified benefits	Stillbrith, low birth weight Smokers have more stillbirth, more low brith weight babies, and more	If smoking is stopped before fourth month of pregnancy, risk to fetus is eliminated	No identified benefit

Mouth Cancer Smokers have 3 to 10 times as many oral cancers as non-smokers. Alochol may act as synergist, intensifying effect	Reducing or eliminating smoking/ drinking lowers risk in first few years. Risk drops to level of non-smokers in 10-15 years	No identified benefit	Peptic Ulcer Smokers get more ulcers and are more likely to die from them; cure more difficult in smokers	Ex-smokers get ulcers too, but they heal faste and more completely than smokers	No identified benefit
Cancer of Oesophagus Smoking increases risk of fatal causes 2 to 9 times. Alochol acts as a synergist	Since risk is proportional to dose, reducing or eliminating smoking/ drinking should lower risk	No identified benefits	Drug and test Effects Smoking changes pharmacological effects of many medicines. It changes results of diagnostic test and increases clots from oral contraceptives	Most blood factors raised by smoking return to normal. Non-smokers on birth control pill have much lower risk of hazardous clots and heart attacks	No identified benefit
Cancer of Bladder Smokers risk is 7-10 times greater. Synergistic with certain occupational exposures.	Risk decreases gradually to that of non-smokers over 7 years	No identified benefits			

Adapted from: "Dangers of Smoking, Benefits of Quitting, prepared by the American Cancer Society, *World Health* of Sept.-Oct.

Source: World Health, Sept.-Oct., 1981.

GENESIS AND GROWTH OF CANCER CONTROL IN INDIA

National Cancer Control Programme

Cancer is an important public health problem in India with nearly 7-9 lakh new cases occurring every year in the country. It is estimated that there are 20-25 lakh cases of cancer in the country at any given point of time. With the objectives of prevention, early diagnosis and treatment, the National Cancer Control Programme (NCCP) was launched in 1975-76. In view of the magnitude of the problem and the requirement to bridge the geographical gaps in the availability of cancer treatment facilities across the country; the programme was revised in 1984-85 and subsequently in

December 2004. There are 5 schemes under the revised programme:

(a) *Recognition of New Regional Cancer Centres (RCCs)*: In order to alugment comprehensive cancer care facilities in regions of the country lacking them, New RCCs are being recognized. A one-time grant of Rs. 5.00 crores is being provided for New RCCs.
(b) *Strengthening of Existing RCCs*: A one-time grant of Rs. 3.00 crores is provided to the existing RCCs in order to further strengthen the cancer treatment facilities in the existing centres.
(c) *Development of Oncology wing*: The scheme aims to correct the geographical imbalance by providing financial assistance to Government institutions (Medical Colleges as well as Government Hospitals) for enhancing the cancer care facilities. The one-time grant has been enhanced from Rs. 2.00 crores to Rs. 3.00 crores.
(d) *District Cancer Control Programme (DCCP)*: The DCCP will be implemented by the Nodal Agency, which may be an RCC or an Oncology Wing. The aim is to strengthen District Hospitals in 2-3 congruent districts for early detection and appropriate treatment or referral. The grant-in-aid has been increased to Rs. 90.00 lakhs spread over a period of 5 years.
(e) *Decentralized NGO Scheme*: This scheme has been devised to promote prevention and early detection of cancers. Non-Governmental Organisations (NGO) will implement these activities under the coordination of the Nodal Agency, which will be an RCC or an Oncology Wing. A grant of Rs. 8000 per camp will be provided for organizing camps for IEC and early detection activities.[6]

Objectives

(i) *Primary Prevention*: Health education and prevention of intake of tobacco;
(ii) *Secondary Prevention*: Early detection of common cancers such as of cervix, mouth and breast, and other tobacco related cancers; and
(iii) *Tertiary Prevention*: Strengthening of the existing institution for comprehensive therapy including palliative care.

To strengthen the National Cancer Control Programme, following steps have been taken:

Regional Cancer Centres

In all, there are 25 Regional Cancer Centres in different parts of the country to provide specialized treatment and undertake research in the field of cancer. For strengthening and upgrading the Regional Cancer Centres as

"Centre of Excellence", approval of competent authority has been obtained for providing additional financial assistance to the nine selected Regional Cancer Centres under the National Cancer Control Programme.

Oncology Wing

As per the revised scheme only Govt. Medical Colleges/Hospitals are entitled for grant-in-aid for development of Oncology Wing under the National Cancer Control Programme. During the year 2006-07 sanction for release of grant-in-aid to 6 Government Medical Colleges/Hospitals has already been issued and it is also proposed to provide grant-in-aid to 8 Medical Colleges/Hospitals under the scheme after completion of necessary formalities. At present, there are 345 Radiotherapy machines located in more than 210 institutions across the country.[7]

District Cancer Control Programme

Under the scheme for District Projects for Health Education, early detection and pain relief measures, one time assistance of Rs. 15 lakhs and a recurring assistance of Rs. 10 lakhs for four years per district has been provided. So far, 40 districts have been provided with the funds under the scheme.

The four most frequent cancers in males in India are of the mouth/oropharynx, oesophagus, stomach and lower respiratory tract (trachea/bronchus/lung). For women, cancers of the cervix, breast, mouth/oropharynx and oesophagus are the most frequent. A number of these cancers are highly amenable to primary and secondary prevention.

Cobalt Therapy Installation

Efforts are being made to further strengthen the programme. Financial assistance for cobalt therapy units is provided upto Rs. 1.00 crore per unit to Non-Government Charitable Organisations and Rs. 1.5 crore for Government Institutions. Financial assistance for mammography unit upto Rs. 30.000 lakhs can be availed by institutions having a cobalt machine.

Financial Assistance to Voluntary Organisations

This scheme is meant for IEC activities and early detection of cancer. Under the scheme financial assistance upto Rs. 5.00 lakhs is provided to the registered voluntary organisations recommended by the State government for undertaking health education and early detection activities in cancer. Detailed guidelines for this scheme are under formulation.

NEW INITIATIVES

Major activities carried out under the National cancer control programme out of WHO funding under the biennium pattern included 16 workshop/training programmes carried out throughout India. The pap Smear Kits and Can scan software were supplied to 12 RCC's. Morphine tablets were also supplied to them. In the WHO biennium 2000-01, following were carried out:

- Outreach activities by medical colleges for early detection and awareness of cancer.
- Training of personnel in early detection and awareness of cancer.
- Supply of Morphine.
- Telemedicine and supply of computer hardware and software.
- IEC activities.
- Modified District Cancer control Programme.
- National Cancer Awareness Day.
- Training of cytopathologists and cytotechnicians in the quality assurance in Pap smear technology.
- Participation in health Melas and distribution of health education material.
- Postage stamp depicting a women carrying out 'self-breast examination' was brought out by Deptt. of Posts on national Cancer Awareness Day.
- Likely telecast of a health magazine 'Kalyani' in the current year, with cancer and anti-tobacco items under the agreement with Prasar Bharti and MOHFW.
- Broadcast of health education audio material developed by CNCI, Kolkata, through FM Radio.

In current biennium 2002-03 the activities are continuing in the similar way. A screening OPD for cancer at Vardhman Mahavir Medical College and Safdarjung Hospital has started functioning out of WHO assistance.

Modified District Cancer Control Programme

Modified District Cancer Control Programme initiated in four states namely Uttar Pradesh, Bihar, Tamil Nadu and West Bengal was concluded on 30.9.2002. Sixty Blocks were covered and 1200 NCD workers, 30 supervisor doctors, and consultants were utilized to conduct the Survey-*cum*-health education drive in which about 12 lakh women in the age group 20-65 years were contacted. Health education about general ailments, cancer prevention and early detection besides 'Self-Breast Examination' was imparted. The data collected is being analysed.

National Cancer Awareness Day

National Cancer Awareness Day was observed on 7th November across the country through the Regional Cancer Centres with a special drive for early cancer detection through camps in Government, charitable, private and corporate hospitals in Delhi and Chennai. A public function was organized at the National Stadium, New Delhi in collaboration with

NCT of Delhi wherein the Union State Minister of Health and Family Welfare, Mrs. Panabaka Lakshmi presided over the function and advocated the need for creating awareness among the general masses and early detection of the cancer. A "Run for Cancer Awareness" was also organized at the function.

SUGGESTIONS

1. Effective Collaboration with Various Countries

Cancer affects people in all countries and on all continents. The term is a collective one and covers over 100 varieties of the disease, each with different clinical manifestations, symptoms, course and prognosis. It is well-known that the prevalence of various forms of cancer differs from one country to another and from one area of a country to another. However, should a tumour of the same origin and the same structure develop in an Australian and a European, the clinical features of the disease, its diagnosis and the sensitivity of the tumour to radiation or chemotherapy will be the same or very similar in both these people, though they are from widely separated parts of the globe. But although the governing principles are the same, they are variously perceived, interpreted and described by physicians in different countries and of different schools. Something must be done to ensure that the successes and failures encountered in cancer control in one country are made known to the rest of the world, for everyone can learn from failure and, of course, from success too.[8]

2. Discourage the use of Alcohol and Tobacco

Recent estimates suggest that 30 per cent of cancers in the USA were caused by smoking. Cancer may be avoidable.

The fight to reduce smoking as a means of ending most forms of lung cancer, and many other diseases may prove to be one of the most significant health victories of the century. Unlike the magnificent conquest of small-pox, it will result from a change in human behaviour. Smoking as a habit produced an epidemic of serious diseases. Ending the habit can point the way to protecting health through decisions made by individuals and communities. It can prove to be a clear example of individual responsibility.[9]

3. Early Detection through Screening

Screening can be very effective way of combat cancer. However, the cost is very high . Therefore screening may be done as a part of integrated health programme. Screening is limited to circumstances in which:

- the disease is a significant cause of morbidity and mortality, the natural history is well understood,
- there is a test that can detect the disease prior to the onset of signs and symptoms, there is an effective treatment,

- there is good evidence that early detection and treatment reduces morbidity and mortality, and
- the expected benefits of early detection exceed the risks and costs.[10]

4. Involvement of Primary Health Care

The primary or front line health worker is in a good strategic position to detect oral cancers at an early stage. Such workers routinely come into contact with large number of people at outpatient clinics and during home visits. Furthermore, they can carry out an examination of the mouth quickly and with simple equipment, for instance, with two dental mirrors in ordinary daylight.[11]

5. Provide Adequate Resources for Research, Screening and Health Education

National cancer organisations can use the mass-media for education, enlisting the help of experts to popularize, for example, news of recent medical progress and its consequences. Other experts can plan person-to-person education, deciding on methods and training key-persons for health centres, schools, and so on. The key persons supported, like the voluntary workers, by the cancer societies can organize educational work at the local level, developing person-to-person communication adapted to their audience. They should be given not only the relevant training but also continuous assistance in their work in the form of educational material and other services.[12]

6. Control Cancer Pain

Freedom from cancer pain is possible with available technology. Relatively simple, inexpensive methods exist that can control the majority of cancer pains and thereby solve this neglected public health problem. Two-thirds of all cancer patients today will die of their disease. Both in developed and developing countries, cancer pain is under treated. Most patients in developing countries are incurable at the time of diagnosis; so before primary prevention will show its effect, before early referral and diagnosis will be implemented, and before adequate manpower for curative therapies have been trained, pain relief is the only realistic and humane alternative for years to come. Yet few countries have any cancer pain relief policies or programmes.[13]

Examples of relevant matters

The natural history of cancer, curability, the smoking problem, sexual hygiene, self-examination of the breasts, smoking cessation, cessation, cancer of the Castro-intestinal tract.

Women: cervical cancer, breast cancer.
Men: prostate, larynx and rectal cancer.

Information on supplementary care rehabilitation, follow up, social support Specific educational campaigns.

Establishment of cancer patients' associations for support and information in all relevant areas.

Examples of Education Activities Communicating Directly with Specific Groups

Environments	*Examples of relevant matters*
School health services	The natural history of cancer, curability, the smoking problem, sexual hygiene,
Screenings for cervical cancer	Sexual hygiene, self-examination of
Maternal health centres	the breasts, smoking ceassation
Health services of the armed forces	Smoking ceassation
Health services at places of work	Smoking cessation, cancer of the castro-intestinal tract Women: cervical cancer, breast cancer Men: prostate, larynx and rectal cancer
Patients at hospitals and in organized groups	Information on supplementary care rehabilitation, follow-up social support
Different organisations (youth, women, men, etc.)	Specific educational campaigns
Voluntary work	Establishment of cancer patients associations for support and information's in all relevant areas

Source: WHO.

7. Develop Epidemiology

The painstaking task of the epidemiologists is to determine how different cancers are distributed—an important first step in finding their causes and planning how to control those causes.[14]

IEC Activities at the Central Level

Health education is an important tool for prevention and early detection of cancers and hence suitable importance is accorded to the same under the NCCP. The programme supports activities of the health magazine "Kalyani" telecast by the Prasar Bharti in eight states. It is an interactive programme which provides an interface to the people with the experts on various health issues. In addition, IEC materials in the form of audio-video sports, posters, leaflets, flipcharts, etc. have been developed for dissemination across the country. DAVP in leading dailies for creating awareness among the general masses and for early detection of cancer.

RECENT DEVELOPMENT

In The Chandigarh Plus, *Tribune News Service* dated Nov. 23, 2007 appears an article "Facility for early detection of cancer at PGI soon." The PGI is all set to have position emission tomography (PET) scan facility at its nuclear medicine department, the technique which is mainly used in the early detection of cancer with a very high sensitivity, long before any structural changes become evident using other imaging techniques.

Expected to be functional soon, the project will include a combined PET and CT scanner and installation of a medical cyclotron with a fully automated system for production and dispensing of the isotopes. Position emission tomography (PET) is a functional imaging modality which is different from anatomic imaging such as ultrasound and CT, said Dr. B.R. Mittal, head nuclear medicine, PGI.

At present PET is available only at a few centres in India, mostly in the private sector and limited to the major metro cities, and that too at a very high cost. The radioisotopes produced by this cyclotron will also be made available to other PET centres which may start in the region in the near future. The nuclear medicine at the PGI is one of the only three institutes in India offering post-graduate (MD) course and second to start M.Sc. in nuclear medicine. The M.Sc. course has been started in collaboration with Panjab University and Dr. Baljinder Singh, faculty member of the department, is coordinating the course.

Dr. Anish Bhattachraya another faculty member, said the department has three state-of-art SPECT gamma cameras being run efficiently to cater to the patients needs. The PET scan facility will definitely prove to be a boon to the patient care, teaching and research activities of the department and the institute, he added.

Explaining about the technique Dr. Mittal said different radioactive compounds of glucose, carbon and oxygen, which are normally used by body tissues, form part of the positron emission tomography and are injected into the body. These compounds are selectively trapped within cancer cells and emit radiations, which are detected as bright spots on a computer screen. A major advantage of this technique is that the whole body can be scanned after a single injection of the radiotracer.

Since the radioisotopes used are very short-lived, they decay within a few minutes to few hours after injection. The radiation dose from this scan is comparable to that from a diagnostic CT scan, and does not cause any harmful side-effects.

However, the information obtained from PET-CT enables the imaging of both structure and function in a single instrument at the same time. This allows more accurate localization of cancer tissues, which exhibit increased clucose utilization.

Apart from oncological indications, PET-CT images are also used for neurological and cardiological diseases. In addition to clinical patient management, this facility will also be used for enhancing the research capabilities of the institute, with the addition of "molecular imaging."

CONCLUSION

If terminal cases of cancer are going to die shortly, then the best technique for dealing with the inevitable must be based on compassion. Strong efforts are needed to bring about this change in behaviour which can restore dying humans to the larger community about them, grant them respite from pain, and offer them the warm touch that they crave and deserve so much.

In an attempt to achieve this goal, one of targets for the WHO cancer control programme is to formulate and disseminate knowledge about efficient pain-relief, from the level of improved personal contacts, via treatments with aspirin/codeine to narcotics and physical interventions. The second step in this programme will be to see to it that recommended drugs will be available, and will be used properly for all cancer patients both at home, around the health dispensary, in district hospitals and in larger hospitals, on all five continents.[14]

We suggests the following:

(1) intensification of IEC activities so that people seek care at the onset of symptoms,

(2) provision of diagnostic facilities in primary and secondary care level so that cancers are detected at early stages when curative therapy can be administered,

(3) filling up of the existing gaps in radiotherapy units in a phased manner so that all diagnosed cases do receive therapy wihout any delay as near to their residence as is feasible, and

(4) IEC to reduce tobacco consumption and avoid lifestyles which could lead to increasing risk of cancers.

We know how to prevent some cancers, and we know how to reduce the number who will die from others. However, much research is still needed. New screening tests are being developed and evaluated, and the accuracy of established tests is being improved. Most important, research is under way to determine the best method for gaining acceptance of the screening tests as part of the health programme in the community.[15]

Notes and References

1. Jan Stjernsward, "Is Cancer Avoidable" in *World Health*, Sept.-Oct., 1981.
2. *World Health*, Sept. Oct. 1981, p. 12.
3. Wedd Wittard, Cigarettes: A Battle We can Win, in *World Health*, *op. cit.*, 1981, p. 154.
4. Jan Sternsward, *op. cit.*, p. 3.
5. Jan Sternsward, *op. cit.*, p. 7.
6. Ministry of Health and Family Welfare, GOI, Annual Report, 2006-07, p. 131.
7. *Ibid.*

8. A.M. Grin, and L. Sabin, "A Common Language", in *World Health*, Nov. 1975, p. 10.
9. Nedd Willard Cigarattes, "A battle we can Win, in *World Health*, Sept. 1981, p. 15.
10. David M. Eddy, Early Detection, *World Health*, Sept.-Oct. 1981, p. 20.
11. *World Health*, Sept.-Oct., p. 1981,. p. 25.
12. Gisela Gastrin, Now Education Helps in *World Health*, Nov. 1975, p. 16.
13. *World Health*, Sept.-Oct. 1988, pp. 7-8.
14. Dying with Dignity, in *World Health*, Sept.-Oct. 1981, p. 34.
15. Annual Report, Ministry of Health and Family Welfare, 2006-07, p. 132.

9

CHAPTER

National Diabetes Control, Cardiovascular Diseases and Stroke

Non-Communicable Diseases

I. NATURE AND MEANING

It is difficult to give an exact etiological, pathogenic and clinical definition of the disease. It may be described as a chronic disorder caused by inherited or acquired impairment of the insulin production in the pancreas—a gland which also discharges digestive juices into the duodenum or first part of the small intestine. This leads to a reduced glucose tolerance, increased concentration of glucose in the blood (hyperglycemia) and other metabolic disturbances which in the long-run, may cause pathological changes in the large and small blood vessels of the body.

Besides the symptoms of diabetes include excessive urination (Polyuria), great thirst, weight loss, despite good appetite, and tiredness. In addition, in some instances, there may be itching and infections of the genitalia and the skin, eye symptoms such as blurred or misty vision, menstrual disorders, impotence, occasionally dehydration and diabetic coma.

Today, on the eve of the twenty-first century, we see that the world health situation is no longer that clear-cut and simple. Many developing countries have made great progress in combating infectious diseases and malnutrition, thereby improving the length and quality of life of their people. But rapid urbanization and industrialization in those same countries, together with the adoption of modern lifestyles that adversely affect health, have brought new problems in the form of chronic non-communicable diseases. In many developing countries these "new" problems are arriving before the 'old' ones are resolved, leading to a double burden of disease. At present, non-communicable diseases are responsible for 70-80% of deaths in the developed countries, and have reached the level of about 40% in the developing world.[1]

Rationale for having a Common Programme for the Prevention and Control of Diabetes, CVD and Stroke

- Diabetes is an important risk factor for both the major forms of cardiovascular disease (coronary heart disease and stroke), especially in India.
- CVD is the major cause of death and disability in persons with diabetes.
- Common risk factors underlie CVD and diabetes: unhealthy diets, physical inactivity and over weight are common to both. Even smoking is a major risk.
- With an increased risk of developing diabetes and a closely associated condition called the 'metabolic syndrome."
- High blood pressure often precedes and predicts the onset of clinical diabetes by several years. This had led to 'hypertension' being regarded as a pre-diabetic condition.
- Clinical trails have shown that, mortality reduction and increased survival are better achieved by blood pressure control than even by blood sugar control, in persons with diabetes.
- Persons with CVDs or diabetes require similar lifestyle therapy and often similar drug therapy for prevention of complications (diet; physical activity; smoking cessation; cholesterol lowering drugs; aspirin; ACE inhibitors; other blood pressure lowering drugs).
- Persons with diabetes frequently need to be screened for CVD and risk factors of CVD.
- Proven lifestyle interventions which can prevent the onset of diabetes (diet and physical activity) are similar to those proven to reduce the risk of developing hypertension, coronary heart disease or stroke.

The strategic approaches and operational elements for prevention and control of CVD and diabetes are thus similar or closely interlinked, whether it is primordial prevention (preventing the acquisition of risk factors in the first place), primary prevention (preventing onset of disease by reducing risk factors which are elevated) or secondary prevention (reducing the risk of complications after the onset of disease).[2]

2. GENESIS AND OBJECTIVES OF THE PROGRAMME

The National Diabetes Control Programme was started on a pilot basis during the Seventh Five Year Plan in some districts of Tamil Nadu,

Jammu and Kashmir and Karnataka, but, due to paucity of funds in subsequent years this programme could not be expanded further.

The Objectives of the programme are:

(i) Primary prevention by identifying high risk subjects at an early stage and imparting appropriate risk reducing health education to them, their family and community by IEC Programme;
(ii) Secondary prevention through early diagnosis and appropriate treatment of the disease to reduce morbidity and mortality with special reference to groups at risk;
(iii) Prevention of acute metabolic and chronic cardio vascular, renal and ocular complications of the disease;
(iv) Provision of equal opportunities for physical attainment and scholastic achievement for the diabetic patients; and
(v) Rehabilitation of those particularly or totally physically handicapped due to the disease.

Recent studies show that upto 10 percent of India's urban population and 2 percent of the rural population above the age of 15 years have diabetes. This number seems to be rapidly increasing and has doubled in the past 20 years, and is fast acquiring epidemic proportions. In 1990, the number of diabetics in India was 1.5 crores and by the year 2000 it will cross the 3.5 crore marks.

Diabetes mellitus is now recognised as one of the fastest-growing threats to public health in almost all countries of the world. A World Health Organisation report notes that it is no longer considered a 'disease of affluence', it increasingly affects Third World Communities and epidemiologic surveys have shown that 10 percent or more of the adult population now suffer from it, and a worldwide total of 100 million prevalent cases are anticipated by the end of the century.

Are Indians more suspect than others ?

Yes, due to a long lineage of poor eating habits and a poor general life-style when it comes to health consciousness, Indian today, particularly those in urban areas, are very likely to develop diabetes at some stage of their lives. Even the median age when an urban Indian is likely to develop diabetes is falling to alarming proportions and there are many men and women in their mid-30s and early-40s who show full-blown symptoms of a type of diabetes that usually occurs only much later.

Diabetes is also called the 'prosperity disease' in India since it is often caused by long-term overeating. Excessive intake of rich food, especially that of sugar and pure ghee taxes the pancreas and reduces its capacity to produce enough insulin to assist the body in burning off the sugar. In villages, it was very common among the opulent zamindars. The probability of developing diabetes due to genetic factors, higher in Indians as it is, can be brought out by an affluent diet. As early as 1907 it was observed: "What gout is to the nobility of England, diabetes is to the aristocracy of India."

But today it is no longer the prosperity disease. In urban as well as in rural India poor eating habits continue to hold sway. Add to this the fact that the many foreign influences in the staple diet of many communities have led them away from a preference of traditional natural organic health-giving foods, to processed products packed with preservatives and calories. Strain, tension, anxiety and the sedentary lifestyle afforded by urban existence only aggravate the disease further.[3]

It is difficult to give an exact etiological, pathogenic and clinical definition of the disease. It may be described as a chronic disorder caused by inherited or acquired impairment of the insulin production in the pancreas—a gland which also discharges digestive juices into the duodenum or first part of the small intestine. This leads to a reduced glucose tolerance, increased concentration of glucose in the blood (hyperglycemia) and other metabolic disturbances which, in the long-run, may cause pathological changes in the large and small blood vessels of the body.

Besides the symptoms of diabetes include excessive urination (Polyuria), great thirst, weight loss, despite good appetite, and tiredness. In addition, in some instances, there may be itching and infections of the genitalia and the skin, eye symptoms such as blurred or misty vision, menstrual disorders, impotence, occasionally dehydration and diabetic coma 10 day, on the eve of the twenty-first century, we see that the world health situation is no longer that clear-cut and simple.

Contrary to popular belief, diabetes mellitus is not a disease that affects only the affluent. It strikes the poor and under-nourished as well. A greater awareness of this fact, as a result to a large mass of epidemiological data, has resulted in the new international classification of diabetes. Malnutrition-related diabetes mellitus (MRDM) was recognized by a recent WHO study group as a clinical class distinct from non-insulin (NIDDM) and insulin dependent diabetes mellitus (IDDM). In several developing countries it may constitute 30 to 70 per cent of all cases of youth-onset diabetes. Indeed, epidemiological data do indicate a low incidence of IDDM and a high prevalence of MRDM in most of the developing world. Clinical features include characteristic leanness with sub-normal body mass, moderate to severe increase in blood glucose, the requirement of large doses of insulin to achieve normalcy in blood glucose, and a frequent history of malnutrition in early childhood.[4]

3. TREATMENT OF DIABETES

(I) Regulated Food Intake

Regulated food intake is essential to control diabetes. 25 per cent of patients can be controlled through diet only. Barbara Milten Posoner and Huda Mura in their Article "Eat Wisely to live longer" rightly suggested on the basis of Food and Nutrition Board of US National Research Council (NRC) the following to improve the control over diabetes.

- Reduce total dietary fat intake to 30% or less of calories. Reduce saturated fatty acid intake to less than 10% of calories and intake of cholesterol to less than 300 mg daily.
- Eat several servings every day of a combination of vegetables and fruit, especially dark green and yellow vegetables and citrus fruits.
- Increase the intake of starches and other complex carbohydrates by eating several daily servings of a combination of whole-grain breads, cereals, and legumes.
- Maintain protein intake at moderate levels.
- Balance food intake and physical activity to maintain appropriate body weight.
- For those who drink alcoholic beverages, limit consumption to the equivalent of less than one ounce of pure alcohol in a single day.
- Limit total daily intake of salt (sodium chloride) to 6 gram or less.
- Maintain adequate calcium intake.
- Avoid taking (unnecessary) vitamin and mineral supplements.
- Maintain an optimal fluoride intake, particularly during periods of tooth formation and growth.

(1) Besides world health organisation has also suggested the wise eating which include:

1. Eat a variety of foods.
2. Maintain a healthy weight.
3. Choose a diet low in fat (30 or less of calories), saturated fat (about 10 calories) and cholesterol (300 mg or less).
4. Choose a diet with plenty of natural fibre.
5. Use sugars in moderation.
6. Use salt and sodium in moderation.
7. If you use alcoholic beverage, do so in moderation.

(2) Physical Exercise can Reduce the Contents of Fats and Carbohydrates

Health agencies must recognize that regular exercise is of Enormous importance to vast number of people. Every individual will benefit greatly in improved health by ensuring adequate regular exercise for himself and his family.

(3) Medicinal Treatment—Serious Patients should be Administered Drugs

The administration of insulin is necessary in diabetes when glucose stability (homeostasis) cannot be achieved by means of diet alone or by diet in combination with oral anti-diabetics. Juvenile diabetics in particular need insulin but so do many sufferers. of more mature age. The percentage of diabetics requiring insulin has decreased with the displacement of the "age pyramid" of the population towards older ages. Today, about 25 to 30 per cent of all diabetics are insulin-requiring; they usually take two injections of insulin daily, using a combination of short and long-acting insulin's to give better blood glucose control throughout the day. In addition, more highly purified pork insulin is now available; its molecular composition is more akin to human insulin than that from other kinds of animals and it is also less immunogenic (that is, less likely to evoke an immune response).

Sufferers in whom the disease develops in adulthood (maturity-onset diabetics) often have a latent secretary capacity in their beta-cells, the cells of the pancreas that normally secrete insulin. The use of drugs known as sulphonylureas to reactivate this capacity has proved extremely valuable, especially for elderly diabetics who are thus spared from needing insulin injections. Because of the neglect of diet therapy, as I have already emphasized, sulphonylureas have been widely used in diabetic therapy. perhaps in as many as 40 to 50 per cent of patients. When properly used, they will continue to play a role in those patients for whom diet alone cannot achieve metabolic balance.[5]

(4) Preventive Approach through Education—The Patients should be Educated about the Disease to Solicit their Cooperation

This will have a lasting effect. One of the aims of education is to involve the patients themselves in the care of their disease. This demands information and instruction which is adjusted to the individual's ability to utilize and follow the advice given. Apart from purely medical problems that are dealt with by a physician, education can best be given by nurses and other health personnel who have been specifically trained for this purpose. Thus, the educational sector in this disease needs to be widened considerably to include all the various categories of personnel who participate in the care of diabetics, whether at home or in clinics and hospitals. Considering the importance of public education in any health activity and especially in primary health care, there have been to date comparatively few such programmes in the field of diabetes, and little is yet known about their potential impact. There is certainly scope for demonstration projects aimed at testing the efficacy of public education campaigns in severely affected communities. Furthermore, several components of the integrated approach for the prevention of non-communicable diseases are also of relevance to diabetes.

Educational activities may be aimed not only at the public, but also at non-specialized and specialized health workers. WHO has provided active support and sponsorship for number of paramedical training courses on diabetes, many of them organized and coordinated by WHO collaborating centers.

(5) Change of Lifestyles—Involving Drinking, Smoking and Leading Sedentary Life

Man today is sick, because, he thinks he is sick. Sickness and disease have no place in the life of a man who does not accept and tolerate the self-limiting thoughts which are the real seeds of our myriad ailments. We stand hypnotized by the belief that disease and illness are our fate and destiny, rather than health and bliss, which are of truly our birthright and heritage. In order to emerge from our mass hypnosis and collective hysteria and to experience health, joy and creative fulfilment, we must make systematic application of yoga in our daily lives. So called modern way of life, social drinking, smoking, etc. resorted to beat stress, perpetuate our ill-health in the long-run.

Non-communicable diseases (NCDs) such as cardiovascular diseases, cancer, chronic lung diseases and diabetes account for 54% of all deaths in the Region. The WHO regional framework for prevention and control of NCDs (formulated in early 2006) provides a step-wise approach to the development and implementation of comprehensive national policies, plan and programmes. The health secretaries of Member-countries of the Region, at their Eleventh Meeting held in June 2006, reviewed the regional framework and reiterated the need to strengthen the integrated epidemiological surveillance and population-based public health interventions that make optimum use of existing health care systems and target the common risk factors and determinants of major NCDs.

The World Health Report of 2002 states that cardiovascular diseases (CVD) will be the largest cause of death and disability in India by 2020. Non Communicable Diseases (NCDs), especially Cardiovascular Diseases (CVD's), Diabetes Mellitus, Cancer, Stroke and Chronic Lung Diseases have emerged as major public health problems in India, due to an ageing population and environmentally driven changes in behaviour. The premature morbidity and mortality in the most productive phase of life is posing a serious challenge to Indian society and its economy. It is estimated that in million diabetes, 2.4 million cancers and 0.93 million stroke. Compared with all other countries, India suffers the highest loss in potentially productive years of life, due to deaths from cardiovascular disease in people aged 35-64 years (9.2 million years lost in 2000). By 2030, this loss is expected to rise to 17.9 million years—940% greater than the corresponding loss in the USA which has a population a third the size of India's.

Non-communicable diseases include Malignant 2005 NCDs accounted for 5,466,000 (53%) of all deaths (10,362,000) in India. In a review published in 1996, it was reported that the prevalence of coronary heart disease (CHD) increased from 1% in 1960 to 9.6% in the year 1995 among urban Indian residents. Similarly, the prevalence in rural residents rose from 2% in 1974 to 3.74% in 1995. The prevalence of CHD is now reported to be 3-4% in rural areas and 8-10% in urban areas among adults.

Based on these data, it is estimated that there were approximately 29.8 million patients with CHD in the year 2003. With an estimated 10%

attrition and event rates they projected an annual new event or death to occur in 2.9 million persons per year with nearly 1.5 million people dying due to CHD every year. The estimated burden of common NCDs are; 2.4 million Ischemic Heart Diseases, 37.8 Neoplasms, Other Neoplasms, Endocrine Disorders, Neuro-Psychiatric conditions, Sense organ diseases, cardiovascular diseases, respiratory diseases, digestive diseases, genitourinary diseases, skin diseases, musculo-skeletal diseases, congenital anomalies and oral conditions).

The word Non-Communicable Diseases (NCDs) in this document is used to refer to Diabetes, Cardiovascular Diseases and Stroke.

Magnitude of Non-communicable Diseases

	2005	*2015*
Total deaths in India	510,362,000	10,949,000
Deaths from NCDs	5,466,000	6458,000
Death from major NCDs		
Deaths due to cancer	826,000	1,06,900
Deaths due to Diabetes	175,000	236,000
Respiratory Diseases	674,000	864,000
Cardiovascular Diseases	2989,000	3,465,000

The causes of NCDs are known and are the same in India as in wealthy countries. The common risk factors are Tobacco, Alcohol, Diet and Physical inactivity and hence the population prevalence levels of these factors can predict the future disease burden. The WHO Stepwise surveillance of NCD risk factors carried out in 5 sites in India showed that only 50% of the population aged 15-64 years, consumed vegetables daily and 60-80% led a sedentary lifestyle.

Tobacco is the foremost cause of preventable death and disease in the world today. In India, 47% of the male and 14% of the female population use tobacco in some form, resulting in nearly 1 million premature deaths annually. The total economic cost of the three major diseases caused due to tobacco use in India was Rs. 308 billion (USS 7.2 billion) in 2002-03. India has played a leading role in the development of Framework Convention on Tobacco Control (FCTC) and was one of the first countries to ratify the convention.

There is evidence-based information that NCDs are preventable through integrated and comprehensive interventions. Cost-effective interventions exist, and have worked in many countries: the most successful strategies have employed a range of population-wide approaches combined with interventions for individuals. WHO estimates that an additional 2% annual reduction in chronic disease death rates in India over the next 10 years would result in an economic gain of 15 billion dollars for the country. India is passing through an epidemiological and demographic transition and the pace of transition varies between states. The policies will have to be flexible to accommodate the differing needs and resources of the states in India.

Multisectoral interventions for providing an enabling environment will have maximum effectiveness in primary prevention. At least 80% of premature heart disease, stroke and type 2 Diabetes and 40% of cancer could be prevented through avoidance of tobacoo products and the adoption of healthy diets and regular physical activity.[7]

NCDs are preventable and manageable using evience-based interventions. Demonstration projects using community-based interventions (CBI) for prevention and control of NCDs were continued with WHO support in Bangladesh, India, Indonesia and Sri Lanka. These projects furnished evidence on the feasibility and appropriateness of applying community-based approaches for integrated prevention and control of NCDs in developing countires. The Regional Office has developed guidelines for monitoring and evaluation of such projects. The project conducted in Depok, near Jakarta, Indonesia gained considerable recognition, paving the way for further sub-national interventions.

Surveillance of NCDs and their risk factors is an important component of national NCD prevention and control programmes. Recent Regional Office initatives helped to strengthen the national capacity to collect, manage, analyse and use relevant data. NCD risk-factor surveillance has been included in the integrated diseases surveillance project of India. Collection of nationality representative data has been initiated in Nepal and Sri Lanka. Datasets, collected in surveys using the STEPS method promoted by WHO, were conducted recently in eight countries and were anlaysed using a standardized approach and format. Technical support was also provided for establishing national NCD databases.

Justification for Phased Implementation

The NPDCS will be implemented in a phased manner with a pilot being done in the Preparatory Phase 2006-07. Subsequently, the programme would be implemented across the country through select institutions over the XIth Five Year Plan. This being a new Programme, the phased implementation would assist us in proper execution of the plan and also evaluation of the strategies for control of NCDs. The programme may be expanded to the rest of the country over the subsequent five year plans.

Aim of the Programme

- Prevention and control of common NCD risk factors through an integrated approach
- Reduction of premature morbidity and mortality from DM, CVD and Stroke

Objectives of the Programme

Long-term goals

1. Reduce prevalence of risk factors of common NCDs.
2. Reduce morbidity and mortality due to Diabetes, Cardiovascular diseases and Stroke.
3. Building capacity of health systems to tackle NCDs and improvement of quality of care.

Immediate objectives

1. Primary prevention of major Non-Communicable Diseases through Health Promotion.
2. Surveillance of NCDs and their risk factors in the population.
3. Capacity enhancement of health professionals and health systems for diagnosis and appropriate management of NCDs and their risk factors.
4. Reduction of risk factors of NCDs in the population.
5. Establish National Guidelines for management of NCDs.
6. Development of strategies/policies for prevention of NCDs in the country through Interministerial collaborations/ coordination.
7. Community empowerment for prevention of NCDs.

Pilot Phase: 2006-07

Preparatory Phase—Pilot Project Cost: Rs. 5.00 crores:

- Establishment of National NCD Cell with the necessary manpower and infrastructure support.
- Establishment of state NCD Cell in 6 states.
- Identification and establishment of 6 Regional Resource Centres
- Identification of one Medical College each in all the regions of the country namely North, South, East, West, Northeast and Central regions.
- Identification of one district under each Medical college for setting up of District Healthy Lifestyle Centres and Strengthening of District and Sub-district health facilities.
- Finalisation of Management Guidelines for NCDs and their risk factors.
- Preparation and Dissemination of IEC strategy.
- Preparation and Dissemination of NCD Resource kits.
  — NCD prevention and management for health professionals,
  — Patient education packages.
- Health Promotion in specific settings.
- Rural/urbani/periurban/schools/workplaces.
- Survey for risk factors/NCDs.

NCD Cell at Centre

For Planning, Coordination, Guidance of National Programme—

- Establishment of Central Hub for NCD to provide the following:
  — Database, and
  — Resources: Training/IEC.
- For Monitoring and Evaluation both Internal and external.

State NCD Cell

- Would be Nodal Office in the state with a Designated Nodal Officer.
- Would facilitate and coordinate NCD control activities in the state.
- Would Monitor and evaluate NCD control activities in the state.[6]

CONCLUSION

One chronic disease, diabetes, figures high among the target diseases of Inter-health since it can lead to such serious consequences as gangrene and amputation, blindness, or early death.

Diabetic patients, if undiagnosed or inadequately treated, develop multiple chronic complications leading to irreversible disability and death. Coronary heart disease and stroke are more Coronary in diabetics than in the general population. Micro-vascular complications like diabetic renal disease and diabetic retinopathy and neuropathy are serious health problems resulting in deterioration of the quality of life and premature death. In fact, diabetes is listed among the five most important determinants of the cardiovascular disease epidemic. Metabolic disorders in pregnant diabetic women as well as those caused by gestational diabetes (diabetes diagnosed for the first time during pregnancy) post: a high health risk, to both the mother and foetus.

Unfortunately, there is still inadequate awareness about the real dimension of the problem among the general public. There is also a lack of awareness about the existing interventions for preventing diabetes and the management of complications. Inadequacies in primary health care systems, that until now were not designed to cope with the additional challenge posed by chronic non-communicable diseases, result in poor detection of cases, sub-optimal treatment, and insufficient follow-up leading to unnecessary disabilities and severe complications, often resulting in early death.

In addition to non-insulin dependent diabetes (NIDDM), which is a rather silent, chronic, often unidentified killer mostly among the adult population, the insulin dependent form of the disease (IDDM) makes an even more dramatic appearance in diabetic children. They develop symptoms of ketoacidosis and often die, since the majority do not have access to adequate medical care, and since the majority often either not available or too expensive. Of the estimated 27,000 deaths of diabetic children aged 0-14 years world-wide in 1990, almost 45% (12,000) occurred in India alone. The projection for the year 2000 remains much the same. Almost all of these deaths would be preventable if free or subsidized insulin and adequate health care services were available.[7]

Notes and References

1. Hiroshi Nakajima, The Health of Nations in Changing, in *World Health*, May-June, 1991, p. 18).
2. Annual Report, 2006-07, Ministry of Women and Child Development, GOI, New Delhi, 154-55.
3. Dr. Shanti, B. Ranjawani, "Diabetes: Understanding the disease", New Delhi, Voluntary Health Association of India, 1997, pp. 2-3.
4. Jasbir S. Bajaj, Diabetes and Malnutrition, *World Health*, Oct. 1988, p. 22.
5. Raff. Luft, Diabetics, The Outlook in Bright, in *World Health*, May 1979, p. 5.
6. Ministry of Health and Family Welfare, GOI, Annual Report, 2006-07, pp. 152-54.
7. WHO: SEARO: Health Situation in South-East Asia, 1994-97, New Delhi, 1999, pp. 145-46.

10
CHAPTER

National Nutrition Programme

NEED

Nutrition is the science of food and nutrients are essential for health. Good health is impossible without adequate nutrition. Poverty and lack of nutrition education are the major causes of malnutrition, which is a serious problem causing a number of diseases. There are large number of diseases caused by Nutritional deficiencies. Nutrition is an important factor in the etiology and management of several of the major causes of death and disability in developing countries. As such the world health organisation has set its objective—'The Health for all by 2000 AD'. All the member-countries endorsed the slogan. More responsibility falls on those who have spent the major part of their lives in the service of mankind in relation to their health.[1]

While going over different projects of various health organisations, it can be seen that all are focussing their attention primarily on family planning and only marginal attention is paid to problems such as Nutrition Anaemia in pregnant, lactating mothers and school going children, preventable blindness and caries teeth in children as well as the malnutrition in vulnerable groups. These are all due to nutritional deficiencies of one or the other kind. The disasterous effect of these factors results in huge child mortality and maternal mortality in our country.

Some efforts are made on the curative side but almost no attempt seems to have been undertaken for prevention. Nutrition plays a major role in prevention and deserves our deep concern. Mental retardation due to early malnutrition in children is an irreversible condition and is a national disaster of high magnitude.[2]

We have to avoid both under-nourishment and malnutrition. Under-nourishment resulting from food scarcity, continues to afflict hundreds of millions of people in developing countries, many of whom have a food intake below the critical minimum level. Increasing the overall food supply and making food regularly available to the community, family and individual therefore remains a top priority for much of the world.

While food availability is undeniably a major concern so far as the promotion of proper nutrition is concerned, malnutrition is not an inevitable consequence of under-nourishment. A key element in this respect is the individual's ability to obtain full nutritional benefit from the food that is consumed.

There is evidence, based on numerous food consumption surveys, to suggest that the average energy intake of an individual in a developing country does not differ all that much from that of a citizen in a developed country. Whatever difference there is depends not so much on food availability as on the absorption and use of nutrients by body. Infection and disease interfere with this process, and untold millions have their potential energy drained away though having to cope with them. The increased need for energy to fight of infection, combined with a decreased appetite for food in the sick individual, can only serve to worsen the effects of malnutrition that occur in food scarce situations.[3]

Malnutrition continues to be a dominant problem in many developing countries or in the Third World. Its manifestations and consequences are diverse and alarming. Over and above the health-related concerns, malnutrition results from deprivation of basic human needs and therefore is treated as a problem in its own right. It is no longer considered as a result of food deficiency alone as there are many inter-related factors leading to problems of malnutrition. It is a national problem interfering with development of human resources. In recent years, the concern over nutrition has centered on organizing and tailoring direct nutrition intervention programmes to specific age-sex population groups. In other words, the vulnerable groups such as infants, young children, pregnant and lactating mothers are regarded as a priority group, who need attention. It is being increasingly recognised that malnutrition being a multifaceted problem needs a multi-sectoral strategy for its control. In fact, it stands as a junction between agriculture, health and social sciences. Therefore, any policy or intervention programme needs a coordinated inter-sectional approach.[4]

MEANING AND SCOPE

Malnutrition is a man-made disease. It is not the only one but in terms of the number of people affected and of its consequences for human well-being, it is the most serious and shameful of them all. It is a social disease which has been with man since he has been a social being. More specifically, it is a disease of human societies.[5]

There is no drug to solve malnutrition, still less a vaccine to prevent it. The real permanent solution entails improving overall living conditions of the people with the greatest need. Five Principal diseases are caused due to malnutrition:

(i) Anaemia

Insufficient red pigment (haemoglobin) in the blood (mainly iron deficiency).

Main symptoms: Pallor of skin and mucous membranes, general fatigue, breathlessness after exertion, palpitation, loss of appetite (anorexia), indigestion, (dyspepsia).

The Foods that prevent them: All kinds of meat, liver fruits, especially citrus fruits, guava, mango, pineapple, berries, green vegetables.

(ii) Endemic Goitre

Enlargement of the thyroid gland resulting from iodine deficiency.

Main symptoms: Deformity of the neck, mental retardation and deaf-mustism; may occur in children born to mothers with goitre.

The Foods that prevent them: Sea foods, such as fish, shellfish and algae, iodized salt.

(iii) Kwashiorkor

Severe protein deficiency.

Main symptoms: Swelling (oedema), apathy and irritability, "flaky-paint" skin, sparse, straight and dyspigmented hair.

The Foods that prevent them: Milk and cheese, meats and fish, eggs, pulses, such as beans, peas and lentils, groundnuts.

(iv) Marasumes

Severe Calorie Deficiency.

Main symptoms: Growth retardation, wasting, no subcutaneous fat, atrophied muscles—"all skin and bone."

The Foods that prevent them: Breast milk for infants, cereals, such as rice, wheat or maize roots and tubers (potatoes, yams or cassava), fats and oils.

(v) Xerophathalmia

Severe Vitamin-A Deficiency.

Main symptoms: Dryness of the eyes (xerosis), night-blindness (nyctalopia), corneal ulcerations, leading to blindness.

The Foods that prevent them: Whole, milk, butter, and cheese, yok of eggs and liver, vegetables, especially carrots and "greens", yellow fruits, such as mango and papaya, red palm oil.[6]

Nutritional Problems.

Nutrient deficiencies, nutrient imbalances, nutrient excesses and presence of food toxins which result from inadequate in-take and improper utilisation are the five types of nutritional problems. Major nutritional problems in India are Protein Energy Malnutrition (PEM), Iodine Deficiency Disorders (IDD), Vitamin A

Deficiency (VAD) and anaemia. Besides, fluorosis is also prevalent and lathyrism is localised to certain regions. The Nutrition Cell in the

Directorate-General of Health Services provides technical advice on all matters related to nutrition. State nutrition divisions set-up in 17 states and union territories assess the diet and nutritional status in various groups of population, conduct nutrition education campaigns, supervise supplementary feeding programmes and other nutritional ameliorative measures. Surveys conducted by state nutrition divisions and National Nutrition Monitoring Bureau under ICMR reveal that malnutrition and other deficiency disorders are found more in young children, pregnant and lactating mothers. To combat these problems, Government has initiated several schemes. The Integrated Child Development Scheme (ICDS) provides a package of services to control nutritional and health problems. To prevent blindness among children due to Vitamin A deficiency, a concentrated dose of Vitamin A is given orally every six months through peripheral health workers. Similarly, to prevent nutritional anaemia among women and children, tablets of iron and folic acid are distributed through health centres. A Pilot Programme against Micronutrient Malnutrition has been initiated in five districts in Tripura, Bihar, Orissa, West Bengal and Assam to assess and improve micronutrients status in school children, adolescent boys and girls, women of child-bearing age and elderly population. The National Institute of Nutrition, Hyderabad and All India Institute of Hygiene and Public Health, Calcutta are the principal organisations for nutrition research and training.

Infrastructure for Nutrition in Govt. of India: As reported in Annual Report of the Ministry of Health and Family 2006-07, is as follows: The Nutrition Cell in the Directorate General of Health Services provides technical advice on all matters related to Policy-making, Programme implementation and evaluation, training modules for different levels of medical and para medical workers. It took up technical scrutiny of standards and labels for foods, proposals, project evaluation, review of research projects, etc.

The Cell has been working on creating awareness regarding prevention and control of micronutrient deficiency disorders, diet-related chronic disorders and promotion of healthy lifestyle through dissemination of various types of IEC materials. Expert committee meetings have been held to examine and finalize scripts with reference to production of video film on lodine Deficiency Disorders and undernutrition and promotion of healthy lifestyles. 10 minutes video film on iodine Deficiency Disorders was produced and released during the Global IDD celebrations.

SUGGESTIONS

We suggest the following to combat malnutrition:[7]

1. Obtain the interest and direct involvement of top decision-makers;
2. Obtain the interest and the involvement at a problem-solving

rather than target-achieving-level of key administrative personnel;

3. Encourage the coordination of all area-level government personnel;
4. Stimulate the active participation and involvement of the community concerned;
5. Train the grassroots-level workers to realize that they are doing a truly important job and are not just and lowest of the low in the government hierarchy; and
6. Inculcate in all concerned a sense of sincerity and dedication.

The following measures are suggested to ensure tackling problem of malnutrition.

1. Popularise Safety Standards of Food

The workers must educate the people about the need and methods of food preservation. Through experience and the communication media, the message has been widely disseminated that food can, and does, get contaminated if it is exposed to flies, if it is handled by people who have not taken care of their personal hygiene, and if it has been improperly stored. What needs to be done is to activate mechanisms that will ensure strict adherence to safety standards on the part of food preparers and food vendors. We all have a responsibility to ensure that our food fulfils the roles it is meant for; to nourish us, to give enjoyment and to sustain life.[8]

2. Educate the People against Wrong Beliefs, Customs, etc.

Food habits and traditions and beliefs affect the endemicity and epidemicity of infectious diseases, and are important primary or secondary causes of malnutrition. When a child becomes ill, traditions, beliefs and taboos may enter into play to influence care and treatment. The result may be recommendations about food suppression or restriction, alterations of the diet or the application of positively harmful "remedies." The indirect effect of infections may thus be more important than the direct one, particularly in traditional societies with a low level of education. The effect of Infection on Nutrition is summarized as follows:

(i) Direct Effect

(a) Anorexia, vomiting, Impaired digestion and absorption Decreased food intake and utilization.
(b) Loss of nutrients and cells, Over utilization, sequestration and diversion of nutrients, Nutrient wastage.

(ii) Indirect Effects

(a) Interaction of infection with socio-cultural factors.
(b) Decreased food intake and nutrient wastage.

3. Encourage Consumers' Associations

Though often inseparable, food borne diseases are now being seen as no less a health hazard than the water borne ones which tend to win bigger headlines in the newspapers. Meeting this challenge will call for the active involvement of groups other than the usual organisations which work alongside government health services, notably the food industry and the consumer associations.[9]

4. Entourage Peoples' Participation

Community participation, within the context of primary health care, is the process by which individuals and families assumed responsibility for their own health and welfare and for those of the community and develop the capacity to contribute to their community development. Such a process is the key to overcoming a high prevalence of malnutrition even in situations where it may be impossible to step up the actual supply of foodstuffs.[10]

5. Integrate with Primary Health Care

In 1978, the International Conference on Primary Health Care held at Alma-Ata. erstwhile, USSR, spelled out the essential elements of Primary Health Care, one of these being the promotion of food supply and proper nutrition. The right kind of food, regularly available, is clearly essential if people are to live socially and economically productive lives. Proper nutrition is no less essential for health and, like health, each contributes to general socio-economic development and in turn benefits from that development.

Several factors have to be considered in the promotion of an adequate food supply and proper nutrition. First of all, food has to be available in sufficient quantities and with the right nutritional content in relation to such factors as age, occupation and climate. However, it must be not only available but also of an acceptable nature, taking into account people's different cultural backgrounds. Most important of all, food has to be safe, which implies that eating it should not give rise to food-borne diseases, either from infection or Intoxication.[11]

A proposal for National Programme for prevention and control of fluorsis was prepared for 11th five year plan.[12]

CONCLUSION

Thus malnutrition continues to be a national problem and its control in India is always linked with a total socio-economic transformations. What is needed is a quantitative and qualitative change in the approach to the problems, based on real issues facing the community. Better coordination between central and state health services for implementing centrally sponsored nutritional and other programmes is essential. Institution responsibilities need to be identified. A concerted and dedicated effort is needed for better nutrition programmes with proper aims and objectives and action plan with a specific target and time frame. A proper implementation, surveillance, monitoring and evaluation are needed for long-term planning and programmed management. The emphasis should be on balanced diet available locally.

Notes and References

1. Ministry of Health and Family Welfare, GOI, Annual Report, 2006-07, p. 142.
2. Dr. R.G. Chitre, Nutrition and Health, in *Health Administrator,* Vol. 5, No. 2, Dec. 1987, p. 1.
3. Albert Pradilla and James Apre, Infection and the Nutrient Drain, in *World Health,* Oct. 1983, p. 22.
4. Dr. Kamla Krishnaswamy, Nutrition and Health, in *Health Administrator,* Vol. 5, No. 2 Dec. 1987, p. 15.
5. Molses Behar, A Man-made Disease, in *World Health,* May 1977, p. 5
6. *World Health,* May 1977, pp. 16-17.
7. *Ibid.,* p. 21.
8. Jitendra Tuli, Safe Food in Good Food, in *World Health,* Oct. 1983, p. 10.
9. Gamini Seneviratne, Is it safe to eat ? in *World Health,* Oct. 1983, p. 21.
10. Alberto Pradilla and James Apre, Infection and the Nutrition Drum, in *World Health,* Oct. 1983, p. 22.
11. Fritz Kaferstein, Safe Food, in *World Health,* Oct. 1983, pp. 2-3.
12. Annual Report 2006-07, Ministry of Women and Child Development, GOI, New Delhi, p. 151.

11
CHAPTER

Oral Health Programme

NATURE AND SCOPE

Oral health has made remarkable progress in most developed countries as a result of prevention programmes that stress the optimum use of fluorides, oral hygiene, and the adoption of healthy eating habits.

However, the situation is beginning to deteriorate in many developing countries, where oral diseases are on the increase and treatment costs are spiraling. Yet oral diseases are not an inevitable corollary of development. We have the means to prevent this health and economic disaster, we have to ensure that these means are implemented for all citizens every where.

Action is urgently needed. In he countries that have achieved sustained improvements, health policies need to be adjusted, staff have to be trained to deal with the new situation, and appropriate services have to be set-up. In particular, care for the elderly should be strengthened to prevent the oral health problems linked with age. At the same time, work among children and adolescents must continue.[1]

In our mouths there are billions of living bacteria. Most of them are harmless, some even helping the digestion of our food. Dental plague is the soft white or yellow layer that sticks to the teeth. Plague is mainly bacteria but it also contains remains of saliva, cells of the mouth tissues, and fibres from food. Some of the bacteria that grow in the mouth cause tooth decay and gum disease. They produce different substances that change the enamel or the tissues that hold the teeth.[2]

Plague builds up where the gum meets the neck of the tooth, in the grooves of the chewing surfaces of the teeth, and in the narrow spaces between the teeth. Plague is found in everybody's mouth, but some have much more than others. These people are more likely to develop gum disease and tooth decay.

CHART 11.1

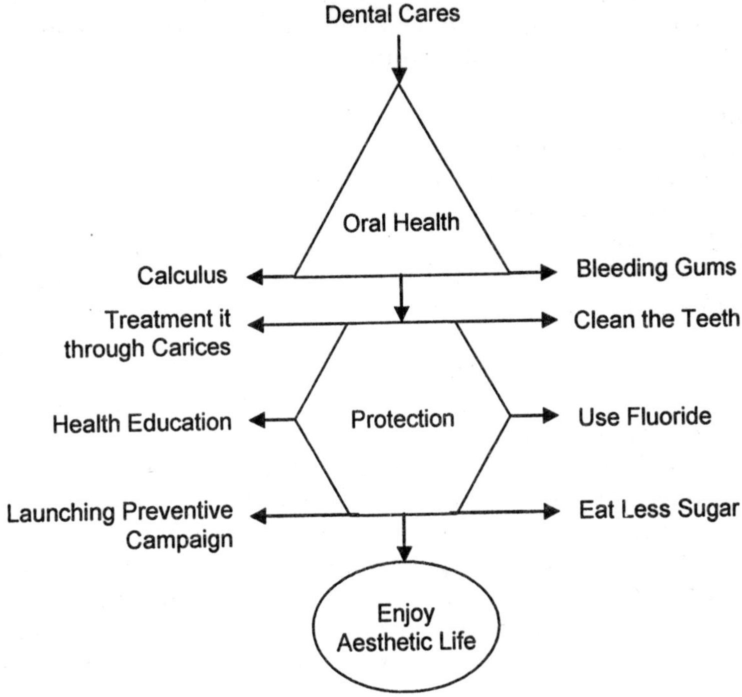

Dental Caries

The bacteria in the plaque produce acids from food we eat; these acids attack the tooth enamel and cause caries. The bacteria grow and produce a lot of acid very quickly if they are supplied with sugar.

If extractions are to be avoided, caries must be prevented from starting or, when present, must be treated with a filling. Most dental caries occurs in children and young adults. Older people mainly have caries of the root and problems with replacement or repairs of fillings.

Inflamed or Bleeding Gums

Gingivitis or inflammation of the gums usually begins in the gums between the teeth. Most people develop gingivitis at some time in their life. Bacteria in the plaque are the cause of the disease. If plague is removed every day thoroughly, the gums will become healthy after one week. Bleeding from the gums is a common sign of gingivitis, period of is a serious bacterial infection of the tissues and bone around teeth. The bacteria attack the fibres that hold the teeth in the jaw. When this happens a gap forms between the teeth and the gum. This gap is called a periodontal pocket. The pocket fills with debris and bacteria which cause further damage. The fibers that hold the teeth are gradually destroyed, and the teeth become loose. Periodonititis is a problem of older adults, but is must less common than gingivitis.

Calculus

If plaque is not removed for a long time it hardens into calculus. Calculus makes cleaning the teeth and gums very difficult so it should be removed by a trained oral health worker.[3]

Prevalence

If the current increasing trends in dental caries countries in the Region will soon have DMFT levels higher than the WHO target. In addition to dental caries, periodontal diseases are widespread. Fair examples, it is reported that 85% of children and 95-100% of adults in India suffer from periodontal diseases. These diseases are initially painless, but they are chronic and lead to gradual tooth loss.[4]

SUGGESTIONS

1. Implement Oral Programmes

Oral health has made remarkable progress in most developed countries as a result of prevention programs that stress the optimum use of fluorides, oral hygiene, and the adoption of healthy eating habits.

However, the situation is beginning to deteriorate in many developing countries, where oral diseases are on the increase and treatment costs are spiraling. Yet oral diseases are not an inevitable corollary of development. We have to ensure that these means are implemented for all citizens everywhere.

2. Involve School Teachers as in Thailand

A national oral health survey in Thailand in 1989 indicated that 12-year-old children had an average of 1.5 decayed, extracted and filled teeth, and 77% of these teeth needed restorative care on occults pits and fissures. So a project was started to treat primary school children in Bangkok—a typical example of a city in a developing country experiencing ever greater caries prevalence. The fact that untreated active fissure caries lesions may result in the total destruction of the affected tooth motivated intensive efforts to solve the problem.

Six primary school teachers were trained by a dentist during a three-day course. The first day dealt with general knowledge of tooth anatomy, caries and oral hygiene instruction. On the second day, the teacher-pupils learnt to handle, mix and apply glass ionomer sealant on plaster casts of teeth. The third day saw the teachers practicing applying the sealants on children, and each teacher treated about six teeth at this session.

The course took place in school rooms, using simple, portable dental apparatus. Air blowers operated by a foot pump sufficed to control excess saliva, in addition to cotton rolls. Two school teachers acted alternately as operator and assistant in mixing and handling the sealant material.[5]

The study demonstrated that school teachers given this brief training could apply the treatment just as well as the dentist. Although only a small percentage of the sealant remained in position when the children's teeth were checked six months later, a significant reduction in caries was observed after two years, particularly among the younger age group. The school teachers who took part enjoyed the training and appreciated being able to give oral care to the children. They also had a better understating of the importance of early prevention of caries. The school-children too cooperated well and took better care of their oral hygiene.

3. Clean your mouth

Do this well once or twice every day. To remove the plaque from your teeth and gums, use a toothbrush or a chewstick—and whenever possible, use fluoride toothpaste. If you have crowns or bridges you also need to use dental floss or interdental brushes to clean between your teeth. These are the basic measures of oral hygiene.

4. Use Fluoride

Fluoride is a mineral found naturally in many foods and in most sources of drinking water, Inhabits the ability of bacteria to produce acids, strengthens the enamel of your teeth, and makes them more resistant to decay. When fluoride levels are below optimal, use fluoridated toothpaste. In addition, either drink fluoridated water or milk or use fluoridated salt in cooking and have it available on the table for use with food. If none of these is available, use fluoride tablets or rinses. Fluoride protects teeth throughout life, but it especially protects the teeth of children.

The use of fluorides in drinking water, salt, milk, toothpaste and mouth-rinses has played a major role in reducing the number of cavities in the teeth of children and young adults throughout the world, especially in the industrialized world. But the problem of cavities is not over. In young people, most cavities develop in the pits and grooves of the chewing surfaces of back teeth, which derive the least benefit from fluorides.

Fortunately, such damaging tooth decay can be prevented by sealing the teeth with a thin plastic coating which will protect them from the acids formed from bacteria and food that cause decay. Unfortunately, dental sealants have been underused by oral health care providers. Too often, they are also unknown to parents and children. Yet youngsters all over the world could suffer significantly less from tooth decay if sealants were used more frequently by dentists, their helpers and community health workers with special training.

The sealing of teeth first started in the mid-1950s, when an American scientist discovered that by etching (putting a very mild acid on the tooth surface to make it rough) a bound could be established between the tooth and the plastic coating. The plastic coating seals the pits and grooves so that food and bacteria cannot get in. Today, Sealants are made to plastics similar to those used in some other dental procedures, such as repairing the broken edges of teeth. They can be applied by dentists, dental hygienists, dental assistants or properly rained community health workers.[6]

5. Eat Less Sugars

Use sugars intelligently. You can safeguard your teeth by eating less sugar-rich food. Or by balancing with other food. Don't let snacks take the place of a well-balanced diet; nutritious food are essential for oral health as well as for overall health. If you really need to nibble between meals, the best snacks are those that contain no fermentable carbohydrates.

6. Affordable Services

The need for oral care is changing. Demand will be greatest when communities perceive services to be rational, affordable, accessible and appropriate.

7. Launching Preventive Campaign

In the countries where the situation is deteriorating this trend must be checked by launching effective prevention campaigns. We must ensure that the adoption of new lifestyles and new eating habits does not lead to an increase in dental caries in populations that have always had healthy teeth. We must find ways to incorporating and encouraging the traditional methods of oral hygiene which have proved heir efficacy, and which are inexpensive and culturally acceptable. Health, well-in and self-confidence are all boosted by a healthy and well-cared-for mouth, which also facilitates communication and human relations.

In devoting World Health Day 1994 to oral health, he World Health Organisation is endeavoring to mobilize member-states, the health professions and the general public so that greater attention is paid to this important aspect of public health. Education and the participation of everyone are the keys to progress in oral health, without which there can be no health for all.

Let us unite our efforts so that the successes already achieved in the field of oral health can benefit everyone.[7]

8. Prevention at a Low Cost

Oral care is costly. Some rich countries spend 5% to 11% of their annual health budges on oral health. It is a price that few Third World countries, if any, can afford to pay.

Prevention rather than repair—and repair when problems do arise—are the real answers. It is estimated that prevention takes much less time and money than treatment and it is better !

Oral health care personnel, such as "dental therapists" or 'dental hygienists', can be trained in two to three years. They undertake oral health promotion and education. They also have the skills to clean teeth, remove tartar deposits, fill cavities and perform ordinary extractions. Dentists can then concentrate on more difficult treatment and carry the overall responsibility for oral health care programmes.

There is a ratio of one dentist for every 1000 population in several rich countries; but only one for over a million people in some poor nations.

When proper mouth care, including prevention, is promoted, these ratios should improve significantly.

Oral health, however, does not depend only on oral health care personnel. It is first and foremost a personal and family responsibility. Children should be brought to a health worker trained in oral care as early as possible. They should learn very early about oral hygiene when they learn about body hygiene, preferably by two years of age. By six years, when the permanent teeth—the teeth of life—are growing, they should have established good oral habits. Parents should take the responsibility for cleaning children's teeth, up to the age of eight years.

The experience of a number of industrialized countries has shown that the cavities dropped by about 80% in the last 20 years as a result of a combination of preventive measures—including health education and information programmes advocating oral hygiene, the optimal use of fluorides, and "prudent" diets. Indeed, it can be said that cleaning teeth and gums, using fluorides, and eating fermentable carbohydrates with meals rather than between meals are the "pillars of prevention."[8]

CONCLUSION

Oral health contributes to a healthy life. Worldwide, oral health has improved greatly in the last decades, although there is still much to be done. And there is a lot that each one of us can do to protect our teeth and keep our mouth healthy.

A cornerstone of the Health for all approach is the focus on prevention. Treatment of dental diseases is both relatively ineffective and beyond the financial resources of much of the world. The effectiveness of prevention has been convincingly demonstrated: it should be allocated the highest priority. Treatment of disease to alleviate pain and discomfort is the next priority. Here WHO's Three Levels Strategy for planning oral health has already had some effect. The strategy emphasizes firstly the use of appropriate technology, that is, simple and inexpensive materials; then simple clinical measures carry out by non-dental personnel or dental auxiliary personnel working in primary health care facilities; finally, specialist personnel to do the more complicated work at the third referral-level.

The strategies available to prevent dental caries and periodontal disease can virtually eradicate them in the near future, and therefore can and should be incorporated into a primary health approach. They include a multi-sectoral food policy to increase the availability of fluoride, where less than optimal levels exist, either as fluoridated water or salt, or in toothpaste, and to develop guidelines for tolerable and adequate levels of refined sugar. A meeting took place in Geneva early in 1989 with the object of tackling this subject. A population approach to improving general hygiene should serve to increase oral cleanliness and thereby reduce periodontal disease.

Dental disease is increasing at a frightening rate in many developing countries, and in some the level is higher than in industrialized countries. An integrated preventive approach offers the only realistic solution to the increasing problem of oral disease in developing countries. For the treatment-oriented dentists in industrialized countries, it may however raise a quite different problem-that of over-manning.

Notes and References

1. Hiroshi Nikajama, Oral Health, For a Healing Life, *World Health,* Jan-Feb. 1994, p. 3.
2. *World Health,* January-Febraury, 1994, p. 11.
3. *Ibid.*
4. SEARO: WHO Health Situation in SEA, 1994-97, New Delhi, 1998, p. 170
5. *World Health,* Jan-Feb. 1994, p. 6.
6. Alice M. Horowitz, Seal out Decay—Seal in a Smile, *World Health,* Jan-Feb. 1994, p. 6.
7. Hiroshi Nakajama, Oral Health, For a Healthy Life, *World Health,* Jan.-Feb., 1994, p. 3.
8. Amsi Tewari, "A Family Care Programme in India", *World Health,* Jan-Feb. 1994, p. 19.

12

CHAPTER

Occupational Diseases

Prevention, Detection and Control

INTRODUCTION

Diseases that arise out of an in the course of various occupations or employment are known as Occupational Diseases. Occupation related diseases are caused by continuous exposure to toxic or hazardous materials or substances used or manufactured in industries. Some other processes and procedures at workplaces also result in occupational diseases.

Occupational Diseases are as old as the occupations themselves, including agriculture. The degree of hazardous exposure may, however, vary from industry to industry. Advanced clinical technology and medical research, in the recent years, have been able to co-relate a number of hitherto lesser-known diseases to a variety of occupations. Early symptoms of most of the occupational diseases are generally mistaken for those of common diseases.

PREVENTION

Interestingly, almost all occupational diseases are preventable. All that needs to be done is, bringing about necessary improvements in working conditions through adequate environmental control and introduction of basic safety measures for the workers exposed to varied risks. Regular health checks up of workers for detection and diagnosis of occupation-related diseases, change of job if necessary, timely and proper medications are the secondary measures that should follow to arrest the trend. The fact to be borne in mind is that most of the occupational diseases are irreversible. Prevention therefore, is, the key to control.

Risk Categories

About fifty percent of the seven million workers, covered under the ESI Scheme of India for health insurance and other integrated social security benefits, are exposed to the risk of occupational diseases and other employment hazards. And, this figure represents only a small percentage of the country's total work force exposed to occupational risks.

An estimated figure of employees, exposed to occupational diseases in some specific industries, presently covered under the ESI Act, 1948 is given below:

Sr. No.	*Industry*	*Employees exposed to risk*
1.	Cotton and Textile	15,00,000
2.	Leather and Rubber	3,00,000
3.	Chemical and Chemical Products	5,20,000
4.	Non-Metallic Minerals	2,60,000
5.	Metallic Minerals	5,20,000
6.	Transport	2,80,000
7.	Paper and Printing	2,77,000

Diseases and Co-relations

Some of the common occupational diseases, prevalent among the workers in hazardous industries in India listed below:

Sr. No.	*Diseases*	*Related Industries*
1.	Byssinosis	Cotton and Textile Industry
2.	Silicosis	Cement, Glass, Stone Crushing, Slate Pencil, Foundaries, Brick Refractories, Ceramic Industries, etc.
3.	Asbestosis	Asbestos Industry
4.	Stanosis	Tin ore mining, etc.
5.	Bagassosis	Agriculture and related industries
6.	Bronchiolitis	Various industries
7.	Siderosis	Electric arc welding
8.	Lead Poisoning	Printing press, ceramic industries, battery storage, alloys, etc.
9.	Chrome ulcer and Perforation	Leather tanning, chrome plating, paint and dye industries
10.	Skin Diseases	Chemical industries, solvents, acids, alkalies, chrome, arsenic and cement industries, etc.
11.	Phosphorous Poisoning	Fertilizer and insecticides industry, etc.
12.	Asthma	Nickel, cotton, wood processing, plastic and rubber industries.
13.	Occupational Cancer	Asbestos and dyes industries, etc.

Personal Protective Equipments

The use of Personal Protective Equipments (PPEs) interpose an effective barrier between a worker and any harmful substance or object, but, do not eliminate any occupational hazard totally. PPEs are not a substitute for basic needs like risk protective engineering inputs or adequate environmental control within the premises besides physically tolerable working hours and good caloric diet. Some PPEs for enhancing personal safety of workers are recommended below:

Body parts exposed to risks	*Equipments recommended*	*For protection against*
1. Protection of Head	Head caps, helmet made of proper materials	Falling objects, flying particles, sparks, hot materials.
2. Protection of Eyes	Safety spectacles, goggles, helmet, eye screen	Dust, Flying particles, splashing liquids, chemicals, gases fumes, glare.
3. Protection of Ears	Ear plugs, ear muff	Noise
4. Protection of Face	Face Shields	Splashes, Flying particles, gases, fumes, chemicals
5. Protection of Arms and Hands	Gloves, sleeves, hand pads, finger guards made of suitable material	Hot and Molten metals, chemicals, corrosive sparks, acids, alkalies, electric shock, flying particles.
6. Protection of Fee and Legs	Safety shoes, gum boots, foot guards leg guards	Flying objects, acids, and alkalies hot liquids, heat sparks, electric stock.
7. Protection of body	Aprons, overalls, jackets, protective suits, coats	Hot materials, heat, spark, flying objects, acids, alkalies.
8. Respiratory system	Respirators and masks	Dust, fumes, smoke, and gases
9. Miscellaneous	Barrier cream, Safety belts	Dermatitis due to chemicals, slip or fall while walking.

Occupational Diseases Centres

Early detection and diagnosis of most of the occupational diseases and adequate evaluation of functional and pathological changes of organ systems is a challenging task that cannot be achieved through ordinary clinical processes. They need a specialized approach that includes detailed analysis of biological materials such as, blood urine for chemicals, perfect evaluation of organ functioning and even audiometry measurements for nerve conduction velocity, etc. The detection of occupational diseases also requires extra special medical equipment, mostly computerized analytical system, for precise results.

It was in this background and keeping in view the increasing number of insured population getting exposed to occupational risks that the Employees' State Insurance Corporation had decided to establish four Zonal Occupational Diseases Centres at New Delhi, Mumbai, Kolkata and Chennai as referral institutions for early detection and prevention of occupational diseases.

(A) OCCUPATIONAL HAZARDS AND HEALTH DISASTER

The interaction between man and his work environment may lead to ill-health, if work hazards are beyond his tolerance, or to better health when his work is fully adapted to the human physical and psychological factors. Occupational diseases have been known for centuries. The Mad Hatter in "Alice in Wonderland", written over 100 years ago, is often cited as an example: the mercury compounds in materials used for making hats were popularly supposed to cause insanity among these craftsmen. Today the picture is not better but worse; occupational diseases are increasing in variety and prevalence.[1]

Among 100 coronary patients, occupational stress proved five times more important as a causative factor than diet, smoking and drinking.[2]

Developing countries are becoming industrialized and industry is continually adding new chemical, physical and psycho-social hazards to health. The situation in agricultural work is not much safer. There is evidence that agricultural accidents from machinery now occupy second place after mining accidents both in frequency and severity, particularly in industrialized countries. The wide use of agricultural chemicals has been associated with episodes of occupational poisoning. From the rather limited statistical information available, it appears that occupational respiratory diseases due to such vegetable and other organic dusts as cotton, flour, wood and tobacco are becoming an important occupational health problem in the agricultural industries of developing countries. In addition, there are the traditional diseases of mining and manufacturing, including pneumoconiosis, poisoning by heavy metals, solvents and other chemicals, occupational allergy and dermatitis, and deafness caused by noise.

In the absence of pre-employment medical screening, general health problems affecting the workers, such as malnutrition and parasitism, are aggravated by occupational hazards. Workers in developing countries may therefore be considered a vulnerable group insofar as the newly introduced work hazards are concerned. Silicosis can be complicated by tuberculosis, liver damage resulting from parasitic infestation is aggravated by industrial solvents, and nutritional anaemia adds to the harmful effects of lead poisoning.

On the other hand, work can be a positive factor in health promotion. Physical activity coupled with an adequate diet maintains a high degree of physical well-being and psychological gratification through work achievement makes a potent contribution to good health. Work is considered as one of the important manifestations of the productive existence of human beings.

Newly developed sciences in ergonomics and humanization of work are capable of realizing an optimum balance between work demands and human capacities. Work management with the guidance of modern occupational medicine can bring about the type of work environment that promotes human motivation and a sense of belonging.

CHART 12.1

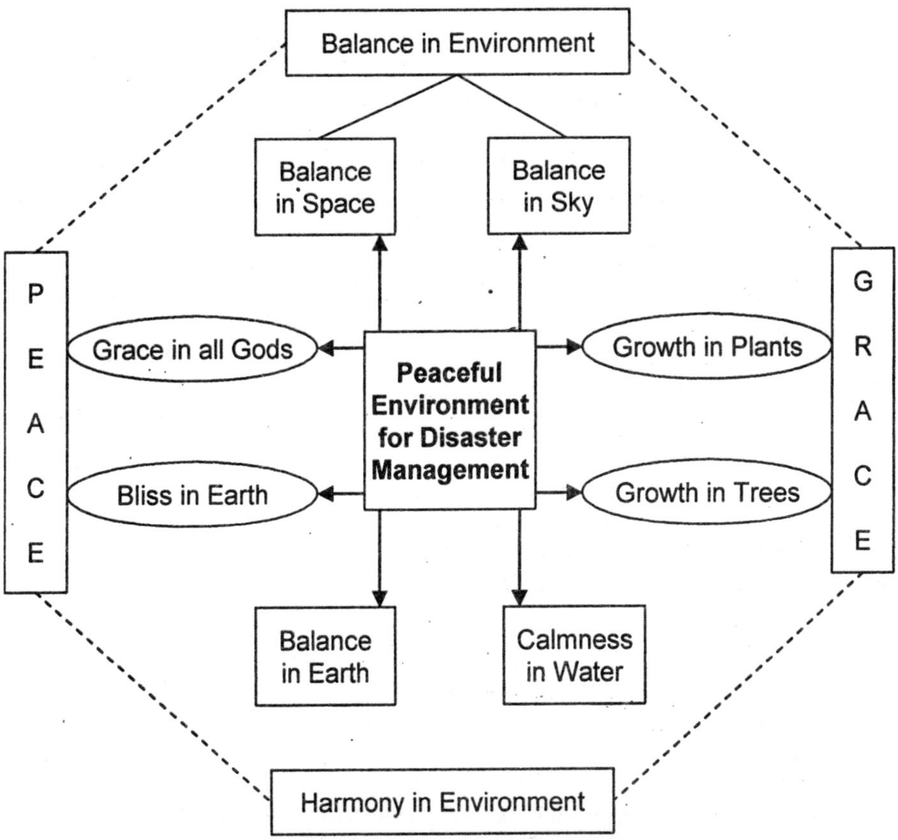

Much has been written about the two main influences of work on health-the negative and the positive, but little reference is made to those health problems in which working conditions and work exposure could be among several causative factors of varying magnitude. We call these problems "work-related diseases."

Epidemiological investigations have shown that certain chronic diseases generally known to occur in middle or old-age may, to a large extent, be the result of work exposure. In the case of such diseases of multiple etiology whose control does not mainly depend on removing one single main causative factor-occupational exposure play a role whose final result depends not only on the type and magnitude of exposures but also on human susceptibility and tolerance. Workers with a high degree of susceptibility, which may be inherited or acquired from general environmental exposure, suffer the most when they are placed in jobs that are not suited to their capacities. Work-related diseases may therefore be an appropriate term to signify those diseases that result from, or are associated with, work hazards acting in combination with other external or hereditary factors. Work-related diseases also lend themselves to control in the working populations by means and measures taken in the work setting and through preventive occupational health and managerial intervention. The following is a brief review of some examples.

Hypertension is one of the disease that affect workers whose job involves concentrated effort, repetitiveness and high responsibility. A study made of air traffic controllers[3] found that hypertension was four times more frequent than would be expected for the same age group, taking into account all other variables, including diet, smoking and alcohol consumption. Heat stress may also play a role in causing or aggravating hypertension.[4] An epidemiological study of workers in steel rolling mills who were exposed to excessive heat from the furnaces showed a significantly higher prevalence of hypertension. The study blamed prolonged exposure and excessive heat as the main causative factor. Medical examination of 2,087 metal workers in Belgrade[5] revealed a prevalence of neurotic manifestations of 38 and 42 per cent respectively, in addition to ulcers and hypertension, all of which were attributed to poor working conditions and work instability.

For many years peptic ulcer has frequently been described in association with occupational factors, usually among workers exposed to a combination of such features as repeated anxiety at work, changing of work hours, irregular shifts, and environmental agents including heat stress and irritant gases.

Studies among seafarers also show an increased frequency of gastritis, indigestion and ulcer accompanied by neurosis and high blood pressure. Polish students at WHO's Pilot Health Centre for Seafarers at Gdynia reported this finding. A study of Indian seamen in 1971 demonstrated that gastritis and peptic ulcer caused the highest morbidity among 26,106 seamen examined between 1695 and 1969.[6] Peptic ulcer alone accounted for 13.6 per cent of the total sickness, and all the other causes of illness occurred at significantly lower rates.

Occupational health intervention aimed at controlling peptic ulcer among workers requires alert epidemiological observation to identify all possible causative factors and to deal with physical, chemical and psychosocial stresses among the workers at risk. It will include a study of their diet (at home and at work), smoking, consumption of alcohol, and whether they were on shift work, night work and so forth.

Arthritis and locomotor disorders are among the common diseases that have been widely described as related to, or caused by, occupational exposures and physical work performance. Of all the rheumatic diseases, only rheumatoid arthritis does not appear to relate to occupation. Joint strain from carrying heavy loads or from unduly heavy physical labour, minor or major injuries to changes in microclimatic conditions (humidity, heat and cold), work posture, and the use of vibratory tools—all these have been described as factors causing degenerative osteoarthritis at the relatively young age of 30 years, low back pain syndrome, and rheumatic diseases of the joints and skeletal system. In many occupations, absenteeism is predominantly due to rheumatism and diseases of the locomotor system. In some countries these diseases are already officially recognized as occupational diseases.

A recent comparative study of lumbar disc degeneration among miners, surface manual workers and office workers found that 43 per cent of the miners examined were affected as compared with 18 per cent of the surface manual workers and 7 per cent of the office workers, though all were of similar ages. This showed clearly that with heavy physical labour, as in mining, the probability of osteoarthritis increases.

Coronary heart disease has often been described as affecting certain occupational groups where emotional stress commonly occurs. From among the multiplicity of etiological factors including diet, obesity, smoking, lack of exercise and alcohol consumption, occupational factors were found in a study of 100 coronary heart disease patients to have played a leading role. After comparing the different factors in these patients, it was found that occupational "stress", described as heavy work of 60 or more hours per week for prolonged periods in tasks requiring mental and emotional reaction, precipitated the disease in 90 per cent of the cases. Occupational stress was five times more important than any of the other factors.[7]

Coronary heart disease was proved to result from exposure to carbon disulphide in the viscose rayon industry. Other studies involving combined exposure to carbon monoxide, heat stress and smoking showed a tendency for susceptible individuals to acquire this disease. Greater safeguards in the work environment and the intervention of occupational medicine should be capable of preventing the occurrence of this disease among high-risk groups.

These are only a few examples of the complex relationship between occupational exposure and certain chronic diseases, which afflict human society. There is no doubt that a multidisciplinary attack on these problems is indicated. While more research is required, determined action in the field or prevention and control is possible. Periodic medical check-ups of the populations at risk should help us to identify in the early stages the biological parameters of any deviation from good health. Bringing about better and more humane conditions of labour is a key element in prevention.

WHO's programme on the criteria for "Early detection of health impairment in occupational exposure to harmful agents" should help to develop methods for the appropriate health screening of workers in different occupations. Complementing this programme is a study of the health effects of occupational exposure to combined hazards, and other studies of the health of vulnerable working groups. All these studies seek to revise the health standards used in places of work, particularly in the developing countries, and to discover better criteria for the early detection of work-related diseases.[8]

Hazards on the Land

Agricultural workers face an entire range of very specific occupational problems because of their exposure to known agents of disease, which may be biological, physical or chemical.

The purpose of occupational health in any type of job is to ensure, firstly, that fit people are engaged and, secondly, that they are not at risk of ill-health by virtue of their occupation. This is equally true of occupational health in agriculture. Since the production of food, which is essential to human existence, is the responsibility of agricultural workers, their health must have a high priority if they are to be able to feed the world's teeming population.

Agriculture has been defined by the Joint ILO/WHO Committee on Occupational Health "as forms of activities connected with growing, harvesting and primary processing of all types of crops, with the breeding, raising and caring for animals, and with tending gardens and nurseries." An agricultural worker is defined as "any person engaged either permanently or temporarily, irrespective of his legal status, in activities as defined above."

The health problems of these workers can be divided into general and specific sub-groups. General health problems include those diseases and afflictions that the agricultural worker, in common with everyone else, is exposed to and suffer from. Many of these arise as a result of poor sanitation, inadequate water supply, inadequate accommodation, malnutrition, and a wide variety of communicable diseases, both parasitic and bacterial, that affect the entire population.

More specific occupational problems occur as a result of worker's exposure to agents of disease associated with agriculture, which may be biological, physical, or chemical.

Biological hazards obviously include zoonoses-diseases of a hich are transmitted to man in handling animals and animal products. The Committee on Occupational Health has compiled a comprehensive list of these diseases, but the most common ones are bovine tuberculosis, anthrax and brucellosis. In addition, certain parasitic diseases are transmitted as a result of contact with polluted water in farmlands. The common ones are schistosomiasis, ankylostomiasis and leptospirosis.

Chemicals are extensively used in agriculture to control insects, fungi, herbs, rodents and so forth, which damage crops. These pesticides and insecticides are harmful to man if not used carefully. Those at risk are mainly workers who are engaged in their manufacture, mixing, transport and application (spraying).

Contamination of food from the use of empty containers has resulted in human poisoning, and so has the accidental consumption of seeds treated with chemicals (mercurial) as preservatives. These chemicals tend to remain long in the environment and may affect birds, fish and other forms of life. The most commonly used are chlorinated hydrocarbons (DDT is the principal member of this group), organ phosphorus (parathion and the less toxic malathion) compounds, carbamates and organic mercury compounds.

Allergic diseases result from inhaling vegetable dusts, pollens and other organic dusts. Some of the conditions encountered include farmers' lung (following excessive inhalation of dust containing fungi), byssinosis from cotton (Gossipium malvaceae), flax (Linum usitatissimum) and soft hemp (Cannabis sativa), allergic conjunctivitis from rubber latex, upper respiratory tract disease due to allergy to wood dust, and dermatitis (also due to certain wood dusts).

As for physical hazards, the most common factors are heat (resulting in heat fatigue and other pathological manifestations including cramps and stroke), noise from machinery, dust, fumes and accidents of all kinds. Cuts from matches and hoes constantly occur among those engaged in subsistence farming. Snake bites and stings from other poisonous insects occur from time to time, especially where farmers go barefoot. On large farms, the main causes of accidents include falling-off tractors, overturning tractors, felling trees and falling from farm buildings.

Considering the importance of agriculture in every country's economy, all efforts made to ensure that those engaged in this occupation enjoy the highest standard of health will pay good dividends. A healthy worker is a productive worker, so providing occupational health for those engaged in agriculture is a worthwhile investment. Such a programme should embrace all activities of health promotion, prevention, treatment and rehabilitation, and it can function through health centres, mobile clinics, or purpose-built occupational health services. Those who operate such centres should have special instruction in how to deal with the special needs of farm workers. Small-organized farms can also make use of mobile clinics and health centres, but these farms need to provide their own first-aid services. Commercial farms, whether owned by individuals, the government or agricultural groups should provide a well-run occupational health ervice for their workers.

Occupational health services for agricultural workers deserve recognition as a priority of the Ministry of Health, which ideally should include an expert (occupational physician) with special responsibility for the health of agricultural workers. There should be close co-operation between the Ministries of Health, Agriculture and Labour in this regard. Ideally, there should be a body made up of representatives from each of the three ministries, under the chairmanship of the occupational physician from the Ministry of Health, charged with looking into various aspects of safety, health, and welfare of those engaged in all forms of agriculture. An improvement in the health of farmers means an improvement in the health of the country, since these are the major food producers upon whom the population depends.

How can their better health be ensured? They need to be advised on all hazardous factors to which they may be exposed. Those at great risk need to be monitored. For example, people who use organic mercury pesticides for seed dressings should have a periodic check-up of their blood or urinary mercury estimation. Where laboratory investigations are not possible, clinical examinations should be done from time to time to detect early signs of toxicity.

Some occupational diseases can be prevented simply by explaining to workers the hazards of every operation they perform. Such instruction needs to be meaningful whether the worker is literate or not. There should be adequate supervision of the use of protective equipment and clothing.

Other measures that can be taken include all kinds of accident prevention, pre-employment, periodic and special medical examinations, provision of emergency services, training of first-aid workers, maintenance of high standards of hygiene in canteens, toilets, and so on for the workers, and provision of facilities for families (schools, maternal and child health services, markets) to ensure good family life. Health education should aim at a high standard of sanitation and healthful living both at work and at home. Statistical data collected periodically should be analysed and the information so obtained used to improve the health and welfare of workers and their families.[9]

Mining is one of the earliest occupational activities of mankind, and has never been far removed from danger and disaster. The first scientific work on occupational health was written by a physician who worked with miners: Georg Bauer, more commonly known as Georgius Agricola, who in 1526 was appointed official doctor to the mining town of Joachimstal, in what is now the German Democratic Republic.[10]

Mining is largely men's work nowadays, but in the past women too worked down the mines, in really shocking conditions. Only the social reforms of the 19th century brought an end to this situation. Curiously enough, in Brazil the miners in general believe that the presence of women underground will cause accidents. The result is that female visitors-and even cassock-wearing priests-are not allowed in Brazilian mines.

Handling, hauling and transporting the material through galleries and shafts entails serious risks. Slips and falls are common. The ceiling of the galleries has to be propped against the risk of collapse, and sudden floods from unsuspected water sources may trap and drown the miners.

In coal mines, there is the risk of exploding "firedamp", the gas methane which exists absorbed in the coal and associated strata, and may be liberated through digging or the use of explosives. The permissible amount of methane in the air should not exceed one to two per cent.

It follows that illuminating the mines poses a particular problem, since candles and torches could trigger-off an explosion of "firedamp." It used to be a common practice to illuminate the galleries with the faint luminescence emanating from a silex stone rubbed against a revolving steel disc. This in turn was the cause of eye disease among the miners since the amount of light was so small.[11]

In the old days of poor illumination, workers suffered from what is called "miner's nystagmus", a rhythmic involuntary movement of the eyes, which is nowadays practically non-existent.[12]

The closed space of the galleries may cause muscular pains or changes in joints, and the presence of machinery results in a tremendous amount of noise, very often leading to hearing problems if the miners are exposed to it for many years. Miners of uranium and thorium are exposed to ionizing radiation coming from the radioactive rocks, and lung cancer is the main risk.

Modernization of the mines has solved many problems in developed countries. Machinery has taken on much of the strenuous work; proper ventilation and exhaust systems reduce the risks of abnormal temperatures and of pneumoconiosis; noise-protected machines and the use of proper precautions prevents occupational deafness. But as the developing countries struggle to extract their natural resources, their economic limitations often preclude the use of modern technology, so that all these mining problems still exist. All the efforts of national and international agencies are needed to improve the conditions of underground mines in those countries, thus protecting that most valuable assets of every miner: his health.[13]

Environmental Health Effects of Endosulfan Spray on Cashew Nut Plantations

A number of reports have appeared in scientific journals and mass media regarding health problems in villages surrounding cashew nut plantation in Kasargode district of north Kerala. Neurological disorders (epilepsy, cerebral palsy and mental retardation), congenital malformations, reproductive disorders and cancers of various organs reported from these areas have been linked with endosulfan, an organ chlorine pesticide sprayed on cashew plantations for more than 20 years to control the tea mosquitoes.[14]

Growing human population, urbanization and large-scale industrialization in the country have lead to environmental degradation, pollution and occupation-related hazards. Environmental pollution is responsible for health hazards such as asthma, cancer, hypertension, etc. Incidence of occupation-related morbidity and mortality too is very high in India. It is estimated that about 17% of the occupational diseases occurring in the world and 18% of the deaths due to occupational diseases take place in India. The Indian Council of Medical Research is engaged in investigating and monitoring the health effects of various industrial toxicants and environmental pollutants through its National Institute of Occupational Health (NIOH) at Ahmedabad and its regional centres at Kolkata and Bangalore.[15]

Analysis of Industrial Accident and Structurization of Database

Nearly 600 fatal and 7500 non-fatal accident cases were recorded from selected industries in Gujarat. Non-fatal accidents from textile industries were included in this study. Detailed analysis of data revealed that younger age group (20-29 years) is the high-risk group for fatal accidents and that head injuries account for nearly 40% of accidents. The severity pattern of non-fatal accidents has a bimodal distribution. Records from textile industries indicate two peaks—the early one at the level of 10% permanent partial disablement and the second one at about 35% disablement.

The remedial measures to minimize man-machine incompatibility and musculo-skeletal stresses and improvement in hazard recognition and safety programmes contributed to the prevention of accidents. Provision of headgear alone could save 207 young lives during the 3 years study period. The average number of days of absence from work were found to be nine per accident. While 92% of the injured could resume work after a considerable period of medical leave, 8% remained away from work due to disability. This remains a serious concern for vocational rehabilitation of injured victims.[16]

Occupational Health Hazards among Automobile Transport Workers

Road transport is one of the major transport systems in Kolkata. The automobile transport workers including drivers, conductors and mechanics are generally exposed to diesel exhaust in the form of diesel particulate matter (DPM), volatile organic compounds (VOCs), i.e. benzene, toluene, p-xylene, and gases like CO, Nox, SO_2 along with heat, humidity and noise. A study was undertaken by Regional Occupational Health Centre at Kolkata to assess the work environment and to identify the health hazards in transport workers.

The environmental monitoring revealed that the exposure to VOCs was higher among the drivers than the conductors. The peak sound pressure level recorded was 90.7 dBA in repair workshop, 117 dBA in tyre changing workshop and 107.4 dBA in the generator room. Some of the automobile workers suffered from hearing problem. Moreover, hypertension was observed in 21.0% conductors, 10.8% drivers and 11.4% mechanics.

The restrictive type (28.4%) of pulmonary function impairment was found significantly higher than the obstructive type (1.71%). The prevalence rates of restrictive impairment in different categories of subjects were: conductors -30.4%, drivers -28.9%, mechanics -27.9% and administration -21.7%. Pain and discomfort in various parts of the body (muculo-skeletal problems) was reported by 71.4% of drivers possibly due to mismatch in sitting posture and steering wheel-leg control interface.

(B) SOIL POLLUTION AND HEALTH HAZARDS

Dr. B.M. Radder, Department of Soil Science and Agriculture, Chemistry College of Agriculture, Dharwad conduded a research studies on persistence and degradation of carlofuran, tenetrothion and eabendogin in some soils of Karnataka.

Introduction

The use of pesticides has become indispensable for modern strategy of crop production. The use of pesticides in health and agricultural programmes in most developing countries including India is relatively very small as compared to the use of pesticides in advanced countries. In India, there are localized zones of heavy pesticides used such as in cotton, tea, coca and in irrigated rice culture, raising problem of environmental contamination. Pesticides residues may constitute a significant source of contamination of air, water, soil, and food and there are reports of undesirable environmental effects of pesticides. Regardless of the method of application, large amounts of pesticides ultimately find their way into the soil which finally acts as reservoir for most of the applied pesticides.

Objective

The project was initiated to study the persistence and degradation of carbofuran and fenitriothion and carbendazine in four selected soils of Karnataka. The behaviour of these pesticides in soils as effected by flooding, autoclaving and the addition of certain organic amendments such as rice straw, FYM (Farm Yard Manure), neem cake and also nitrogenous fertilizers like urea and ammonium sulphate was studied. The leaching loss, movement and distribution of carbofuran and fenitriothion were estimated. The persistence in soil and uptake of carbofuran by rice plant under different methods of application was investigated.

Result

The results indicated that the degradation of added pesticides occurred in all the four soils and the rate of degradation was high in saline soils. The degradation of carbofuran and fenitrothion was related to initial pH of the soil. Alkaline condition favoured the hydrolysis of carbofuran to carbofuran phenol. Fenitorthion was hydrolyzed to 3-methyl-4 nitrophenol. Soil flooding was reported to enhance the rate of degradation. Addition of organic amendments to flooded soil resulted in more rapid degradation of both the insecticides. Application of rice straw and FYM were more effective than neem cake for fenitrothion while neem cake and rice straw were more effective for carbofuran. Application of nitrogenous fertilizers such as urea, ammonium sulphate showed no significant effect on the degradation process. The leaching loss, movement and distribution of both the insecticides due to leaching was more in coarse-textured (red and laterite) soils than in fine-textured (black and saline soils). Bulk of the insecticides was retained in 0-7 cm. And the concentration decreased with the depth. Among the different methods of application of carbofuran to rice, the root zone application and soil incorporation were found superior to paddy water broadcast.[17]

Usefulness of the Findings and their Application

The study suggested that root zone application of insecticide is a better practice for increasing efficiency of the applied chemical. Flooding and addition or organic matter to soil are helpful in removal of toxic pesticides from the soil environment.

The information generated will be useful to the State Pollution Control Board. The same is happening in Punjab and Rajasthan in cotton belt.[18]

Dr. B.D. Tripathi, Coordinator, Environmental Science, Department of Botany, Banaras Hindu University, Varanasi, Uttar Pradesh in a Research on Long Terms of Treaded and Un-Treaded sewerage irrigation on the soil charodiastes of wheat and paddy crops.

Objectives

1. Quantification of some important heavy metals, i.e. lead, cadmium and chromium in treated and untreated sewage of the Varanasi city.
2. Assessment of micro and macro-nutrient status of soil under long-term repeated sewage irritation.
3. Eco-behaviour and mineral composition of wheat and paddy crop plants grown in long-term repeated sewage irrigated soil.
4. Distribution and accumulation behaviour of some important persistent chemicals from sewage to plant parts through soil.

Results

Study was conducted to evaluate the impact of repeated sewage irrigation on soil properties and productive behaviour of wheat and paddy crops. During the investigation period the tubewell water, treated and untreated sewage were analyzed for various physiochemical properties. Paddy and wheat plants were analyzed every year for various eco-behavioural properties and experimental soils were analyzed before the start of investigation and after three years of continuous cropping of paddy and wheat crop. Statistical analysis was also done to check the significance and validity of observed data. On the basis of present observation following important conclusions may be drawn:

(i) More than 320 acres of agricultural land is being irrigated with treated and untreated sewage water at Varanasi.

(ii) High organic carbon content, BOD, COD, sulphate, chloride, micro and macro-nutrients were recorded in untreated sewage, while, nitrate was found highest in treated sewage.

(iii) An increasing trend of pollution load in the city sewage was observed during the investigation period. However, slight variation in the toxic metals like lead, cadmium and chromium was noted in every year.

(iv) After repeated sewage irrigation of paddy crop 2.4-3% increase in grain yield was observed without application of chemical fertilizers. However, this increase was about 2.6-3.2% in case of wheat crops.

(v) Increase in straw yield after three years of repeated irrigation with sewage water were recorded 4.2 and 5.5% in paddy and wheat crops respectively.

(vi) Accumulation of toxic metals like Pb, Cd and Cr were noted highest in roots of untreated sewage irrigated plants followed by plants irrigated with treated sewage. Concentration of metals in grains was well below the prescribed limits.

(vii) The NPK content of soil were increased by 2.11-2.94%, 2.31-3.37% and 2.42-3.52% respectively in sewage irrigated samples.

(viii) After repeated sewage irrigation, total lead content of soil was found increased on 0-9.37 ug/g in treated sewage irrigated soil and 0-9.57 ug/g in untreated sewage irrigated soil.

(ix) After repeated sewage incorporation total cadmium content of soil had increased from 0-8.12 ug/g in treated sewage irrigated soil and 0-9.06 ug/g in untreated sewage irrigated soil.

(x) After repeated sewage incorporation total chromium content of soil also increased from 0-6.54 ug/g in treated sewage irrigated soil and 0-6.83 ug/g in untreated sewage irrigated soil.

Usefulness of the Findings and its Application

The results of the study are useful to all Government and Non-Governmental organisations and research institutions related to pollution monitoring, impact assessment, sewage management and urban planners.[19]

(C) SOLID WASTE MANAGEMENT

Thermal Flyash from Thermal Power Plants: A Health Hazard

Urban Solid Waste Management

The level of urban wastes being generated in different cities poses a serious threat to the environmental quality and human health. Approximately 36.5 million tons of solid waste is generated annually. Many cities generate more solid wastes than they can collect or dispose-off effectively. Even when there are adequate resources available by way of public provisions to the municipal authorities, the safe disposal of urban solid wastes often remains a major problem. The problem is made worse by unscientific waste disposal systems used. Dumping and uncontrolled land filling are the two options that municipal authorities resort to. These methods of waste disposal are the primary cause for the breeding of bacteria and viruses that cause diseases. Due to inadequate collection, improper disposal and lack of proper storage facilities, solid wastes get into open drains and obstruct the free flow of water, which in turn becomes on ideal breeding ground for diseases.

The Municipal Solid Waste sites often receive industrial and hazardous waste including those from hospitals and laboratories adding to serious consequences for the environment and the health of individuals. The system of disposing non-biodegradable urban solid waste is a very nascent stage in the country.

As is evident then, there is tremendous scope in the country for improving the technological inputs for urban waste management and institutionalization of responsible social practices that will facilitate an efficient and environmentally safe method of waste disposal.

A major problem in urban solid waste management relates to sewage disposal. With inadequate and often inappropriate and malfunctioning systems of sewage disposal, the mounting threat of the availability of safe drinking water is quite serious in most urban areas of the country. There is an urgent need for revamping and maintaining sewage systems in most cities and more importantly, increasing its coverage to slums and the shanties that are entrenched around most metro cities of the country.

Combating Poverty

The importance if sustainability of livelihoods of the poor is a pre-condition for sustainable development. People's enterprise, micro-credit, their participation in resource management and focused intervention in poor areas and investment in poor people have shown positive results in the nineties. The target for the end of Tenth Five Year Plan is to bring down the poverty ratio by 5% points by 2007 and by 15% points by 2012. Since income is only one of the dimension of poverty, a concerted effort to invest in social sectors for improvement in the living conditions of the poor is a critical element of this strategy.

Putting People First

Devolution of power to people through constitution of amendments, in the nineties, is already showing remarkable results in a number of areas. By transferring management powers of 29 sectors of economy to village councils and allowing them to raise resources through taxation, the first major step in empowering people including women to manage their resources has already been taken. The steps contemplated for the future are, sharing of state and central revenue with village councils and their direct involvement in management of social sector activities and village infrastructure. Moving beyond the elected representatives of village councils, a number of initiatives for management of natural resources seek direct involvement of the whole village, for example, Joint Forest Management, Watershed Development Committees and Participatory Irrigation Management to mention a few. Clearly the emerging strategy is to empower people to manage their resources to establish sustainable livelihoods.

Harnessing Scientific and Technological Process

India has the third largest pool of scientific manpower in the world. Efforts since Independence have also ensured a well-established scientific and technological institutional base. Institutions of higher learning continuously replenish the stock of trained personnel of highest caliber. Strategically, this process is being used to solve not only the complex issue to clean technologies for power, coal and oil sector but also for clean drinking water, eradication of disease and improved food availability by using biotechnology. A mutually beneficial relationship between large public financed laboratories and the private sector and usage of information technology to bridge the rural-urban and poor-rich gaps in access to knowledge are other key elements of this strategy.

Setting Standards, Institutions and Legislations

In the last ten years, a substantial progress has been made in setting environmental standards for various sectors. The range of standards cover effluent discharge standards for industries, fuel standard for vehicles, rules for disposal of solid waste and bio-medical waste, etc. Regulatory and implementing institutional infrastructure is rapidly being set-up which includes an important role for the private sector. The environmental standards that have been set for the ambient air, water quality and waste disposal. It also gives a brief account of the progress made and the remaining challenges. The developments in the natural resources sector and economic sectors respectively in terms of objective setting, progress and challenges.

Target

The commitment of the government to the above mentioned strategy is clearly reflected in the targets that have been set-up for the Tenth Five ear Plan (2002-07) in the social and natural resources sectors. Thus, apart from aiming to achieve an 8% growth rate in GDP during the Tenth Five Year Plan, the nation has set specific and monitorable targets for a few key indicators of human development and conservation of natural resources.

Target for Sustainable Development

- o Reduction of poverty ratio by 5 percentage points by 2007 and by 15 percentage points by 2012.
- o All children in school by 2003; all children to complete 5 years in school by 2007.
- o Reduction in gender gaps in literacy and wage rates by at least 50% by 2007.
- o Reduction in population growth between 2001 and 2011 to 16.2%.
- o Increase in literacy rate of 75% by 2007.
- o Reduction of Infant Mortality Rate (IMR) to 45 per 1000 live births by 2007 and to 28 to 1 by 2012.
- o Increase in forest cover to 25% by 2007 and 33% by 2012.
- o All villages to have sustained access to potable drinking water by 2007.
- o Cleaning of major polluted rivers by 2007 and other notified stretches by 2012.[20]

Waste Disposal

Municipal Services and industrial waste disposal facilities have not been able to keep pace with the growing population and rapid Industrialization. As a result, India faces serious challenge of disposal of municipal solid waste, hazardous waste, bio-medical waste and radioactive waste in environmentally sound manner. In the last ten years a framework of laws, rules, research and institution is emerging that attempts to meet this challenge. Environment (Protection) Act has been used to issue notification to tighten the rules of management of waste, fix institutional responsibility, enhance resources for waste disposal and specify standards for land fill sites and treating of pollutants. The following notifications issued by MoFF under the Environment (Protection) Act lay down the guidelines for management of various types of wastes:

Municipal Wastes (Management and Handling) Rules, 2000, aims to enable municipalities to dispose municipal solid waste in a scientific manner.

Biomedical Waste (Management and Handling) Rules, 1998, lay down guidelines for proper disposal, segregation, transport, etc. of infectious wastes.

Hazardous Wastes (Management and Handling) Rules, 1989, brought out a guide for manufacture, storage and import of hazardous chemicals and for management of hazardous wastes.

Hazardous Wastes (Management and Handling) Amendment Rules, 2000, a recent notification issued with the view to providing guidelines for the import and export of hazardous waste in the country.

In addition, the Atomic Energy Act of 1982 deals with radioactive waste.[21]

Water

India is considered rich in terms of annual rainfall and total water resources available. However, there are problems of uneven distribution of water resources and inequitable access, further compounded by deterioration in water quality. Improvement of water quality and conservation of water resources is therefore one of utmost concern.

Standards

Specific standards have been set for drinking water, discharge of industrial effluents, coastal water, and marine outfalls and effluent discharge from selected specific industries. While the drinking water standards developed by Indian Council of Medical Research bear a close resemblance to WHO standards, discharge of industrial effluents is governed by Indian Standard Codes, which take into account the specificity of Indian conditions. There are specific standards for effluent discharge from industries such as, iron and steel, aluminium, pulp and paper, oil refineries, petrochemicals and thermal power plants.

Institutions

The Central Pollution Central Board (CPCB) monitors water quality of national aquatic resources in collaboration with State Pollution Control Boards (SPCBs). It has a network of 507 monitoring stations, covering rivers, groundwater, lakes, annals, creeks, drains, ponds, etc. The Central Water Commission also has a network to measure flow and monitor water quality at about 369 field stations. In addition, the Central Groundwater Board (CGWB) monitors groundwater quality at 15355 stations. In an effort to assess the health of a water body, the CPCB has also initiated a bio-monitoring project under the Indo-Dutch collaboration Programme on Environment and selected 215 locations for the purpose.

Monitoring Results

The water quality monitoring results obtained during 2000 a recent notification issued with the view to providing guidelines for the import and export of hazardous waste in the country.

In addition, the Atomic Energy Act of 1982 deals with radioactive waste.[21]

The water quality monitoring results obtained during 2000 indicate that organic and bacterial contaminations continue to be critical pollutants in Indian aquatic resources. This is mainly due to the discharge, from urban centres, of domestic wastewater in untreated form. This situation leads to spread of water borne diseases and has a particularly adverse effect on the poor as they are not in a position to make private investment in water filtration/treatment for domestic use.[22]

The water quality monitoring results were analyzed with respect to indicator of oxygen consuming substances (bio-chemical oxygen demand) and populations at risk. Other factors include access to safe drinking water and sanitation in rural and urban areas, air quality (especially in urban areas), indoor air pollution (especially in poor rural and urban households), solid waste management and agro-industrial pollution. The health effects measured in terms of Disease Adjusted Life Years (DALY) lost.[23]

Air Pollution

Air pollution poses a major health hazard. It has been a subject of major debate in media, environmental circles and judiciary.

Standards

National Ambient Air Quality Standards (NAAQS) for major pollutants notified by the CPCB in 1994 are deemed to be levels of air quality necessary with an adequate margin of safety, to protect public health, vegetation and property. The NAAQS prescribed specific standards for industrial, residential, rural and other sensitive areas. Industry specific emission standards have also been developed for iron and steel plants, cement plants, fertilizer plants, oil refineries and the aluminium industry. The NAAQS are similar to those prevailing in many developed and developing countries.[24]

The National Human Development Report, 2001 (Planning Commission) mentions that the ambient air quality recorded for 23 major cities in the country revealed that the Suspended Particulate Matter (SPM) levels are critical in many cities in the country. What is most startling is the fact that in smaller and medium towns of the country, the SPM levels are far higher than the larger metropolitan cities. Also, in addition to the common air pollutants like sulphur dioxide and the oxides of nitrogen, several toxic and carcinogenic chemicals are being detected in urban air.

In the rural areas, the burning of unprocessed cooking fuels in homes is a major source of pollution. Rural households rely mostly on bio fuels like cow dung, fuel wood, and crop residues and in some cases low grade coal for meeting their fuel and energy requirement. The indoor pollution on account of pollutants released in closed and unventilated places is perhaps more harmful than outdoor air pollution. It is estimated that indoor air pollution in India's rural areas is primarily responsible for 50,00,000 deaths annually, mostly of women and children under 5. This accounts for 6 to 9% of the Disease Adjusted Life Years. These estimates make the health impact of indoor exposure larger than the burden from all but two of the other major preventable risk factors-malnutrition (15%) and lack of clean water and sanitation (7%).

An integrated approach focused on civic amenities, appropriate technology and efficiency of public systems has become an imperative for public policy and administration in most of the urban and rural areas of the country. An additional requirement, especially in the rural and semi-urban areas, is in the urgent need to make it possible for the people to quickly move up the energy ladder with a view to address the health impact of indoor pollution on account of the use of unprocessed cooling uels.[25]

The Municipal Solid Wastes (Management and Handling) Rules, 2000, the Flyash Notification, 1999 and the Recycled Plastics Manufacture and Usage Rules, 1999 constitute the regulatory framework for the management of solid wastes in the country.

To further streamline and improve the utilization of flyash generated by the thermal power stations, the Notification of 16th September, 1999 has been amended and notified on 27th August, 2003 vide S.O. 997 (E). The salient features of the amendment are:

- o The geographical coverage of the Notification has been extended from 50 to 100 kms from Thermal Power Stations.
- o Responsibility has been placed on construction agencies to use flyash-based bricks/products in a time bound manner.
- o Time limits have been specified for State Pollution Control Boards to take decision on the applications for manufacture or flyash-based bricks/products.
- o Flyash has been included in the guidelines/specifications of road/building construction projects.
- o Provision has been made for filling up low-lying areas with pond ash.
- o In the year 2002-03, out of about 103 million tonnes of ash generated, 26 million tonnes were utilized. In 2003-04, the ash generation was about 108 million tonnes and utilization was about 31 million tonnes. The major users were cement manufacturers, land fills road embankments, back filling of mines and britals.

A Notification amending the Recycled Plastics (Manufacture and Usage) Rules, 1999 was issued on 17th June, 2003 vide S.O. 698(E). The salient features of the amendment are as follows:

- o Manufacture, sales, distribution and use of virgin and recycled plastic carry bags, which are less than 8x20 inches in size, is banned.
- o Registration of manufacturers of plastic carry bags with State Pollution Control Boards has been made mandatory.
- o Exemption provided to exporters of plastic carry bags.

The status of implementation of the Municipal Solid Waste (Management and Handling) Rules, 2000 was reviewed during the year. All the State Pollution Control Board/Committees have been requested to take up the matter with the relevant local authorities/civic bodies for preparation of time bound action plans for management of Municipal Solid Waste in accordance with the rules. During the year, financial assistance has been provided to Kozhikode city in Kerala for developing and implementing a model system on solid waste management.[26]

(D) ORGANISATION AND ROLE IN PREVENTING ENVIRONMENTAL DISASTERS, MINISTRY OF ENVIRONMENT AND FORESTS

The Ministry of Environment and Forests is primarily concerned with the implementation of policies and programmes relating to conservation of the country's natural resources including lakes and rivers, its biodiversity, forests and wildlife, ensuring the welfare of animals and prevention and abatement of pollution. While implementing these policies and programmes, the Ministry is guided by the principle of sustainable development and enhancement of human well-being. The Ministry also serves as the nodal agency in the country for the United Nations Environment Programme (UNEP), South Asia Co-operative Environment Programme (SACEP), International Centre for Integrated Mountain Development (ICIMOD) and for the follow-up of the United Nations Conference on Environment and Development (UNCED). The Ministry is also entrusted with the issues relating to multilateral bodies such as the Commission on Sustainable Development (CSD), Global Environment Facility (GEF) and of regional bodies like Economic and Social Council for Asia and Pacific (ESCAP) and South Asian Association for Regional Co-operation (SAARC) on matters pertaining to environment.

The broad objectives of the Ministry are:

- o Conservation and survey of Flora, Fauna, Forests and Wildlife.
- o Prevention and Control of Pollution.
- o Afforestation and regeneration of degraded areas.
- o Protection of the Environment.
- o Ensuring the welfare of animals.

These objectives are sought to be fulfiled by the Ministry primarily through:

- o Environmental impact assessment.
- o Eco-regeneration.
- o Assistance to organisations implementing environmental and forestry programmes.
- o Assistance to organisations including animal welfare programmes.
- o Promotion of environmental and forestry research, extension, education and training.

- o Dissemination of environmental information.
- o International cooperation.
- o Creation of environmental awareness among all sectors of the country's population.

These objectives are well supported by a set of legislative and regulatory measures, aimed at the preservation, conservation and protection of the environment. Some of them are the Water (Prevention and Control of Pollution) Act, 1974, the Air (Prevention and Control of Pollution) Act, 1981, the Environment (Protection) Act, 1986, the Public Liability Insurance Act, 1991, the National Environment Tribunal Act, 1995, the National Environmental Appellate Authority Act, 1997, the Wildlife Protection Act, 1972 and Forests (Conservation) Act, 1980. The main legislations relating to protection of animals is the Prevention of Cruelty to Animals Act, 1960. Besides the legislative measures, a National Conservation Strategy and Policy Statement on Environment and Development, 1992, National Forest Policy, 1988 and a Policy Statement on Abatement of Pollution, 1992 have also been evolved.

The organisational structure of the Ministry indicating various divisions, subordinate officers and autonomous institutions is given in Annexure 12.1.

Notes and References

1. WHO: Valery Abramov, One man's meat, another man's becquerel, *World Health*, June 1988, p. 10.
2. WHO: Mostafa El Batawi, Work-related diseases, *World Health*, June 1978, p. 10.
3. Cobb, S. and Rose, R.M. (1973), *Journal of the American Medical Association*, 224(4), 489-92.
4. Kloetzel, K. and others (1973), *Journal of Occupational Medicine*, 15(11), 873-83.
5. Milosevic, V.M. and Savicevic, M. (1971), Industrial Hygiene and Faculty of Medicine, Belgrade, 10(2), 373-80.
6. Bhattacharjee, S.C. and others (1971), *Indian Journal of Public Health*, 15:2.
7. Russek, H.I. (1967), Diseases of the Chest, No. 1, Vol. 52.
8. WHO: Mostafa El Batawi, Work-related Diseases, *World Health*, June 1978, pp. 10-13.
9. WHO: S.E. Asogwa, Hazards on the land, *World Health*, November 1981, pp. 14-15.
10. WHO: Diogo Pupo Nogueira, Danger Underground, *World Health*, November 1981, p. 10.
11. WHO: Diogo Pupo Nogueira, Danger Underground, *World Health*, November 1981, p. 11.
12. WHO: Diogo Pupo Nogueira, Danger Underground, *World Health*, November 1981, p. 13.
13. WHO: Diogo Pupo Nogueira, Danger Underground, *World Health*, November 1981, p. 13.
14. Annual Report, 2001-02, Indian Council of Medical Research, New Delhi, "Environmental and Occupational Health", pp. 100-01.

15. Annual Report, 2001-02, Indian Council of Medical Research, New Delhi, "Environmental and Occupational Health", p. 100.
16. Annual Report, 2001-02, Indian Council of Medical Research, New Delhi, "Environmental and Occupational Health", pp. 106-07.
17. Annual Report, 2001-02, Indian Council of Medical Research, New Delhi, "Environmental and Occupational Health", p. 108.
18. Environmental Research in India, M/o Environment and Forests, GOI, March 2003, pp. 77-78.
19. Environmental Research in India, M/o Environment and Forests, GOI, March 2003, pp. 81-82.
20. Empowering People for Sustainable Development, M/o Environment and Forests, 2002, pp. 7-8.
21. Empowering People for Sustainable Development, M/o Environment and Forests, 2002, p. 29.
22. Empowering People for Sustainable Development, M/o Environment and Forests, 2002, pp. 27-28.
23. Empowering People for Sustainable Development, M/o Environment and Forests, 2002, pp. 50-51.
24. Empowering People for Sustainable Development, M/o Environment and Forests, 2002, p. 28.
25. Empowering People for Sustainable Development, M/o Environment and Forests, 2002, pp. 6-7.
26. Annual Report, 2003-04, M/o Environment and Forests, GOI, pp. 125-26.

ANNEXURE 12.1

Allocation of Business

- Environment and Ecology, including environment in coastal waters, in mangroves and coral reefs but excluding marine environment on the high seas.
- Environment research and development, education, training, information and awareness.
- Environmental Health.
- Environmental Impact Assessment.
- Forest Development Agency and Joint Forest Management Programme for conservation, management and afforestation.
- Survey and Exploration and Natural Resources particularly of Forest, Flora, Fauna, Ecosystems, etc.
- Bio-diversity Conservation including that of lakes and wetlands.
- Conservation, development management and abatement of pollution of rivers which shall include National River Conservation Directorate.
- Wildlife conservation, preservation, protection planning, research, education, training awareness including Project Tiger and Project Elephant.
- International co-operation on issues concerning Environment, Forestry and Wildlife.
- Botanical Survey of India and Botanical Gardens.
- Zoological Survey of India.
- National Museum of Natural History.
- Biosphere Reserve Programme.
- National Forest Policy and Forestry Development in the country, including Social Forestry.
- All matters relating to Forest and Forest Administration in the Andaman and Nicobar Islands.
- Indian Forest Service.
- Wild Life Preservation and Protection of wild birds and animals.
- Fundamental and applied research and training including higher education in forestry.
- Padmaja Naidu Himalayan Zoological Park.
- National Assistance to Forestry Development Schemes.
- Indian Plywood Industries Research and Training Institute, Bangalore.
- Afforestation and Eco-development which shall include National Afforestation and Eco-Development Board.
- Desert and Desertification.
- Forest Survey of India.
- Indian Institute of Bio-diversity, Itanagar.
- Central Pollution Control Board.

- o G.B. Pant Institute of Himalayan Environment and Development.
- o Wildlife Institute of India and Indian Board for Wildlife.
- o Indian Institute of Forest Management.
- o Central Zoo Authority including National Zoo Park.
- o Indian Council of Forestry Research and Education.
- o Andaman and Nicobar Islands Forest and Plantation Development Corporation Limited.
- o Prevention of cruelty to animals.
- o Matters relating to pounds and cattle trespass.
- o Gaushalas and Gausadans.
- o The Prevention of Cruelty to Animals Act, 1960 (59 of 1960).
- o The National Environment Tribunal Act, 1995 (27 of 1995).
- o The National Environment Appellate Authority Act, 1997 (22 of 1997).
- o The Water Prevention and Control of Pollution Act, 1974 (6 of 1974).
- o The Water (Prevention and Control of Pollution) Cess Act, 1977 (36 of 1977).
- o The Air (Prevention and Control of Pollution) Act, 1981 (14 of 1981).
- o The Indian Forest Act, 1927 (16 of 1927).
- o The Wildlife (Protection) Act, 1972 (53 of 1972).
- o The Forest (Conservation) Act, 1980 (69 of 1980).
- o The Environment (Protection) Act, 1986 (29 of 1986).
- o The Public Liability Insurance Act, 1991 (6 of 1991).

1. Activities of Natural Resources:
   (a) Flora
   (b) Fauna
   (c) Forests
2. Conservation on Natural Resources including Forestry and Wildlife:
   (a) Biosphere Reserves
   (b) Wetlands, Mangroves and Coral Reefs
   (c) Bio-Diversity Conservation
   (d) All India Coordinated Project on Taxonomy (AICOPTAX)
   (e) Assistance to Botanic Gardens
   (f) Forest Conservation
   (g) Wildlife Conservation
   (h) Animal Welfare
   (i) Environmental Impact Assessment
3. Prevention and Control of Pollution
4. Hazardous Substances Management
5. Regeneration and Development
6. National Afforestation and Eco-development Board
7. Research:

(a) Forestry Research
(b) Wildlife Research

Organisational Chart of the Ministry of Environment and Forests

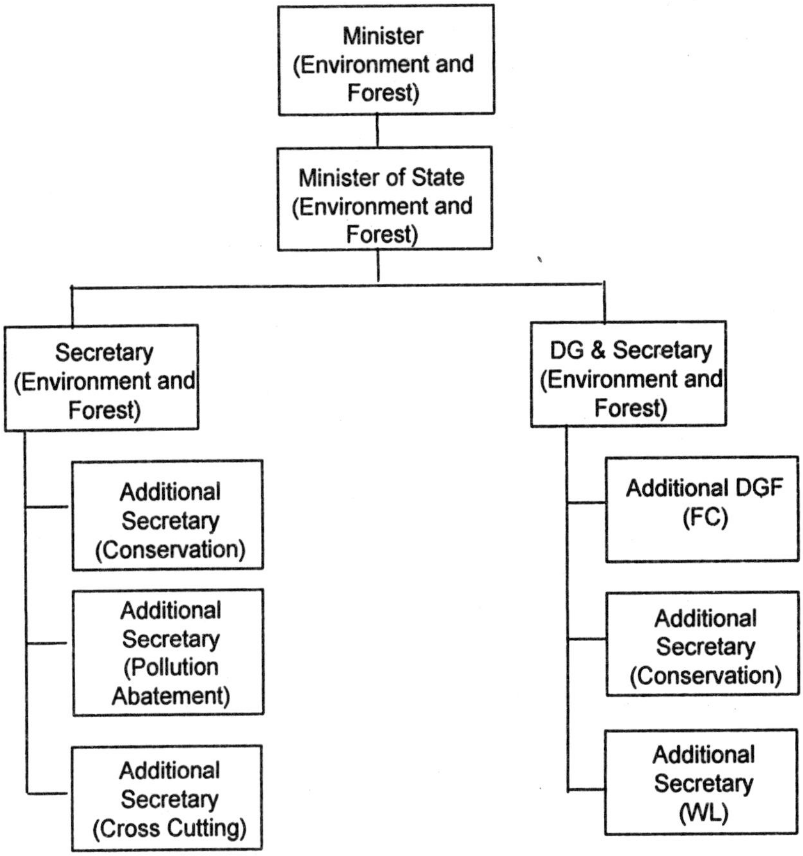

8. National Natural Resource Management System (NNRMS)
9. Education, Training and Information Forestry Education, Training and Extension
10. Wildlife Education and Training
11. National Museum of Natural History (NMNH)
12. Fellowship and Awards
13. Environmental Education, Awareness and Training
14. Strengthening Environment Education in Indian Management Schools
15. Non-formal Environment Education and Awareness
16. Centres of Excellence
17. Environmental Information
18. Legislation and Institutional Support
19. Women and Environment

20. International Cooperation
21. Climate Change
22. Ozone
23. Administration, Civil Construction, Plan Coordination and Budget
24. Civil Construction Unit
25. Plan Coordination and Budget.

13

CHAPTER

Women's Health and Development

DEMOGRAPHY AND STATISTICS

Women Population

There has been a slight increase in the total female population of the country, from 407.1 million (48.1 percent of total population) in 1991 to 495.7 million (48.3 per cent) in 2001. While the percentage increase of 0.2 is very marginal, increase in term of absolute numbers was 88.6 million as against 77.1 million between 1981 and 1991. The grown rate of female population for the 1991-2001 decade was 21.79 percent, which was 0.86 percentage points higher than that of the total population. Yet, the demographic imbalances between women and men continue to exist till date. (Refer Table 13.1)

TABLE 13.1

Sex Ratio (1981-2001)

Census	*Sex Ratio*
1981	934
1991	927
2001	933

Note: Sex Ratio Females percent and males

Source: Census 01 India, 2001, Provisional Population Totals, Registrar General and Census Commissioner, GOI, New Delhi

If demographic balances were affected by economic factors, then poor states of Orissa, Bihar or Madhya Pradesh would have recorded the worst sex ratios. On the contrary, it is the prosperous states of Haryana, Punjab and Delhi that are among the worst. Better sex ratios are noted among the southern states, some hill regions and states with large tribal populations. Kerala (1071), Pondicherry (1007) are the only States/UTs where sex ratio is tilted in favour of the females.

Comparison over the decade 1991 to 2001 based on rank analysis shows that ranks of Maharashtra, Madhya Pradesh, Punjab, Goa, Gujarat and Himachal Pradesh have dropped by 2 or more places, while it has improved in the States of West Bengal, Manipur, Arunachal Pradesh, Mizoram, Meghalaya and Nagaland. (Refer Table 13.1) This clearly points to the fact that economic growth may not necessarily bring about an improvement in the status of women. This, in turn, can be attributed to the discrimination the girl child faces and the consequential problems of poor health and nutritional status. Added to these at the problems of female foeticide and female infanticide, the incidence of which is on an increase.

Expectation of Life

The life expectancy at birth among females has been steadily improving over the years from 23.3 in 1901 to 65.3 in 2001 and has surpassed that of men since the eighties. Male life expectancy in 2001 is 62.3 years. The urban female life expectancy is higher at 68. The rural-urban difference is the highest in Madhya Pradesh (8.6) and the lowest in Kerala (1.0). (Refer Table 13.2)

The life expectancy indicator highlights that number of older women will be on the rise. Many of them will be widows and living alone given the increasing tendency of nuclearisation of families. The absence of social security measures for them on the one hand and the declining Support structures from family and society on the other, indicate the plight of these already low status aged women.

TABLE 13.2

Sex Ratio in 6+ Age-group Ranks in 1991 and 2001 and Decadal Differences (1991-2001) among States

Rank	*States/UTs*	*Adult 2001*	*Sex Ratio 2001*	*Rank 1991*	*Differences 2001-1991*
1.	Sikkim	858	860	2	2
2.	Haryana	869	862	3	7
3.	Punjab	886	883	6	3
4.	Arunachal Pradesh	888	829	1	59
5.	Uttar Pradesh	895	867	5	28
6.	Nagaland	899	865	4	34
7.	Bihar	916	899	7	17
8.	Madhya Pradesh	917	926	12	-9
9.	Maharashtra	923	931	12	-8
10.	Rajasthan	925	908	9	17
11.	Assam	926	910	10	16

12. .Gujarat	927	936	14	-9
13. West Bengal	929	907	8	22
14. Mizoram	932	911	11	21
India	934	923	—	11
15. Tripura	947	940	15	7
16. Goa	964	967	19	.3
17. Karnataka	966	960	18	6
18. Meghalaya	974	947	16	27
19. Orissa	976	972	20	4
20. Andhra Pradesh	980	972	21	8
21. Himachal Pradesh	981	980	23	1
22. Manipur	981	955	17	26
23. Tamil Nadu	992	978	22	12
24. Kerala	1071	1049	24	22

Source: Annual Report of Women and Child Development Department, Ministry of HRD (Government of India)

Female Infant Mortality Rate

In many States, the number of infant deaths among girls exceed that of boys due to discriminatory child care practices. The worst case is that of Haryana, where the gender difference in IMR is 19. This is followed by Punjab, Rajasthan and Tamil Nadu. Contrarily in Orissa, where infant mortality rates are the highest (96), girls have marginally higher chance of survival than boys.

TABLE 13.3

Life Expectancy at Birth (1981-2001)

Year	*Females*	*Males*
1981-85	55.7	55.4
1989-93	59.7	59.0
1996-2001	65.3	62.3

Source: Ibid. Estimates.

Maternal Mortality Rate

In India the Maternal Mortality Rate (MMR), which is calculated as the number of maternal deaths per 100,000 live births, is among the highest in the world and therefore a matter of great concern. It has come down from 468 in 1980 to 407 in 1998. (Refer Table 13.4)

There is wide range of variation in MMR across regions and Statesœfrom 28 in Gujarat to 707 in Uttar Pradesh.

Mean Age at Marriage

The effective mean age at marriage for females has also increased from 18.3 years in 1981 to 19.5 years in 1997. The Child Marriage Restraint

TABLE 13.4

Maternal Mortality Rate (1990-98)

(Per lakh live births)

Year	*Maternal Mortality Rate*
1980	468
1993	437
1998	407

Source: Ibid.

Act, 1976 which raised the age of marriage for girls from 15 to 18 years has no doubt, helped reduce child/early marriages and the consequent early pregnancies and birth of premature babies at the same time, education and employment of women/girls has also played a very important role in raising the age of marriage. (Refer Table 13.5)

TABLE 13.5

Mean Age at Marriage (1981-97)

(in years)

Year	*Females*	*Males*
1981	18.3	23.3
1991	19.5	23.9
1997	19.5	N.A.

Source: Sample Registration System Bulletins for respective years, Registrar General and Census Commissioner, GOI, New Delhi.

Women's Health and Family Welfare

Lack of adequate resources prevents women belonging to poorer households from availing health services for themselves. Undernourished, ill-fed and over-worked, most women from such households are extremely vulnerable to ailments and diseases, which do not get properly diagnosed and treated. Poor sanitation, unhygienic surroundings, difficulty in procuring safe drinking water are some of the factors that affect the general health of women. Every second woman in India suffers from some degree of anaemia 2 percent of them are severely anaemic, while 35 and 15 percent have mild and moderate anaemia levels respectively. Here again, the inter-State differences are very pronounced.

While the Birth Rate has declined by 7.8 points from 33.9 in 1981 to 26.1 in 1990, the Death Rate has also declined by 3.8 points from 12.5 in 1981 to 8.7 in 1999. (Refer Tables 13.6 and 13.7) However while the female

Death Rate has come down by 4.4 points from 12.7 in 1981 to 8.3 in 1999, the male death rate has come down by 3.4 points, i.e. from 12.4 in 1981 to 9.0 in 1999.

Female Literacy

Literacy or the ability to read and write is the first step towards formal education. Female literacy has been steadily improving over the years. The proportion of women who are literate has increased by percent over the last decade from 39.29 percent in 1991 to 54.16 percent in 2001. Yet, even today, 193 million women are illiterate in India. Gender gap in literacy continues to be very high at 22 percentage points. The gaps are even more glaring among disadvantaged groups such as scheduled castes and tribes. Among scheduled castes (STs), 41 percent males are literate while only 24 percent females can read and rewrite. Similarly, among scheduled tribes (STs), 41 percent and 18 percent, males and females respectively are literate.

TABLE 13.6

Birth Rate (1981-99)

(per thousand)

Year	*Birth Rate*
1981	33.9
1991	29.5
1999	26.1

Source: Ibid.

TABLE 13.7

Death Rate (1981-99)

(per thousand)

Year	*Females*	*Males*	*Total*
1981	12.7	12.4	12.5
1991	9.7	10.0	9.8
1999	8.3	9.0	8.7

Source: Ibid.

Urban-rural differences are significant, with urban females almost matching up to rural male literates, especially among SC/STs. The female literacy rate for rural areas is only 47, while it is 73 in urban locations. Bihar and Jharkhand, the two poor literacy states in rural areas (30) perform relatively better in urban areas. They are at third and eighth ranks respectively.

The gross enrolment ratio for girls both at primary and middle levels have also increased from 64.1 in 1980-81 to 85.2 in 1999-2000 in respect of primary level and from 28.6 to 49.7 in respect of middle level during the same period. Between 1990-91 and 1999-2000, the GER of girls at the middle level has also increased from 47.8 to 49.7.

TABLE 13.8

(In Percent)

Census	*Females*	*Males*	*Persons*	*Male-Female gap in Literary rate*
1981	29.76	6.38	43.57	26.62
1991	39.29	64.13	52.21	24.84
2001	54.16	75.85	65.38	21.69

Note: The literacy rates relate to the population aged seven years and above. The 1991 census rates exclude Jammu and Kashmir.

Source: Census of India, 2001, Provisional Population Totals, Registrar General and Census Commissioner, GOI, New Delhi.

TABLE 13.9

Enrolment of Girls in Graduate/Post-Graduate/Professional Courses (1990-91 to 1999-2000)

(Figures in Million)

Levels	*1991-91*		*1996-97*		*1999-2000*	
	Women	*Total*	*Women*	*Total*	*Women*	*Total*
Graduate (B.A./B.Sc./B.Com.)	1.14 (34.7)	3.29	1.82 (37.4)	4.87 (40.9)	2.66	6.51
Post-Graduate (M.A./M.Sc./ M.Com.)	0.12 (32.8)	0.35	0.17 (30.5)	0.54	0.22 (39.6)	0.55
Ph.D./D.Sc./D.Phil.	0.01 (26.2)	0.03	0.01 (29.2)	004 (35.4)	0.02	0.05
B.E./B.Sc. (Eng./ B. Architecture	0.03 (10.9)	0.24	0.05 (14.9)	0.33	0.08 (22.0)	0.36
M.B.B.S.	0.03 (34.3)	0.08	0.04 (35.4)	0.12	0.05 (37.8)	0.14
Total	1.32 (33.0)	3.99	2.09 (35.3)	5.90	3.03 (39.8)	7.61

Source: Selected Educational Statistics for respective years, Department of Education, Ministry of Human Resource Development, GOI, New Delhi.

The number of women in higher education which includes colleges, universities, professional colleges of engineering, medicine, technology, etc. has also increased from 1.32 million (33.0 percent) in 1990-91 to 3 million (39.8 percent) in 1999-2000 (Table 13.9). The number of women enrolled has shown an increase in both absolute and relative terms

TABLE 13.10

Work Participation Rates by Sex (1981-2001)

(In per cent)

Census	*T/R/U*	*Females*	*Males*	*Persons*
1981	Total	19.7	52.6	36.7
	Rural	23.1	53.8	388
	Urban	8.3	49.1	30.0
1991	Total	22.3	51.6	37.5
	Rural	26.8	52.6	401
	Urban	9.2	4.89	30.2
2001	Total	25.7	51.9	39.3
	Rural	31.0	52.4	42.0
	Urban	11.6	50.9	32.2

Source: Census of India, 1991, Series 1 and Census of India 2001; Provisional Population Totals, Registrar General and Census Commissioner, GOI, New Delhi

Work and Employment

While the female work participation rate increased from 19.7 per cent in 1981 to 25.7 per cent in 2001, still it is much lower that the male work participation rate in both urban and rural areas (Table 13.11). There are wide regional variations amongst the major states, ranging from as high as

TABLE 13.11

Women in the Organised Sector (1998-99)

(Figures in Million)

Year	*Women*	*Men*	*Total*
1981	2.8 (12.2)	20.1	22.9
1991	3.8 (14.1)	23.0	26.7
2001	4.8 (17.2)	23.3	28.1

Source: Director-General of Employment and Training, Ministry of Labour, GOI, New Delhi.

34 per cent in Mizoram to as low as 4 per cent in Punjab, as per the 1991 Census. (State-wise data for the 2001 Census is not yet available). (Table 13.11)

Women's share in the organised work-force has also shown an Increasing trend, from 2.8 million (12.2 per cent) in 1981 to 4.8 million (17.2 per cent) in 1999. Between 1991 and 1999, rise in the percentage points of women was 3.1 in contrast, the share of men has been declining. However, women's participation in the organised sector is still very low, as compared to men. (Table 13.11)

Similarly, women's employment in the public sector has also recorded an increase from 1.5 million (9.7 per cent) in 1981 to 2.8 million (14.5 per cent) in 1999 (Table 13.12). However, it is still much lower than that of men. (Table 13.12)

TABLE 13.12

Women in the Public Sector (1981-99)

(Figures in Million)

Year	*Women*	*Men*	*Total*
1981	1.5 (9.7)	14.0	15.5
1991	2.4 (12.3)	16.7	19.1
2001	2.8 (14.5)	16.6	19.4

Source: Director General of Employment and Training, Ministry of Labour, GOI, New Delhi.

Just as in the case of women in Public Sector, they also hold a low-key with only 14.6 per cent of the total 10.7 million employees in Government in 1997. No doubt, there has been an increasing trend in the representation of women in Government, as it rose from 11.0 to 14.6 per cent between 1981 and 1997, but at the same time, their representation can be rated as very low, when compared to the number of educated women. (Table 13.12)

REPRESENTATION AT DECISION-MAKING LEVELS

(i) Administrative

The representation of women in the decision-making levels through the Premier Services viz., the Indian Administrative Services (IAS) and Table 13.13 Indian Police Services (IPS), which stood at only 5.4 per cent in 1987 increased marginally to 7.6 per cent in 2000. However, the figure is still very low, requiring not only affirmative action but also special interventions to help raise the number of women at various decision-making levels. (Refer Table 13.13)

TABLE 13.13

Women in the Government (1981-97)

(Figures in Million)

Year	*Women*	*Men*	*Total*
1981	1.2 (11.0)	9.7	10.9
1997	1.6 (14.6)	9.1	10.7

Source: Director General of Employment and Training, Ministry of Labour, GOI, New Delhi.

TABLE 13.14

Representation of Women in Premier Services (1987-2000)

Service	*1987*		*1997*		*2000*	
	Women	*Total*	*Women*	*Total*	*Women*	*Total*
	339 (7.5)	4204	512 (10.2)	4991	535 (10.4)	5159
IPS	21 (0.9)	2418	67 (2.2)	3045	110 (3.3)	3301
Total	360 (5.4)	6622	579 (7.2)	8036	645 (7.6)	8460

Source: Department of Personnel and Training, GOI, New Delhi.

(ii) Political

The 73rd and 74th Constitutional Amendments in 1993 have brought forth a definite impact on the participation of women, in terms of absolute numbers, in grass-root democratic institutions viz. Panchayati Raj Institutions (PRIs) and Local Bodies. In fact, these amendments have helped women not only in their effective participation but also in decision-making in the grass-roots democracy. Of the 475 Zilla Parishads in the country, 158 are being chaired by women. At the Block Level, out of 51,000 members of Block Samitis, 17,000 are women.

In addition, nearly one-third of the Mayors of the municipalities are women. In the elections to PRIs held between 1993 and 1997, women have achieved participation even beyond the mandatory requirement of $33^1/_3$ per cent of the total seats in states like Karnataka (43.45 per cent), Kerala (36.4 per cent) and West Bengal (35.4 per cent). However, the all India figure for women show that their representation in 2001 is still low.

Although the number of women in Parliament has increased from 59 in 1998 to 70 in 2001, their share continues to be very low. representing only 8.5 per cent (Table 1.3.16) of the total members in Parliament in 2001.

TABLE 13.15

Women in Panchayati Raj Institutions (1995-2001)

(Figures in Thousand)

Year	*Women*	*Men*	*Total*
1995#	318 (33.5)	630	948
2001@	725 (26.6)	1997	2722

Source: Ministry of Rural Development. GOI. New Delhi.

TABLE 13.16

Representation of Women in Parliament (1998-2001)

Year	*Females*	*Males*	*Total*
1998	59 (7.2)	761	820
1999	67 (8.5)	723	790
2001	70	750 (8.5)	820

Note: Figures within parentheses indicate percentage of total.
Sources: 1. Election Commission of India
2. National Information Centre, Parliament House, New Delhi

The number of women in the Central Council of Ministers continues to remain extremely low, but with a marginal increase of 0.8 percent between 1995 and 2001. Of these, 2 are of Cabinet rank and 6 are of the rank of Minister of State, and of these, 2 are holding Independent Charge. These trends point out very clearly to the need for affirmative action besides addressing these issues in a systematic and expeditious way so that women's concerns gain political prominence and a fairly representative number of women are in position not only at grass-root level, but also at the state and national levels.

Table 13.17 presents the status of women including that of the girl child along with the progress made by them over a period of two development decades (1981-2001) as reflected in the 21 Selected Gender Development Indicators.

A quick review of the progress made by women has not only focussed light on the gains but also brought forth to surface certain critical areas of concern relating to women by Draft Tenth Plan requiring attention of the Government during the Tenth Plan. They include: increasing burden of

TABLE 13.17

Representation of Women in the Central Council of Ministers (1985-2001)

Year	Females	Males	Total
1985	4 (10.0)	36	40
2001	8 (10.8)	66	74

Source: National Information Centre, Parliament House, New Delhi.

poverty; unequal access to primary health care, under/malnutrition, high rates of illiteracy and lack of training; lack of access and control on assets and resources; inequalities in sharing of power and decision-making; lack of access to information and media; increasing violence against women, adolescent and the girl child, persisting discrimination against the girl child, etc. Keeping these issues/concerns in view, the Tenth Plan suggests the following approach not only to strengthen, but also to speed up, the on going process/efforts of empowering of women.

Health is both an important factor in the achievement of status as well as an indicator of social status, particularly for women, whose health is conditioned to a great extent by social attitudes. The health status of women includes their mental and social condition as affected by prevailing norms and attitudes of society in addition to their biological and physiological problems. Societies delineate women's roles partly according to their biological and physiological problems. Societies delineate women's roles partly according to their biological functions and partly from prevailing attitudes regarding their physical and mental capacity. These social attitudes also influence the provision and use of preventive and curative health care, including maternal care. The health care facilities offered by a community in the form of medical particularly maternity services for women, is a significant index of the emphasis that community places on the health of its women. Some studies in both the developed and developing countries have shown a definite link between low status of women and deficiencies in the knowledge and utilisation of preventive health services.[1]

We cannot hope to solve the increasing international problems of economic and social development and improve the quality of human life while leaving aside half the resources of humanity.

The impact of maternal mortality on the individual, the family and society at large is like a pebble dropped into a pond, where the ripples of action and reaction reach out to all shores. Women's concern for health and their ingenuity in ensuring good health for themselves, their families and their communities, often in the face of great odds, marks them out as a leading force for development and peace.[2]

TABLE 13.18

Selected Gender Development Indicators: 1981-2001

S. No.	Indictors	Women	Men	Total	Women	Men	Total
Demography and Vital Statistics							
1.	Population (in Million in 1981 and 2001)	330.0	353.4	683.4	495.7	531.3	1027.0
2.	Decennial Growth (1981 and 2001)	24.93	24.41	24.66	21.79	20.93	21.84
3.	Sex Ratio (1981 and 2001)	934	—	—	933	—	—
4.	Life Expectancy at Birth (in years in 1981-85 and 1999-01)	55.7	55.4	—	65.3	62.3	—
5.	Mean age at Marriage (in years in 1981 and 1991)	18.3	23.3	—	19.5	23.9	—
Health and Family Welfare							
6.	Birth Rate (per thousand in 1981 and 1999)	—	—	33.9	—	—	26.1
7.	Death Rate (per thousand in 1981 and 1999)	12.7	12.4	12.5	8.3	9.0	8.7
8.	Infant Mortality rate (per thousand live births in 1988 and 1999)	93.0	96.0	94.5	70.0	69.8	70.0
9.	Child Mortality Rate (per thousand live births under 5 years of age in 1985 and 1997)	40.4	36.6	—	24.5	21.8	—
10.	Maternal Mortality rate (per one lakh live births in 1980 and 1998)	468	—	—	407	—	—

Literacy and Education						
11. Literacy Rates (1981-2001)	29.78	56.38	43.57	54.16	75.85	65.38
12 Gross Enrolment Ratio (1980-81 and 1999-2000)						
Class I-V	64.1	95.8	80.5	85.2	104.1	94.9
Class VI-VIII	28.6	54.3	41.9	49.7	67.2	58.8
13. Drop out Rate (1980-81 and 1999-2000)						
Class I-V	62.5	56.2	58.7	42.3	38.7	48.3
Classes VI-III	79.4	68.0	72.7	58.0	52.0	64.5
Work and Employment						
14. Work Participation Rate (1981 and 2001)	19.7	52.8	26.7	25.7	51.9	39.3
15. Organised Sector (No. in Million in 1981-1999)	2.80	20.05	2285	2.83	23.28	28.11
16. Public Sector (No. in Million in 1981 and 1999)	1.5	14.0	15.5	2.8	16.6	19.4
17. Government (No. in Million in 1981-1997)	1.2	9.7	10.9	1.6	9.1	10.9
Decision-Making						
18. Administration (No. in IAS and IPS in 1987-2000)	360	6262	6622	645	7815	8460
19. PRIs (No. in Thousand in 1995 and 2001)	318	630	948	725	1997	2722
20. Parliament (No. in 1998 and 2001)	59	761	830	70	750	820
21. Central Council of Ministers (No. in 1985 and 2001)	4	36	40	8	66	74

Source: Census of India, 1991, Census of India, 2001.

The impact of maternal mortality on the individual, the family and society at large is like a pebble dropped into a pond, where the ripples of action and reaction reach out to all shores. If a society does not have an adequate mechanism to manage or absorb the costs, and most importantly to care for the children involved, each persons and the society quality of life will decline as will their health, livelihoods and the nation's developmental prospects.[3]

That society would be highly developed and prosperous where women have their rightful place expounds Manu. The woman is the pivot around which the family, the society and humanity itself revolves. It is well said that the hands that rock the cradle, rule the world. Women play a significant role in the development of their offspring. Truly, if a man is educated, one person is educated but if the woman is educated, the whole family is educated. One of India's greatest poets, Rabindranath Tagore, had expressed the pain and inequity of the situation more than half a century ago, thus:

"O Lord Why have you not given woman the right to conquer her destiny?
Why does she have to wait head bowed,
By the roadside, Waiting with tired patience
Hoping for a miracle in the morrow?"

National Perspective Plan for Women, 1988 spell out the following activities for better health to girls and women:

(i) Change our attitudes to provide prompt and adequate medical care for girls.
(ii) Prepare girls for better motherhood.
(iii) Reduce infant and child mortality of girls.
(iv) Reduce maternal mortality.
(v) Ensure adequate maternal health care—pre-natal, natal and post-natal.
(vi) Ensure proper knowledge and services for family planning.
(vii) Provision of basic health and nutrition services for girls and women.
(viii) Raise the level of literacy and education among women.[4]

Beijing UN International Conference emphasized a life span perspective for health of women. A lifespan approach addresses the health issues of women—a conception and birth, in infancy and childhood, during adolescence, throughout the reproductive years, into old-age-within the context of their biological and social vulnerabilities and their status in society. It also takes into account both the specific as well as the cumulative effects of poor health and nutrition.

There is increasing evidence that health problems that begin in childhood and adolescence affect the health status of women during their reproductive years and beyond, as well as the health of their newborns. Discrimination against the girl child as seen in some countries of the Region can also significantly retard her growth and development.[5] Ninth Five Year Plan stresses holistic approach to health of women. The Ninth Plan recognises the special health needs of women and the girl-babies and the importance of enhancing easy access to primary health care. There are many indicators to point out that the neglect of health needs of women especially that of the pregnant women, adolescent girls and girl-babies, is responsible for the present high rates of IMR/CMR/MMR. Therefore, a holistic approach with Reproductive Child Health (RCH) measures will be adopted in improving the health status of women by focusing on their age-specific needs.[6]

Today, technological advancements and, in general, development in every sphere and the race against time have compelled women to come out of the confines of the house and contribute more to the main stream. It is a pity that a large majority of Indian women are still steeped in ignorance and have not been able to break themselves away from the clutches of old rituals, traditions and beliefs. Only a microscopic minority of womenfolk have been able to utilise the rights enshrined in the constitution. The time has come for women to march side by side with men. To shoulder this new responsibility effectively, women have to be better equipped and qualified.

National development depends a great deal on the welfare of women, who are the real architects of a nation. The program for women welfare aims at raising the economic and social status of women, so that they can play an important role in building a strong and prosperous nation. The reason for poverty and misery in the developing countries is not essentially the lack of potentialities or resources, whether human or material, but under-utilization of these resources. Today, developing countries are not utilizing more than 15 per cent of the potential capacity of this manpower. A plausible remedy to increase the GNP and improve the standard of living, it appears, is the maximum utilisation of more than 51 per cent of the world population on a bigger scale in the task of development. National reconstruction and social change.[7] As Helvi Sipila, a Finnish lawyer, who is the UN's Secretary-General for the International Women's Year says:

> "We cannot hope to solve the increasing international problems of economic and social development, and improve the quality of human life, while leaving aside half the resources of humanity."[8]

There is need to harness stagnant and unexploited potential female energy. The Economic and Social Survey of Asia and the Pacific, 1976 also stresses the same view.

> "The wastage of human resources that results from the exclusion of women from the development process is something that developing

countries can ill-afford. This wastage can take the form of the use of a large part of women's time in carrying out domestic tasks amenable to increased efficiency through some investment."[9]

We should not think that we can conceive of women development independently of the socio-economic development of the country. Women development could contribute to the development and modernization of the world. A similar message was conveyed by the UNESCO that women can play an important part in the process of development. They represent the means through which the changes in attitudes and behaviour necessary for adaptation to the modern world can be achieved. Their responsibility for bringing up new generations means that they must also attend to the education of children and supervise their scholastic progress and critical faculty. As home managers, they have the task of improving the conditions of the family life while as household administrators, they must balance the financial budget. A UN report also supported this view:

"The exclusion of women from many aspects of the development process also has important indirect effects. First, there is the effect on the nature of their influence on the education and socialisation of their children, because by and large, women will pass on their own experience and attitudes. Secondly, there is the indirect effect on population growth. This is an extremely complex subject. Though it is not easy to isolate the factors affecting fertility, many of the relevant factors can be combined under the heading of Exposure of women to modernization."[10]

Changing Status of Women: Constitutional and Legal Provisions

In the ancient India, women held a high place of respect in the society, as mentioned in Rigveda and other scriptures.[11] Volumes can be written about the status of our women and their heroic deeds from the Vedic period to the modern times. But later on, because of social, political and economic changes, women lost their status and were relegated to the background. Many evil customs and traditions stepped in which enslaved the women and tied them to boundaries of the house. The untold miseries and sufferings of women of the 19th century awakened the conscience of mankind. Many reformers like Raja Rammohan Roy, Swami Dayanand, Justice Ranade, Mahatma Gandhi, and others championed the cause of the emancipation of women. The Constitution of India also prohibits any discrimination on grounds of sex.[12] Many laws have also been enacted by the Government of India to protect the rights of women.[13]

The Constitution of India not only grants equality to women but also empowers the State to adopt measures of positive discrimination in favour of women for neutralising the cumulative socio-economic, educational and political disadvantages faced by them. The Preamble to the Constitution resolves to secure to all its citizens, justice, social, economic and political, liberty of thought, expression, belief, faith and worship, equality of status and of opportunity and to promote among them all, fraternity, assuring the dignity of the individual and the unity and integrity of the nation.

Article 14 confers equal rights and opportunities on men and women in the political, economic and social spheres while Article 15 prohibits discrimination on the grounds of religion, race, caste, sex, etc. a provision under Article 15(3) enables the State to allow affirmative discrimination in favour of women. Article 16 guarantees equality of opportunity in public employment. The State also imposes a fundamental duty on every citizen to renounce practices derogatory to the dignity of women.

To uphold the Constitutional mandate, the State has enacted various legislative measures intended to ensure equal rights, to counter social discrimination and various forms of violence and atrocities and to provide support services especially to working women.

- The Employees State Insurance Act, 1948.
- The Medical Termination of Pregnancy Act, 1971.
- The Indecent Representation of Women (Prohibition) Act, 1986.
- The Equal Remuneration Act, 1976.
- The Immoral Traffic (Prevention) Act, 1986.
- The Dowry Prohibition Act, 1991 (amended in 1984 and 1986).
- The Child Marriage Restraint (Amendment) Act, 1976.
- The Special Marriage Act, 1954.
- The Hindu Marriage Act, 1955.
- The Hindu Succession Act 1956.
- The Family Courts Act, 1954.
- The Criminal Law (Amendment) Act, 1983.
- The Factories (Amendment) Act, 1986.
- The Plantation Labour Act, 1951.
- The Contract Labour (Regulation and Abolition) Act, 1976.

The legal edifice thus effectively affirms and promotes the principles of equity and equality of women and takes care of their special needs. Much that has been granted to women by law is yet to be within the reach of them all, in reality. Continual large-scale effort is needed to liquidate the limitations still suffered by women to work shoulder to shoulder for improving the standard of living of the Indian masses so that opportunities for living a richer and fuller life would be available to both women and men.[14]

Institutional Framework for Implementation of Women Programmes

Efforts towards women welfare started with the establishment of the Central Social Welfare Board in 1953. A Department of Women and Child Development was set-up in 1985 under the newly created Ministry of Human Resource Development. The National Commission for Women was set-up by an Act of Parliament in 1990 which came into operation in 1992 as a national apex statutory level body to review the constitutional and legal safeguards for women. These have been supplemented by concreted efforts of the women 's movement and the voluntary sector. The progress in the last few decades has been noteworthy. In areas relating to women's rights, education, employment and health significant gains have been achieved. More women are literate, there is a better understanding of rights and responsibilities, there is greater awareness and gender sensitivity, better access to health services and income generation has become available to many women.

The 73rd and 74th Constitutional Amendment Acts of 1993 constitute a watershed for the advancement of Indian women. They ensure one-third of the total elected seats and positions of Chairpersons in rural and urban local elected bodies to women. About 1 million women are estimated to emerge as leaders at the grass-root levels in the rural areas alone. Of these 75,000 are to be Chairpersons.

POLICIES AND PROGRAMMES

In order to ensure the benefits to women, many programmes have been initiated. Some of these are given below for reference.

- National Perspective Plan for Women (1988).
- Shramshakti—the Report of the National Commission for Self-Employed Women and Women in the Informal Sector (1988).
- Report of the National Expert Committee on Women Prisoners (1986).
- The National Plan of Action for the Girl Child (1991-2000).
- Reservation for Women in Grass-root Level Democratic Institutions (1993).
- Poverty Eradication Programmes.
- Mahila Samriddhi Yojana (MSY) (1993).
- National Credit Fund for Women (1993).
- Support to Training and Employment Programmes (STEP).
- Training-*cum*-Employment-*cum*-Production Centres.
- Socio-Economic Programme (SEP).
- Condensed Courses of Education and Vocational Training for Adult Women (CCE and VT).
- Monitoring of Beneficiary Oriented Schemes (BOS) for Women.
- Gender Sensitisation and Awareness Generation.
- Gender Sensitisation of 1991/2001 Census.
- Support Services.
- Legal Literacy Manuals (LLMs).
- National Resource Centre for Women.
- Domestic Violence Act, 2005.

PRESENT SOCIO-ECONOMIC SITUATION IN RESPECT OF WOMEN AFFECTING THEIR HEALTH

The health situation pertaining to women can be assessed from a number of socio-economic factors affecting the women in the developing world. We already know that health affects and is affected by socio-economic factors. We shall discuss some of these factors.

1. Unfavourable Sex-ratio in Respect of Women

The sex-ratio was 972 females per thousand males in 1901 and has declined to 927 in 1991. The decline has been more or less steady over the decades, except for a marginal rise between 1941 and 1951 and a small rise, more recently, between 1971 and 1981. The adverse sex-ratio for females and its decline since 1991 is attributed mainly to higher mortality among females, as compared to males, in all age groups right from childhood through child-bearing ages. Limited access to the health infrastructure contribute to high maternal mortality and relative deprivation of the female child from nutrition. Health and medical care have been identified as some of the other contributory factors.

The adverse sex-ratio for women needs to be seen against other indicators of falling mortality rates for both men and women, higher child survival rates and the improvement of life expectancy, which is more significant for women than for men. The improving health care in India should contribute to a more favourable sex-ratio for the country in the years to come. Among the factors that would remain to be resolved however, would be the persistent bias in favour of the male child.

2. Lower Literacy Rate

Despite intensive efforts of the State during the last four decades to improve the literacy levels, the achievement has not been completely satisfactory. Literacy has shown substantial increase from 18.33 in 1951 to 52.51 in 1991. The sex differentials in literacy, however, have been throughout consistent and pronounced. Over the four decades (1951-91), female literacy has gone up five times, i.e. from 8.86 in 1951 to 39.29 in 1991. During the decade 1981-91 in particular, female literacy increased at a relatively faster pace (9.6%) than male literacy (7.5%).

Females are generally disadvantaged in the ESCAP region, both in access to education and in continuation of their education relative to males. It was stated in a UN report that:

> "Lack of training and education affects their skill and employability and relegates the majority of women to the burdens of home-related chores or to the jobs that carry the least status and the lowest pay. It also greatly reduces any possibility of valid aspiration on the part of girls for viable or self-fulfiling roles in society."[15]

The National Plan of Action for Women mentioned the following causes responsible for the low literacy among women in India:

(a) General indifference to education of girls.
(b) Social resistance arising out of fears and mis-conceptions that education might alienate girls from traditions and social values and lead to maladjustments, conflicts and non-conformism.
(c) Early marriage and social inhibition against girls pursuing education after marriage.
(d) Prevalence of child labour among girls belonging to weaker sections and the hard domestic chores which some of the unmarried girls especially from middle and lower-middle class families are required to perform.
(e) The prevailing notion that the sole occupation of women is to bear children, look after her husband and children, and thus be restricted to domestic work.
(f) Discrimination effected by employers against women labour in both organised and unorganised sectors in matters of recruitment, training and promotion.
(g) Many girls and their parents find that the school curriculum does not conform adequately to their needs and interests.
(h) Unsuitable and inflexible school timings and inadequate facilities for girls in schools, particularly in the co-educational schools.[16]

3. Age at Marriage

Traditionally, attainment of puberty has played an important role to determine the age at marriage for girls. By the age of 25-29 years, more than 90% of women were married in 1992. About 300/0 females, who were married off at younger ages, were still in their teens (i.e.15-19 years).

The mean age at marriage for females which was around 13 years at the beginning of the century rose to 18.3 years by 1981. The mean age at 'effective marriage' for females was 19.5 years in 1992. The Child Marriage Restraint Act, 1976 raised minimum age at marriage of girls to 18 years from 15 years and for boys to 21 years. This was intended to prevent child marriages, early marriage of girls and consequent early pregnancies and thereby curtail fertility at young ages and birth of premature babies. Acquiring higher education and greater employment by women have also played a role in raising their age at marriage.

4. Poor Economic Status

Women contribute greatly to the economy. Employment of women is an index of their economic status in society, specially with reference to equality. According to the Census data, the work participation rate (i.e., the proportion of employed or total workers to population) of females steadily rose from 14.22% in 1971 to 19.67 in 1981 and to 22.27 in 1991. The rise in work participation of rural females has been even steeper from 15.92 in 1971 to 26.79 in 1991. The rise in work participation of urban femalès over the two decades is somewhat less impressive. During the 1991 Census, conscious efforts were made to count women workers more completely and remove their invisibility. This could be one of the reasons for the increase reflected in the work participation rates between 1981-91. Women's employment in the organised sector has revealed significant increase from 1.9 million in 1971 to 4.0 million in 1993, constituting 14.6% of the total employment of 27.18 million. Of these 2.47 million women, i.e. about 62% were employed in the public sector and 1.6 million, i.e. 38% in the private sector.

The ILO report underlines the main causes of this structural imbalance—

> "the only ways to lessen or remove these differentials between men's and women's earnings, however calculated, are changes in the structure and character of women's education, training and employment and in the cleavages between 'men's work' and women's work-changes aimed at removing persisting inequalities and discriminations and overcoming the stereotyped sex roles acquired by women over the ages in the world of work."[17]

One of the reasons why women are sometimes discriminated against in regard to employment is that fringe benefits such as the provision of crèches, maternity leave and other medical amenities have to be provided for women. The employer is naturally unwilling to engage women when he has to provide such amenities. The solution is to provide these facilities at State expenses for the first two children of the women workers. In developing countries the most pressing need is to improve the education of girls and to wipe out illiteracy as well as to encourage all types of training facilities that can help women to become self-employed, since wage earning employment will be limited for both women and men in coming years.

5. Women in Decision-making

As they are half the population. women must be in decision-making in all socio-economic and political organisations. If more and more women are associated at different levels, it is sure to affect public policy. Women' issues will be transformed into societal issues. The most critical role for women will be to resist inequality and injustice, nor merely for women, but for all. At present the number of women in the positions of power is significantly very less. In Parliament it has been varying from 2.8% to 7.2%. Women in IAS 7.5%, IPS 9% and Indian Foreign Service 9%. These need to be stepped up to provide them better opportunities.

PROVISION OF HEALTH SERVICES

1. Adequate Health Facilities

Health facilities are undoubtedly inadequate, especially in rural areas. The women services have four components: care of general medical problems; care of gynaecological problems; obstetric care and family problems. The purpose is to provide planned maternal and child health services to ensure that expectant and nursing mothers maintain good health, have a normal delivery and bear healthy children. It is a service planned for the promotion and restoration of health of mothers and children and provision of safe confinement. The following suggestions may be considered to improve the health services for women:

(a) Since a major part of our population stay in villages, where dais playa significant role. we should accelerate the training programme for them. This would reduce greatly the maternal and infant mortality rates.
(b) Arrangements may be made for special identifiable services for women in all types of institutions, especially in the PHCs.
(c) At present, one PHC is provided for 30,000 population. It is suggested that one PHC be provided for not more than 25,000 population.
(d) Cooperation of the private practitioners of the indigenous system of medicine should be sought for identification and referral of high risk pregnancies and for delivery and expansion of family-welfare services.
(e) Blood transfusion services may be streamlined to provide blood to women, who are likely to lose their lives due to haemorrhage.

There is a need of increasing women's access to appropriate, affordable and quality health care throughout their lifespan and strengthening preventive programmes that promote women's health. A gender perspective to health must also take into account the differences between men and women relative to their access to health services and the quality of care they receive. This can only be done through an analysis of health service utilization statistics obtained from facilities along with community-based statistics, which include population groups not using health facilities.

2. Provision of Nutritional Services

The nutritional status of women especially that of the rural poor is far from what is desired. Inspite of the prophylactic programmes against nutritional anaemia targeted at the expectant and lactating mothers, these women continue to suffer from acute anaemia. It has been pointed out that much wasting and stunting of growth takes place during young age. With early and multiple pregnancies, women miss the opportunity of attaining full bodily growth. The low nutritional status of women in India applies to all the age groups but is more acute in the cases of young girls, pregnant and aged women. While in the lowest socio-economic groups, the low nutritional status of women is mainly due to poverty and the burden of family responsibilities, in the lower middle income groups, it is aggravated by general neglect and is the indirect result of stronger gender discrimination.

Women in developing countries are generally more malnourished than men. The additional biological demands due to menstruation, pregnancy and lactation have made nutritional deficiencies the most widespread and disabling health problem among women. For example, low birth weight in newborns is partly a reflection of poor maternal nutrition the proportion of net weighing less than 2500 gram; ranged from 13% to 50% in countries of the South-East Asia.

Iron deficiency anaemia is more common in women than in men. About 55% of pregnant women and 44% of all women suffer from anaemia in developing countries. At ages between 15-44 years, the burden of iron deficiency anaemia in developing countries in 1990 in terms of thousands of DALYs per year was 4898 for men and 7135 for women. Anaemia lowers the physical work capacity of women and their ability to cope with various infections. It also has serious repercussions on their reproductive health, with maternal mortality being significantly higher in anaemic women.[18]

The most serious problem affecting women is lack of adequate nutrition. Girls and women generally get the leftovers because of the social customs, poverty and their poor social status. A pleasant and healthy diet, not necessarily an expensive one. is one of the most satisfying and stimulating activities of family life. It contributes to the physical, the mental and social well-being of all the members of the family. Man does not always instinctively choose the right nutrition for maintaining his health. He is influenced in his food habits by religion, culture, social status, traditions and beliefs. Nature abounds in good nutritious foods within reach of the economically under-privileged families. A balanced diet does not mean an expensive diet. With proper education, families with limited financial resources can take better care of their nutritional needs. It is, therefore, essential for the health department and voluntary organisations to impart this type of education as this can go a long way in promoting the health and well-being of family members.

Health institutions do not provide, at present, any special nutritional services. There is a need to plan well-equipped and staffed nutrition clinics attached to all hospitals and PHCs. There may be arrangements to educate the women about the nutritive value of locally available foods and also teach methods of cooking that would retain food value. The properties of medical herbs and medicines and traditional cures can be analysed and popularized among mothers.

3. Planning and Development of Health Personnel for Women's Health

We have already discussed the various aspects of health manpower planning. We may suggest here some methods which can help in making more women health personnel available to cater to the health needs of women:

(a) More reservation of seats for women in medical colleges till a sufficient number of qualified lady doctors are available.

(b) More women may be encouraged to undergo training in ISM through the reservation in service as well.

(c) In order to encourage self-employment among women doctors, financial assistance may be provided to set-up clinics, etc.

(d) Community Health Workers' Scheme must include at least fifty per cent women to deal effectively with the women health problems.

4. Planning Adequate Facilities for Reproductive Health

The greatest burden of reproductive health problems, however, falls on women. It is they who face the risks from complications of pregnancy and childbirth, from unwanted pregnancies and from unsafe abortions. Over one-third of all healthy life lost in adult women in the developing world is due to reproductive health problems, as compared to only 12% in men. And yet large number of women remain ill-informed about basic facts related to their reproductive health.[19]

A country's level of maternal mortality is a sensitive index of the provision and quality of health and obstetric services. India's maternal mortality ratio, usually estimated at 400-500 per 100,000 live births, is fifty times higher than that of many developed countries and six times higher than that of neighbouring Sri Lanka (Ascadi and Johnson-Ascadi, 1990 in Meshram and Heaver,1995). The lifetime risk of a woman in a country like India dying from pregnancy ranges from 1 in 25 to 1 in 40, which contrasts sharply to the fact that only one in several thousand women run a similar risk in England. France, or the US. (Saran. 1994). According to the National Family Health Survey (NFHS). the maternal mortality ratio in 1992-93 was 420 per 100,000 (International Institute of Population Studies, 1995). This survey estimated that close to 1,10,000 women die every year in India from causes related to pregnancy and according to Bhatia (1993). 88 to 98 percent of these deaths are avoidable and 78 percent of maternal deaths can be prevented by timely action. Maternal mortality is just the tip of the iceberg of the obstetric health problems of women. Many women suffer from severe pregnancy-related morbidities during the ante-natal, delivery and post-natal periods. However, information on reproductive morbidity and maternal mortality is either fragmentary or inaccurate and the causes are also not clearly given. This vital information is not being collected/reported due to improper/irregular/inadequate home visits, lack of supervision and follow-up, under-reporting and mis-classification of deaths and also due to inaccessibility of interior rural areas.[20]

Women must be encouraged to adopt family planning. In rural areas women start their reproductive life when they are barely out of adolescence and may have four or five children by the time they are thirty. This adversely affects their health and well-being. Women in the rural and urban areas have hardly any say in family planning. It is men who decide matters, but among the educated women, some mutual understanding is evident. The education of women, population change and overall development are closely inter-related. Women have a crucial role to play in all these areas still uncovered. A study of the inter-relationship between the status of women and family planning was conducted in accordance with the Economic and Social Council Resolution. The report affirmed:

"(a) The right to decide freely and responsibly on the number and spacing of their children is a fundamental right of individuals which facilitates the exercise of other human rights especially by women;

(b) Adequate information, education and services enabling individuals to exercise this right are essential pre-requisites for the promotion of the status of women, and for ensuring their complete integration in social and economic development at all levels; and

(c) Family planning which should constitute an integrated and essential part of development plan and programmes, in countries suffering from over-population can only succeed in concert with other measures which also improve the status of women."[21]

The establishment of a close doctor-patient relationship is an absolutely essential requirement for the success of the programme. Careful follow-up by doctors of vasectomy and tubectomy cases is as necessary as the operation itself. for the psychological rehabilitation of the patient, as well as for the assurance of potential acceptors. A maternal death is defined as the death of a woman while pregnant or within 42 days of the termination of pregnancy, irrespective of the duration and site of the pregnancy, from any cause related to or aggravated by the pregnancy or its management but not from accidental or incidental causes.

Most maternal deaths are preventable. The medical interventions necessary to prevent them are trained assistance at delivery, a well established primary health care infrastructure with a good referral system. and referral facilities (e.g. at district level) for managing complications. Most women do not receive the services of a skilled attendant (midwife, nurse or doctor) at the time of delivery. For example, the report of a three-year study covering a population of 686,000 in a rural area of India showed that "delay in seeking care and too many and inappropriate referrals through lower levels of the health system not capable of dealing with the problem, significantly increased the risk of dying. Similarly, residence in the village proper (which has better transport facilities) as compared to the hamlets had a protective effect. A trained attendant at delivery, presence of an ANM (Auxiliary Nurse Midwife) in the village, an educated husband (the usual decision-maker) and the social custom of migrating to the natal home for delivery all had a protective effect."[22]

5. Planning Women Education for Family Health

Healthy families make healthy people. The family is the primary unit of healthy care, a front line in the sequence of education, prevention, diagnosis, treatment and rehabilitation of its constituents. "Health begins at Home" was the theme chosen for World Health Day (1973) on 25th Anniversary of WHO in recognition of the important role of the family in promoting and protecting the health of its members. Women occupy an important place in shaping the lives of its family members. The mother is still the best teacher on life and health. The education imparted by her remains with children as long as they live. Government should provide health education to women as notions of health and hygiene given at home to children would help them to be good citizens. Women, if properly educated, can really help in the socio-economic development of the country. This would release the potential energy of the women and help in channelizing it for the welfare of the family and ultimately national development.

6. Planning for HIV/AIDS and STDs, Infertility and Gynaecological Disorders

Acquired immuno deficiency syndrome (AIDS), unknown eve 15 years ago, has now become a major challenge to public 'health is important to educate women about STDs and HIV infection. It even more important to empower them to say "NO" to unsafe sex, STDs in women are not easily identified or cured because over 50% of STDs in women are asymptomatic, diagonsis is difficult, an women's access to services for STD treatment is poor. Sills in pregnant women cause complications such as seplis, spontaneous abortion, premature birth, still-birth and congentia infection. Almost two-thirds of cases of infertility among women an 35% of cases of post-pactum morbidity are attributable to STDs.

Worldwide, the disease burden of Sills in women is more than five times that in men.[23] During the Ninth Plan, attempts are being made to provide for screening for syphillis, gonorrhea and HIV infection at PHC/CHC level wherever possible. Utilising the microscope and laboratory technician available at PHCs vaginal/cervical smears in women with symptoms of RTI are to be screened for identifying organisms responsible and appropriate treatment provided.

Infertility

It is estimated that between 5 to 10% of couples are infertile. While provision of contraceptive advice and care to all couples in reproductive age group is important, it is equally essential that couples who do not have children have access to essential clinical examination, investigation, management and counselling. The focus at the CHC level will be to identify infertile couples and undertake clinical examination to detect the obvious causes of infertility, carry out preliminary investigations such as sperm count, diagnostic curettage and tubal patency testing. Depending upon the findings, the couples may then be referred to centres with appropriate facilities for diagnosis and management. By carrying out simple diagnostic procedures available at the primary health care institutions it is possible to reduce the number of couples requiring referral. Initial screening at primary health care level and subsequent referral is a cost-effective method for management of infertility both for the health care system and those requiring such services.

Gynaecological Disorders

Women suffers from a variety of common gynaecological problems including menstrual dysfunctions at peri-menarchal and peri-menopausal age. Facilities for diagnosis of these are at the moment available at district hospitals or tertiary care centres. During the Ninth Plan period the CHCs. with a gynaecologist, have started providing requisite diagnostic and curative services. Yet another major problem in women is prolapse uterus of varying degrees. The PHCs and CHCs refer women requiring surgery to district hospitals or tertiary care centres.

Cancer Cervix is one of the most common malignancies in India and accounts for over a third of all malignancies in women. Cancer Cervix can readily be diagnosed at the PHCs and CHCs. Early diagnosis of Stage I and Stage II and referral to places where radiography is available will result in rapid decline in mortality due to cancer cervix in the country in the near future.

7. Environment and Work-Related Health Problems

Health problems that are work-related or those arising out of adverse environment conditions, cover a broad range of illnesses and disabilities. Such problem arise out of injuries, infections, exposure to dust, chemicals and gases, from psychological stresses, and from the harmful effects of a degrading environment Women often work long hours, increasing their exposure to illness and injuries. A large proportion of women are engaged in agricultural work. This can expose them to worm infestations, which aggravate anaemia, to injuries, snake bites and insecticide poisoning as well as to disorders resulting from extreme climatic conditions. Exposure to pesticides and chemical fertilizers can also result in abortion and stillbirth. The health department must provide facilities against such risks.

8. Violence against Women

Many women face violence throughout their lives, like rape and domestic violence. Although national statistics on violence against women are not readily available. the problem is serious, Domestic violence is relatively common. Available evidence suggests that thousands of cases of domestic violence are reported directly to police stations each year like dowry deaths are regularly reported by the media. However, domestic violence is often regarded as a private family matter and many cases may therefore go unreported. Fear and shame also contribute to the non-reporting of domestic violence.

9. Increasing General and Functional Literary for Good Health

Education is the most potent factor for changing women's position in society. We must correct the imbalances by encouraging the education of girls. We can use the adult education or non-formal education system. What can be the future of a country where general illiteracy, especially among women, is very high? Besides, the women have also to handle the new generation, i.e. the child who is the future hope.

All this would remain a dream unless women are themselves enlightened. Education is the key factor in elevating the status of women. It equips them to contribute in different fields more meaningfully. Dr. (Mrs.) P.K. Devi, Professor of Gynaecology, in PGI, Chandigarh, has rightly stated on the basis of her critical examination of the various states of the Indian Union, that "Literacy, especially of women seems to be a significant factor in differences in the mortality and morbidity rates between various Indian states and infant mortality rates coincide with a very low female literacy rate." In India, planners, statesmen, educationists and administrators have come to realise that the pace of development cannot accelerate unless women are also properly qualified. So to improve the education of women quantitatively and qualitatively, the following steps are submitted for consideration:

(a) Expansion of the facilities of women education including adult and vocational education tremendously so that the literacy in respect of this group may be increased.

(b) Removal of disparity between rural and urban literacy by (i) provision of good institutions in villages to avoid the attraction for cities; (ii) to bring awareness towards hygiene among women through community development programmes; (iii) preference in employment to rural people; (iv) setting up of professional and other training institutions in the villages; (v) setting up of rural-based industries in village; (vi) training of women in modern methods of agriculture; (vii) encouraging the formation of mahila mandals to exchange information on various problems facing the nation; and (viii) setting up of model villages.

(c) The contents of women education may be somewhat different from men as women have to devote a lot of their time in homes as well. Jobs in the country are limited and hence the women education (general) can create more frustration rather than prove an asset. Hence along with general education, some course like Home Science, Agriculture, Music, etc. may also be imparted.

(d) Involvement of women at the policy-making, planning and implementation of all the programmes aimed at national reconstruction, e.g. Family Planning, Rural Planning, Rural Development, etc. This would give the impetus to women education.

(e) The share of the women in the Government jobs is very limited at present as the men presume without any justification that women cannot be effective in good administration. The State must employ more and more women if eligible and even. I would suggest that preference may be given till they are properly represented. Strangely, when one sees the University results, the girls are surpassing the boys but the same is not true in Government jobs. More and more women may also be assigned gazetted jobs of responsibility. Women may be encouraged even to take up part-time jobs.

(f) Women may be imparted education in the fields like management, marketing, etc. so that they can actively participate in cooperative organisations. They can make the cooperative movement a success.

(g) Incentive like mid-day meals, scholarships, free school uniforms, free books and study material, stipends, awards, etc. should be extended to all girls in the rural areas and urban slums.

(h) Scheme to activate the reduction of drop-outs may be planned.

It may be concluded that women education can help in nation building. Napoleon once said, "Give me good mothers, I will give you a good nation."

Illiteracy is a great obstruction in the path of development and education is the backbone of democracy. The Director-General of UNESCO has described illiteracy as "the most monstrous of all the many instances of wasted human potential which still at the present time keeps more than one-third of the human race in a state of hopelessness-below the level of modern civilisation." Therefore, in order to translate the essence of the Preamble and the Directive Principles of the State Policy enshrined in the Constitution of India in to practical life, it is imperative for us to increase the literacy rate in general and of women in particular.

10. Collecting Accurate Data for Improving Health Status of Women

A lot of difficulty has been experienced with regard to data pertaining to the status of women. Lack of data in quantity and quality would impede effective planning. The action plan suggested that there is a need to augment the information available in the field of health, family planning and nutrition through the following research studies.

1. The data available at present regarding maternal morbidity and mortality are based on hospital statistics and hence are of limited value. The system of registration of vital events is also incomplete. It is suggested that periodic special surveys be undertaken to study the pattern and, causes of mortality and morbidity among women and female children. The studies should cover different communities and different regions. Such studies would also provide information on the relative value of age-structure, parity and other "High Risk" factors in the delivery of maternity services.
2. Practical service-oriented field studies should be undertaken to assess the felt needs of the community and their attitudes towards the services offered, with a view to providing guidelines for framing health policy decision relating to the delivery of maternal care and family planning services.
3. Studies be conducted on the inter-relationship between pattern of family formation, nutrition, health and causes and incidence of sterility.
4. Studies of attitudes, beliefs and practice of traditional birth attendants (dais) should be made, to improve upon the training programme now designed for them and to obtain their greater participation in maternity and family planning services.
5. The base-line data will have to be established first against which the impact of this plan of action would be measured.[24]

The World Plan of Action has also emphasised that "A scientific and reliable data base should be established and suitable economic and social indicators urgently developed which are sensitive to the particular situation and needs of women as an integral part of the national and inter-national programme of statistics.[25]

11. Planning Women's Participation in their own Welfare

Women should themselves exert pressure to get the due benefits for their welfare. They should unite to form voluntary organisations to help themselves and ultimately the nation. It was rightly stated in the National Plan of action for women that:

> "Women voluntary organisation are best suited for motivation in the field of health, family planning and nutrition. There is therefore, every need for creating a conducive climate, so that they can render the needed service effectively."[26]

The women's voluntary organisation in the form of Mother's Club in the Republic of Korea has been quite useful in raising the status of women. By mid-1977, nearly 70,000 such clubs had been organised. The clubs provide opportunities for village women to get together to talk about health, education of children and improvement of environment. The club helps in family planning, vaccination and treatment of emergency cases. The mother's clubs are a genuinely grass-root community network, which owes little to outside administrators or planners. J.C. Abacde, in his article on "Women Power in Korea" observes that mother's clubs are helping to change age-old social attitudes towards women. He says: "The growth of women's clubs in Korea has coincided with considerable changes in social attitudes towards women. The trend is towards greater recognition between husband and wife, and more open discussion of family planning matters. It seems clear that the enhanced status of women and the growth of mothers clubs have gone hand-in-hand and are contributing significantly to the development of rural communities in Korea."[27]

Such clubs should be set-up in other countries as well. These would help mobilise voluntary resources lying idle and if not used can be a source of destruction. In the developing countries like India. voluntary organisations are urban-based and serve the urban area. These organisations must create a strong base by setting up such clubs and diffuse information to them to be passed on to the members of the community. This would bring about a socio-economic revolution and contribute substantially to modernisation and development.

The planners, policy-makers and administrators responsible for the improvement of the status of women should not be satisfied only with effective planning and policy-making, but should think of the vehicle or administrative structure through which plans and policies are to be implemented. Myron Weiner has rightly pointed out:

> "India's forte is one of the crisis management. Instincts of leadership are to cope, rather than innovate, and to work within an existing framework not only of institutions but of ideas as well."[28]

Thus, with the help of well designed administrative machinery using modern management methods we should try 10 put the policy into action.

In this implementation process, women themselves will have to be the most forceful agents for change and active participants in the development effort, wherever they have the opportunity to play a dynamic role. The contemporary social situation of women in India should not be frustrating and disheartening but should be rather challenging and it is the men and women of India, particularly the women who have to face the challenge. It has been demonstrated by the women in the field that they are as capable and efficient as men in carrying out various kinds of work and have even much more endurance for hardships than is commonly believed. All of us who are associated with the development of the country in any capacity, must renew our dedication to the cause of women which would eventually lead to national development and modernisation. Inspite of these singular policies, programmes and achievements, there are certain critical areas, which call for immediate attention, as following:

- Inadequacy of institutional mechanisms for the advancement of women.
- Persistent and institutionalised discrimination against the girl child.
- Feminisation of poverty.
- Gender blindness in macro-economic policies.
- Invisibility of women's contribution to the economy and environmental sustenance.
- Poor participation by women in decision-making structures and processes.
- Gender gaps in literacy, education and health.
- Growing trend of violence against women.
- Barriers encountered by women in accessing legal entitlements.
- Gender biased societal norms.
- Negative portrayals and perpetuation of gender stereotypes by mass media.

Prevailing ill-health among women is a major concern. These are being addressed through several programmes, such as nutrition, RH, MCH and WHD. Inspite of realisation that it is women who die in the process of reproduction, who pay the highest toll for untreated sexually transmitted disease, who bear the largest brunt of poverty, and yet who are conditioned to remain silent. Accordingly, investment in women's health bas been one of the actions identified in the Declaration for Health Development in the South-East Asia Region in the 21st Century. It has been recognised in the Declaration that since women's health is integral to development, a multi-sectoral approach would be needed through the development of partnerships with other relevant sectors.[29]

There is a need of increasing women's access to appropriate, affordable and quality health care throughout their lifespan and strengthening preventive programmes that promote women's health. Investing in women's health has strong synergistic effects on other dimensions.

We may conclude in the words of Pt. Jawaharlal Nehru: "To awaken people; it is the women who must be educated. Once she is on the move, the family moves, the village moves, the nation moves."

The Govt. of India enunciated that a holistic approach to women's health which includes both nutrition and health services will be adopted and special attention will be given to the needs of women and the girl at all stages of the life cycle. The reduction of infant mortality and maternal mortality, which are sensitive indicators of human development, is a priority concern. This policy reiterates the national A demographic goals for Infant Mortality Rate (IMR). Maternal Mortality Rate (MMR) set out in the National Population Policy, 2000. Women should have access to comprehensive, affordable and quality health-care. Measures will be adopted that take into account the reproductive rights of women to enable

CHART 13.1

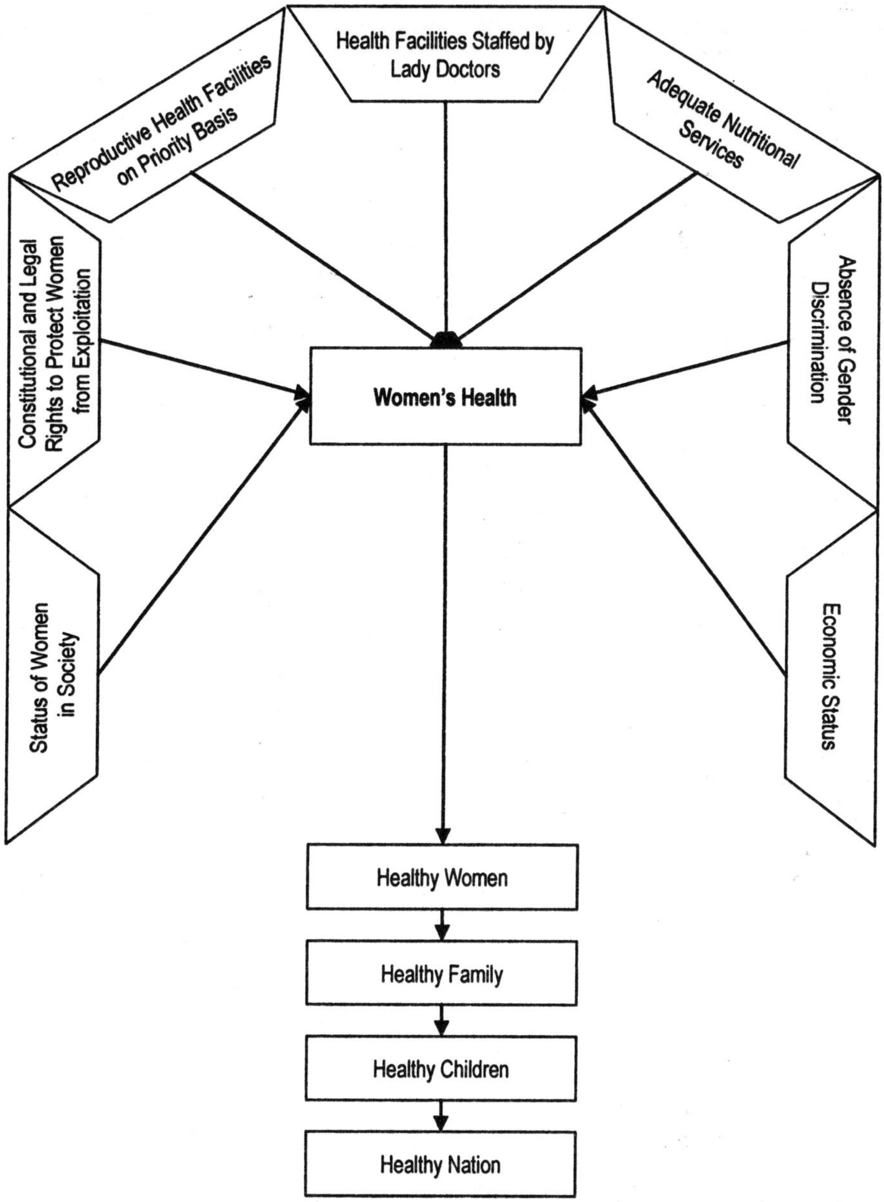

them to exercise informed choices. their vulnerability to sexual and health problems together with endemic, infectious and communicable diseases such as malaria, TB and water-borne diseases as well as hypertension and cardio-pulmonary diseases. The social, developmental and health consequences of HIV/AIDS and other sexually transmitted diseases will be tackled from a gender perspective.

In view of the high risk of mal-nutrition and disease that women face at all the three critical stages viz.. infancy and childhood, adolescent, and reproductive phase, focused attention would be paid to meeting the nutritional needs of women at all states of the life cycle. This is also important in view of the critical link between the health of adolescent girls, pregnant and lactating women, and the health of infant and young children. Special efforts will be made to tackle the problem of macro and micro-nutrient deficiencies, especially amongst pregnant and lactating women as it leads to various diseases and disabilities.

Intra-household discrimination in nutritional matters *vis-a-vis* girls and women will be sought to be ended through appropriate strategies. Widespread dissemination of nutrition education would be made to address the issues of intra-household imbalances in nutrition and the special needs of pregnant and lactating women. Women's participation will also be ensured in the planning, superintendence and delivery of the system.[30]

Notes and References

1. GOI, Deptt. of Social Welfare, Ministry of Education and Social Welfare, Towards Equity, Reports of the Committee on the Status of Women in India, Dec. 1974, New Delhi, p. 310.
2. Aleya, E.I. Bindari Hammad, Improve Our Health, Improve the World, in *World Health*, Sept. 1995, p. 4.
3. Uruali Ravyajin and Bencha, Yoddumnen Attig, Social Cost of Maternal Deptt., *World Health*, Sept. 1995., p. 19.
4. GOI, Deptt. of Social Welfare, Blue Print for Action, Points and National Plan of Action for Women, New Delhi, 1988.
5. WHO: SEARO, Regional Health Report 1998, Focus on Women, New Delhi, 1998, p. 7.
6. GOI, Planning Commission, Ninth Five Year Plan, 1997-2000, Vol. II, New Delhi, p. 22.
7. UNDP, 12th Session of the UNDP-Governing Council, 7.23 June 1971, pp. 112-14.
8. *The Tribune*, Chandigarh, June 22, 1975.
9. UN: ESCAP: Economic and Social Survey of Asia and the Pacific, 1976, Bankok, 1976, p. 56.
10. *Ibid.*, p. 56.
11. Rigveda: 2/17, p. 122.
12. Ariticle 1.5(1), Constitution of India.
13. Speccial Marriage Act, 1954: Hindu Marriage and Divorce Act, 1955, Hindu Succssion Act, 1956, The Hindu Guardianship Act, 1956.
14. Raksha Sen: Status of Women, Encyclopaedia of Social Win in India, Vol. II, p. 374.
15. UN 1974, Report on the World Social Situation, New York, 1975, p. 224.
16. Govt. of India: (Deptt. of Social Welfare) Blueprint of Plan and National Plan of Action of Women, pp. 1-2.
17. ILO: "Workers in Changing World", Preliminary Report, Chapter-6.
18. WHO: SEARO, Regional Health Report, 1998, Focus on Women, New Delhi, 1998, p. 8.

19. *Ibid.*, p. 10.
20. H.Basker, DFID, Karnataka Watershed Development Society, Karnataka, 2005, p. 95.
21. *Ibid.*
22. WHO: SEARO; Regional Health Report, 1998, Focus on Women, New Delhi, 1998, p. 13.
23. *Ibid.*, pp. 21-23.
24. *Ibid.*, p. 26.
25. World Plan of Action, Para 166.
26. National Plan of Action for Women, p. 71.
27. WHO: *World Health*, May 1979, p. 19.
28. ICSSR: Programme of Women's Studies, New Delhi, 1977, p. 10.
29. WHO: SEARO: Highlights of the World of WHO in the South-East Asia Region, 1st July 1997-30th June 1998, New Delhi, SEARO, 1998, p. 37.
30. H. Basker, Practicing Gender of the Field, DFED, 2005, p. 43.

14 CHAPTER

Youth Health and Development

One may be tempted to call this period as that of extended childhood. But the interests, attitudes, characteristics or worries of the youth do not resemble those of children. Youths even have some illnesses which are peculiar to those years or which demand special consideration at this time of life. One immediately thinks of such conditions as acne, epiphysitis, athletic injuries, growth and development disorders. the psychologic conflicts, dysmenorrhea, amenorrhea, and menorrhagia, hypertension, obesity, duodenal ulcer, cerebral palsy, epilepsy and ulcerative colitis (which are absent during childhood).

It was recognized that the policy perspectives on Adolescents in the period upto the Ninth Plan have been piece meal, with various sectors referring to this age group as part of the overall approach and no specific focus was given in most cases. The Draft National Youth Policy, 2001 provided a comprehensive overview of youth issues and concerns and comes closest to a policy for adolescents. The draft policy "Working with youth and not merely for youth" highlighted several areas of concern for adolescents and youth in the country and emphasized an intersectoral approach. The policy laid stress on providing youth with more access to the process of decision-making and implementation of these decisions. The Draft Youth Policy actually made a distinction between the age of adolescence (13-19) and the age of attainment of maturity (20-30 years). By marking the age of adolescence, the policy facilitated advocacy efforts for focus on adolescents in government programmes.

PROGRAMMES FOR ADOLESCENT GIRLS

Apart from the two schemes for Adolescent Girls implemented by the Ministry of Women and Child Development, Kishori Shakti Yojana and the Balika Samriddhi Yojana other departments were also implementing programmes for a Adolescent girls, which had a bearing on their well being and developmental opportunities. Nehru Yuva Kendras undertook activities for Health Awareness to educate and enable people to adopt health and family welfare programmes. The Ministry of Social Justice and Empowerment implemented a scheme for providing educational facilities including scholarships and hostels for tribal girls. The Department of Family Welfare provided for maternal care including safe motherhood and nutrition facilities, prevention of unwanted pregnancies, and safe abortion facilities to all women. The Directorate General of Employment and Training, Ministry of Labour facilitated registration in employment exchanges for job placements and career counselling and vocational guidance for adolescents.[1]

For many years the health of young people has been neglected because these were considered to be relatively free from diseases and less vulnerable than young children or older people. However, they are highly vulnerable to social conditions which have changed so markedly in contemporary times and their health is threatened in many ways by new lifestyles. They have to face such hazards as unwanted or too early pregnancies, sexually transmitted disease and AIDS, tobacco, alcohol and drug use, and accidents and injuries stemming in part from risk-taking behaviours. At the same time, the enormous competitive pressures for economic and educational opportunities may be leading them to more psychological disorders and even to suicidal behaviour.

But, just as hazards are unprecedented, so is the willingness of young people to give their time and energy to improving the surrounding world, and in many instances the health of their families and communities. Such commitment to social development and to promoting the health of other people is a value that deserves to be capitalised upon more than any other. It improves the well-being of young people by enhancing their self-esteem and the rewards that come from a sense of accomplishment, it offers a constructive rather than a descructive channel for their energy, and it provides an opportunity to experience healthy and responsible interactions among generations.

Young people are willing and able to take greater responsibility for their health and their lives, but whether they do so is heavily dependent on the behaviour of others. How well we listen, how well we respond to their needs, how much we trust them, how much we facilitate their action; that is the urgent choice which those who are past youth must make. The purpose must be to focus the attention of the world on how we can help youth to choose health and in so doing give health to all.[2]

WHAT IS YOUTH?

It has been defined as the period between the onset of puberty, i.e. when the person enters the gateway of manhood or womanhood; with the appearance of secondary sex characters to the completion of 24 years of age.

CHART 14.1

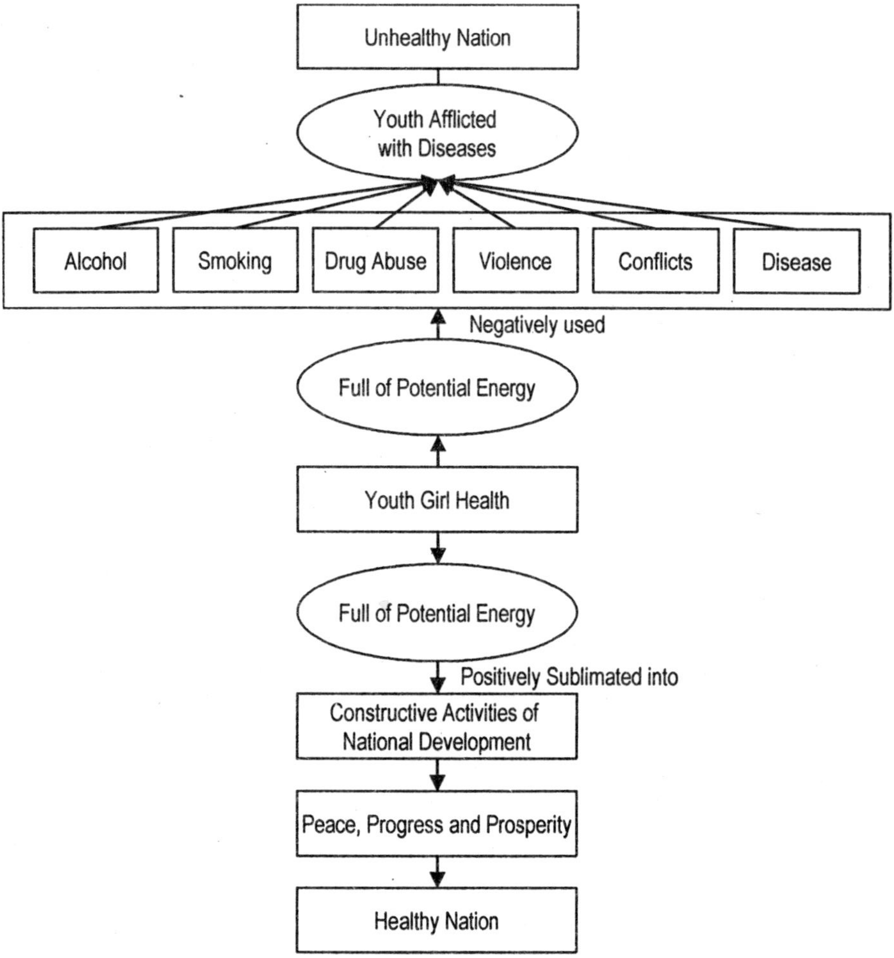

This is the period when the young person completes his physical growth (adolescence) as well as social and cultural growth (early adulthood). This is the period when he attains maturity, gets employed. may get married, develops financial and psychological autonomy, stability, wisdom, reliability, integrity and\compassion (Craig, 1980). WHO considers the period between 15-24 years age as youthood.

Young people of today are not sick human beings but they maybe made "sick" by the society. Then they become sick of life, and in my opinion this creates physical and mental health problems. The period from 14 to 24 is the age of adolescence and young adulthood when there are physical and mental changes? Nagging, scolding, yelling and abusing are not the methods of helping a young person, who needs to be understood, recognised, listened to and encouraged towards a healthy sharing of human relations with parents, teachers and society.

Without all this, young people get sick, confused and angry, start to dislike parents and others, feel lonely and aimless, and eventually may become physically and mentally sick. Some take to drugs, alcoholism and sex-and-violence. We strongly feel that youths must be saved and we need teamwork to help them.

Mother Nature has given us a miraculous and tremendous system to protect ourselves; let us take care of this human system to the best of our ability, and with actions not just words. Youth is not a stage in life that deserves to be destroyed but a time that should be treasured as the jewel of society.[3]

In the space of a few decades, there have been remarkable reductions in morbidity and mortality due to infectious and parasitic diseases in most developing countries in all regions of the world. However, other threats to health in the form of the so-called "Western degenerative" or "lifestyle" diseases are emerging at rates that far outstrips what would be expected from the fact that people are living longer. In many developing nations, already beset with economic, social and other health problems, the rate of heart disease, diabetes and hypertension are as high as or even higher than in major developed nations. These chronic diseases impose a destructive drain on communities through their association with sickness and premature death.

Primary preventive activities will focus on behavioural and structural changes related to smoking, healthy nutrition, and levels of physical activity in the community. Secondary prevention target include improved case detection, expanded health education services, and an upgrading of follow-up and rehabilitation facilities.[4]

HOW DO THEY DIFFER FROM CHILDREN?

They differ in their interests, talk, dress, daily life; in their needs and worries; in their size and shape. 'They do not chase cats or play dolls any more, and they are not yet concerned with housekeeping. In contrast, they are concerned about becoming sexually mature, about popularity among peers and the members of opposite sex. They want recognition, and they relentlessly seek the approval and applause of their own peer group.

Anything which keeps them from active participation will be resented and, if possible, ignored. In childhood sex mattered little; now, in one form or another, it is just on their minds. How to reconcile this drive and their behaviour. Their growth and development may now become a source of anxiety. How tall, how bearded, how full-bosomed, now are very important. To acquire independence is a paramount matter for them and they vacillate both in their desire and ability to do without their parents. Thus, four major developmental tasks are accomplished during this period. The first is to become emancipated from parents; the second is to acquire an academic degree or a professional skill for future economic independence; the third is to learn heterosexual role; and the fourth is to acquire stable, and positive adult self-identify (Gallagher, 1976).

South-East Asia Regional office of world health organisation in its report of Regional Health Report, 1998 (Focus on women) suggests the additional problems of female youth. With the onset of puberty and with learning new ways of behaving that may lead to experimentation with sex, drugs and alcohol, adolescents find themselves exposed to a host of factors which can adversely affect. Maternal mortality is estimated to be three to four times higher in adolescent women than in adults, and pregnancy-related complications are the leading cause of mortality among adolescent girls in many countries. In addition, infants born to adolescents are more likely to have low, birth weight, to be premature, to be injured at birth, or to be stillborn.

Adolescent girls are both biologically and socially more vulnerable to sexually transmitted diseases (STDs) including HIV infection. Unwanted pregnancies in single adolescents are of increasing concern and could lead adolescent girls to seek abortions. Often such abortions are sought from illegal and unsafe sources and may lead to serious complications and even death.

CHARACTERISTICS

Youth is a time of great and rapid physical growth: this brings with it not only increased nutritional needs but also the emotional needs and the needs to adjust to new attitudes and responsibilities. Many youths, suddenly presented with a large body, handle it awkwardly, are self-conscious about it and wish to behave as though they were adults. Others in their anxiety seek attention in socially inept or even in unacceptable ways.

Youth represents a tremendous potential for society. Provided it is channeled in the right direction, the enthusiasm, initiative and idealism of young people can help others, including the elderly, the handicapped, the poor, and in so doing can create a hapapier and more balanced society. Young people's participation in community activities—particularly in primary health care is a key precondition for Health for all. The year of the healthiest third of the world's population—those who have survived the risks of childhood diseases and who are not yet threatened by the ills of mature years and old age. Their health is a key element for development. It requires special services that young people themselves must demand. As they enter the reproductive age, they need services that can guard them against the risks of sexually transmined diseases. And they must demand access of family planning services so that they can make their own choices about marriage and parenthood.[5]

On World Health Day, 1985, in the drive towards health for all, every community should take stock of its youthful resource and nurture it for all its promise. The joyous and explosive energy of youth and its natural curiosity are there to be exploited to build a better world.[6]

CHALLENGES OF HEALTH FACED BY YOUTH

Unprecedented challenges face the youth of today, said Dr. Hiroshi Nakajima, Director-Genera I of WHO, in a message to the World Assembly of Youth. And he added that young people may be given opportunities "to demonstrate their creativity, energy and commitment to solving their own problems and helping to build a healthy future for the entire community in which they live."

1. Sexual Needs Lead them to Sexually Transmitted Diseases and Conception: Need of Advance Planning

Young girls today, generally present an appearance of blooming health. But in the domain of sexual relationships, a whole series of fearful choices may lie before the growing girl. Whatever choice she makes demands a high degree of maturity, and the risks of making an error of judgement are all the greater if she is at a younger age, or is less knowledgeable about sexual matters. It is time for the health professionals to show sufficient imagination and initiative to ensure that adolescents prefer contraception to abortion; and it is up to medical science to discover vaccines against syphilis and gonorrhoea and thus make a significant contribution towards the battle to control these diseases.[7]

2. Search far Identity: Need of Providing Special Status

It is not altogether surprising then, that a so-called generation gap should have emerged to further emphasize the marginality of the adolescent from the core of the social framework or that adolescence shows an inclination, albeit an unnecessary one, to become a problem period of growth. It is, after all, this fact that has contributed to adolescence attracting the attention and concern that it has today. But it is perhaps ironic that—in an age when so much is known about the needs of human beings with respect to personal and social life—more is not actually done to structure the context in which adolescents function in such a way that meaning and identity would be easier to define and, once defined, would show more consistency with the society concerned.

3. Drug Abuse: Need of Change in the Habits and Practices of Community

The psychic craving for any chemical substance licit or illicit, which results in an individual's physical, mental, emotional or social impairment is called drug abuse. The problem is not the drug, but the impulse to use the same. All the drugs of addiction are harmful drugs. Once one admits anyone into his life, one becomes completely dependent on the drug and hence becomes its slave. With increasing surrender to chemical comfort and dependence with resultant rise in Crime, with attendant social degradation, is causing anxiety in developing countries like India.

According to a recent study 50 million people in the world have become hopelessly addicted to drugs. According to an estimate of WHO 30 million people smoke marijuana, 7.8 million use cocaine, 1.7 million consume opium, 7 lac heroin and the remaining other chemicals. Even in India it is catching up, where it has been glorified by the wandering hippies. While the possibility of acute cardiac arrest, asphyxiation, accidents and organ failure are reason enough to cause alarm, recent findings also suggest that chronic uses may suffer neuropsychological impairments.

Why Drug Abuse?

Adolescents may use drugs either for experimentation or as a method of dealing with stress. It is usually a group activity. Problems with family, school, various relationships; chronic anxiety and depression; poor self-esteem; ready access to drugs; parents as models (who frequently use drugs including alcohol) are the factors that predispose to drug abuse.

The young man or young girl will initially deny his drug-taking behaviour but eventually will become out-spoken about his habit. Various demanding activities such as school work and jobs will deteriorate. Secrecy and privacy, a part of any adolescent's normal development, will increase, and signs of intoxication may be seen. Money and ornaments may start disappearing from the home, and materials like glue-soaked rags, pills, needles, syringes may be found hidden. Parents often fail to react until matters are out of control. Drug-abusing behaviour may be directly related to the abuser's family and the issues of separation and individuation. However, parents should not over-react and they should remain available to the adolescent despite denial and often rejection by the adolescent. Activities undertaken in an effort to prevent drug problems are often boring, irrelevant, impractical and ineffective. Why do they fail? Boring approaches are mostly those which set out to warn young people of the alleged dangers, harm or evil of drugs, coupled with recommendations to be good boys and girls. Young people tend to respond much better to approaches that involve them and allow them an active role.

We have to try to change the beliefs, rituals and habits that now make drug use appear pleasurable, glamorous or special. There has to be a change in the community's perception of drug use too. If the community begins to see it as rather a flat, boring and silly experience, the efforts can be successful. Eventually, the community can hope to reach the stage where even habitual users recognize that they are stuck in a fixed and limited routine, and therefore less able to enjoy real life.[8] We need to educate communities, particularly the young, on how to cope in a society where drugs proliferate. This is only possible if political leaders, law-makers and society at large recognize the many dimensions of the drug problem and all work together to support the response of health professionals.[9]

We have to take more care of drug abuse in women. In most countries, psychoactive substance use has traditionally been a problem affecting males. But with the rapid social and economic changes over the past few decades, there has been a dramatic increase in this problem among women in both developed and developing countries.

Women and men respond differently to alcohol and drugs, women having a lower tolerance to most substances. Since many women substance users are of child-bearing age, the effects on the developing fetus are of serious concern. Especially women and their partners should be made aware of the risks when alcohol, tobacco and other legal substances are used during pregnancy. The use of psychoactive substances facilitates the spread of HIV infection through sexual contact or needles shared by injecting drug users. In many societies drug use, drug dealing and prostitution are closely connected; consequently the women involved are at high risk of infection with HIV and other sexually transmitted diseases. To deal with these problems the focus must be on both men and women, taking into account the effects on the family and children. Women who do not use substances can suffer from their use by a partner or other family members; for instance, a family's income for food, health care and education may be spent on alcohol, tobacco or drugs. Domestic violence is often associated with alcohol or other drug use.

At all levels—international, national and local the issue of women and substance use is increasingly being recognized, as is the important role of women. Women assume the major responsibility for health care within the family, and are often concerned about the social and health situation in the community. Thus, women, especially if training and education can be provided, are instrumental in preventing substance abuse and its potential harmful consequences.[10]

4. Lifestyles Glamour: Need of Education

Unwise lifestyles pose the biggest threats to young people's health. Innovative judgements, a tendency to show off, or the desire to keep up with their feeling that these incline them towards risk-taking behaviour. This may include experimenting with dangerous substances like alcohol or drugs, driving too fast on the highway, or simply defying adult society.[11]

In many cases, the cigarette is the very first contact young people have with the lifestyles of adulthood. This first encounter often occurs at a very early age: by the time they reach their teens, they may already be unable to break the smoking habit. It is vital that they should be aware of the short-term and long-term risks that smoking represents to their health.

Fitness is a lifestyle, it does not require much time. To protect against physical deterioration, you have to adopt an exercise progranune, spending 20-30 minutes exclusively in the morning or evening. In addition to that one can perform exercises like jogging, yoga asanas, stretching, etc. Whenever there are a few minutes free waiting for a bus, during recess, at mid-day tea, soon after you have finished your study or office work. There are exercises to perform while travelling in a car, sitting in your study chair or just waiting to receive your guest. Then one has to be honest to oneself in keeping an account of the exercises input. Having a leisurely stroll for 10-

15 minutes may be just an apology for exercise but it is still better than not taking any exercise at all. In the race for health everyone is a winner was theme of WHO in 1986. So one has to be aware of the importance of fitness first of all and then one has to be on the job religiously. Straight back and flat tummy (and not a protruding one) can be the envy of your friends. Exercise programme should be made compulsory in every school, college, office, factory and other places to improve the performance in study, business, etc.

To reassure the youth and to evaluate his potential to undertake fitness programme it would be necessary if his growth and development, viz. physical, sexual and emotional is monitored under medical supervision (Frarco Columbus, 1982).

5. Use of Risk-taking: Need of Education

The risk destroying their most important assets; the health and physical fitness through laziness and lack of exercise, rash driving and traffic accidents. suicide or attempts to suicide, slow suicide through the use of alcohol, smoking, drug abuse, excessive intake of tea and coffee, unprotected sexual encounters, sexual misadventures like rape, sexually transmitted diseases, teenager pregnancies and abortions or unwed child births. The ill-effects on their health can extend far into later life. Accidents are estimated to disable permanently three times as many as they kill, smoking and alcohol can store epidemics of respiratory diseases, liver damage and cancer. Teenager pregnancy can kill mother or child or else leave them physically and mentally handicapped. Needless to conclude that in some countries youth is the only age-group in which mortality and morbidity rate is rising, due to these ills of modern society. Alcohol and unemployment is behind alarmingly large number of deaths through accidents and suicide (Jerome, 1980).

We need, for a start, to be clearer about levels of drinking and situations in which drinking causes harm, and to recognize that some alcohol consumption will indeed take place, among young people. Then it may be much easier to devise strategies. We may try to provide alternatives to alcohol and promote healthy lifestyles, of which avoiding alcohol abuse may be a part. Treatment is also important, in the sense that early intervention may prevent problems which, if ignored, could become more serious later in life. Legislation may also be used to control young people's opportunities for drinking, and an important measure may be to control the advertising of alcoholic drinks. Young people themselves should be made aware of the problems related to alcohol and participate in programmes to reduce them. With alcohol, little may be too much. The instinct of risk-taking is natural for the youth. But if youth energy could be guided to positive form of risk-tackling and violence such as mountaineering, swimming, competitive games, NSS, NCC, and forces, fighting of natural calamities like floods, famine, earthquakes, epidemics of disease, environmental control, social evils like dowry and child marriages, learning of various arts such as painting, titing, public speaking, and their emotions sublimated to creative arts, gainful employment and socially useful activities, they could be made a resource. Unfortunately, most of our youth population, which is about 1/3rd of our total population remains unutilized, why?

6. Traffic Accidents and Violent Behaviour: Need of Review

A leading cause of mortality and morbidity among the youth is the traffic accidents, for which the well-established vogue for mopeds and motor-cycles coupled with alcoholism, psychological stress and speed are largely to blame. The mortality rate of boys in such accidents is much higher than in girls. But should we accept this loss of human life as inevitable, as a price of speed? Are we vitally concerned with the fact that every year around a quarter of a million people must die and a millions must be injured. Quite apart for the loss in human terms, the financial costs involved are incalculable. We need not accept massive death and injury as the price of progress. Transport practices which have been developed elsewhere are not to be super-imposed on the developing countries where the conditions are different. Following the guidance of WHO, we can stop categorising traffic death and injury as a transportation problem. We can look at it for what it truly is a major public health problem. We can attack it—through the entire community—as we would do, if it were cholera, typhoid, plague, yellow fever, enteritis or birth defects (Paul, 1982).

What is sure is that aggression and violence intrude more and more into our daily lives; the instantaneous and world-wide coverage by the media makes sure of that. Another certainty, which daily observation and statistics confirm, is that adolescents and young adults more than any other age group are at one and the same time the instigators of violent behaviour and its victims, in the industrialized world, and in many Third World countries. Violent death which includes suicide, murder and accidental death—heads the list of causes of death among those aged 15 to 24, especially young men.[12]

7. Unemployment: Need of Creating Jobs

Today, most of the problems mentioned above inmate from the fact that the youth is not productively employed. We must use their potential for development.

8. Loose Control of Social Values: Need of Strengthening

Young people are not following the social norms, values and traditions, resulting in alienation. There is no control over them by the senior family members. Family health is more than just the sum total of the health of all its members. It also involves interpersonal relations and the social environment.

Throughout history the family has played a unique and fundamental role. With relatively few exceptions, it has provided, for example, the most effective and socially appropriate milieu in which procreation could take place, and in which the physical and emotional development of children could be ensured.[13] Through the routine responsibilities and interaction of its adult members, it has constituted an environment in which offspring could be gradually exposed to, and instructed in the values and customs considered necessary for integration into society; at the same time it has provided a source of informal control over their activities. For older members it has represented a source of emotional and economic support as they themselves pass through their life phases.

CONCLUSION

Adolescence is long—but it can be treated. Read a recent headline in a health magazine. The article added: "They eat at any time, they behave badly, they have pimples or puppy-fat, they are irritable and irritating, and their symptoms are so special that nowadays there are 'adolescentologists.' One thing is certain: during this period of their life, young people are passing through a physical and psychological crisis from which they must emerge victorious, once they have mastered their immediate problems and adopted for the future ways of life and habits of physical and mental hygiene which should ensure their full subsequent development.

All this makes it necessary to communicate successfully with them. At that age, human contacts are extremely important, and those with the task of informing and educating have to respect this concept of a homogeneous group in a particular social class. The constant refrain is: "For us young people today; things are not the same as they were for you adults in your time"

Consequently, lectures on morals or wisdom will not help adults to penetrate this closed society. The health of youth needs some to show young people whom to be loyal to, somebody of good standing and good character. Then the fruits of loyalty will be love and the fruit of love will be obedience. Everybody would like to leave the world a better place than he or she found it.

Every homeless child in the street is the product of a broken home, and the fact of being homeless is a reflection on his or her family background. When we look at the special health problems of the young, the mortality rates for accidents. The problem of sexually transmitted diseases, and the various nutritional, psychological, recreational and health service needs of the adolescent, it must not be forgotten that all these are intimately related to the fundamental, social and cultural context in which the adolescent lives, the adolescent and youth population in the country is increasing. There are at the moment no specific health or nutrition programmes to address the problem of this important group. In the past teen age pregnancy and its attendant problem were the main focus of attention. Over the years there is a significant rise in age at marriage. Efforts to educate the girl, her parents and the community to delay marriage will continue to receive attention during the Ninth Plan. There is an urgent need to mount programmes for early detection and effective management of nutritional (under-nutrition, anaemia) and health (infections, menstural disorders) problem in adolescent girls, health and nutrition education to this group is essential. Adolescent pregnancies are still common in India. Adolescent girls are at high risk of anaemia, HDP and infections. They will receive appropriate care throughout pregnancy and institutional delivery to ensure safety of both the mother and the baby.[14]

The General Assembly of the United Nations recognised the "...profound importance of the direct participation of youth in shaping the future. ..." In the WHO global strategy for Health for All by the Year 2000, one of the key factors to reaching this goal is described as "community involvement in shaping its own health: and socio-economic future, including mass involvement of women, men and youth, ..."

It is obvious, then, that there is an explicit appeal to young people to be actively involved in all aspects of development, of which health is an integral part. However simple this concept may be, the implications are multiple and complex. An essential prerequisite is the political and social acceptance of young people as equal and responsible partners in the process of development. But circumstances differ, not only from country to country, but even from locality to locality, and there can be no blueprint for a plan of action that will have universal application.

Before a dam was constructed on Satluj River, at Bhakra, the water resource was not only wasted, but it resulted in floods, leading to loss of life and property. The same is true for youth resource. The idle youth is not only a waste, but also the tide of this unutilized energy can result in negative development wasted in the field of health and economy. The youth can be our best resource if they are healthy and if their joyous energy is channelised for building a better society. The potential energy of youth has to be converted into kinetic energy with understanding, support and technological know and its use should be made to build modern India. Much needs to be done both for and by young people. It is not sufficient merely to have activities directed towards youth. If the aims and objectives of International Youth Year, 1985, and of the WHO Global Strategy for Health for All by the year 2000 are to be achieved, serious efforts of collaborative action by everyone—young and old—are needed. The youngsters of today, with their capabilities. Energy and commitment, represent a vital resource; they must be partners in the quest for a just future.

It was recognized that the policy perspectives on Adolescents in the period up to the Ninth Plan have been piecemeal, with various sectors referring to this age group as part of the overall approach, and no specific focus was given in most cases. The National Policy on Education (1986, modified in 1992) lays emphais on the eradication of illiteracy especially for the 15-35 age group and universalization of primary education and the Adolescents age group are considered as part of children to be provided

CHART 14.2

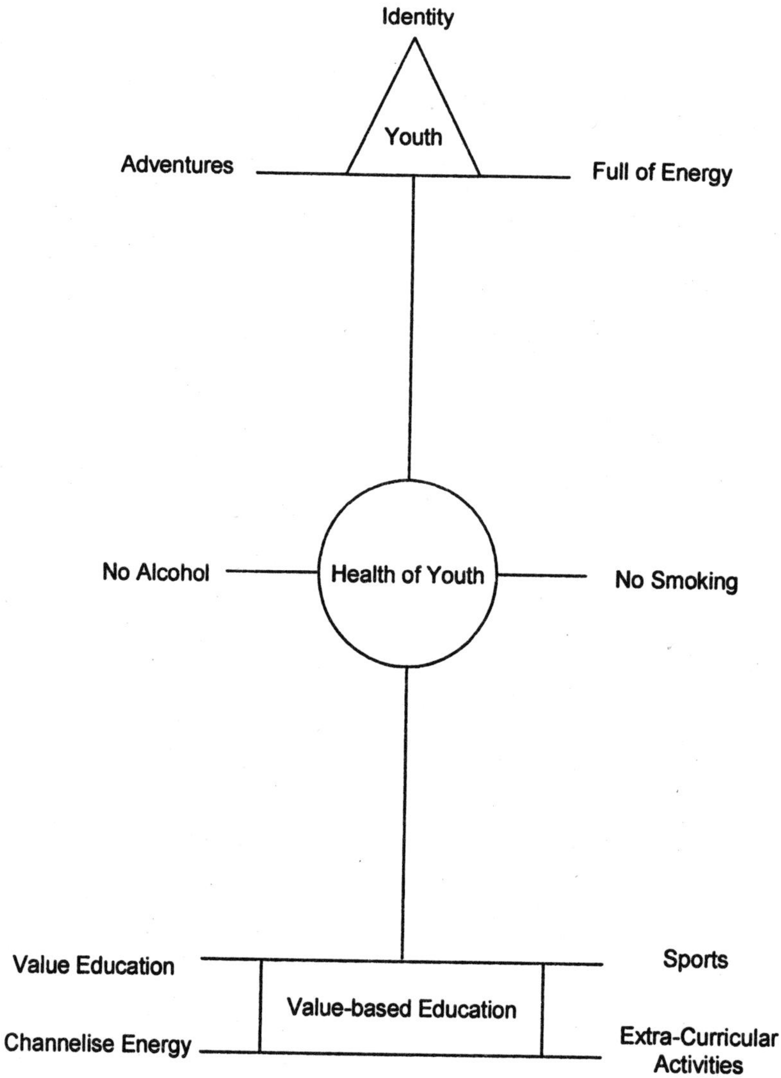

primary education and adults who are participants of adult literacy activity. To some extent, the employment-related educational needs are addressed through vocational education at the higher secondary level. The policy also talks about meeting the non-formal and need-based vocational needs of youth (15-35 years). "Education for Women's Equality" has special relevance for education programme for adolescents. Mahila Samakhya Progarmme which aims inter alia, at ensuring equal access to educational facilities for adolescent girls and young women responded to a growing demand from adolescent girls for opportunities to complete formal education and also acquire leadership and vocational skills.[15]

Notes and References

1. Ministry of Women and Child Development, Sub-Group on Child Protection, For the Eleventh Five Year Plan, 2007-12, pp. 77-78.
2. Herbert Friedman, Youth of Today, in *World Health*, 3/89, March, 1989, p.3
3. Mauritius Non-Communicable Disease Study Group, Lifestyle Hazards, *World Health*, June 1989, pp. 18-19.
4. *Ibid.*
5. *World Health*, Janury-February, 1985, pp. 10-17.
6. Dr. H. Mahler, Healthy Youth Our best Resource in *World Health*, January-February 1985, p. 5.
7. Sub-Group Report on Child Protection, 11th Five Year Plan (2007-2012), Ministry of Women and Child Development.
8. *Ibid.*, pp. 98-99
9. Oblivier Jeannert, That Awakened Age, in Worlth Health, Dec. 1976, p. 11.
10. Manual Carballo, Search for Identity, in *World Health*, Dec. 1976, p. 9.
11. Diyanath Samarasinghe, Removing the Glamour, in *World Health*, July-August, 1995, p. 5.
12. Dr. Hiroshi Nakajama, Substance use is a Health Issue, in *World Health*, July-Aug., 1995, p. 3.
13. Pia Bergendahi and Lee Nath, HSW, Women and Substance Abuse, in *World Health*, July-Aug. 1995, p. 12.
14. *Ibid.*
15. Ministry of Women and Child Development, Sub-Group Report on Child Protection, For the Eleventh Five Year Plan, 2007-12, pp. 76-77.

15

CHAPTER

Children's Health Development and Protection

Child development is integral to over all socio-economic development of a nation. "Children's health-tomorrow's wealth" the theme affords an occasion to convey to a world-wide audience the message that children are a priceless resource, and that any nation which neglects them would do so at its peril. World Health Day, 1984 thus highlighted the basic truth that we must all safeguard the healthy minds and bodies of the world's children, not only as a key factor in attaining health for all by the year 2000, but also as a major part of each nation's health in the twenty-first century.[1]

There is an old saying, attributed to Jesuit teachers: "Give me the child for seven years and 1 will give you the man for life." Regarding the welfare of the children, Mahatma Gandhi said very rightly that Prayer of the Nation is child's smile and fortune. Pt. Jawaharlal Nehru said: "Nation marches on the tiny feet of the children." IYC slogan of India was Happy Child is Nation's Pride. Children's health is linked to many inter-sectoral factors, e.g. health, environmental and nutritional needs, social and psychological needs, educational needs and special attention of girl child. (Chart 15.1) The potential in the children can be harnessed and kindled if the developing countries provide congenial socio-economic environment for their children to develop sound personality so that they in turn can contribute for accelerating the development of the country. This would bring in dynamism and promote the socio-economic development of the country. Thus, there is a need of planning for the needs of children for the better future of mankind.

Despite the overwhelming needs for orienting planning towards children, it is a sad fact that the needs of the children have been ignored or shelved in the plans and policies of the developing countries. One of the

Chart 15.1

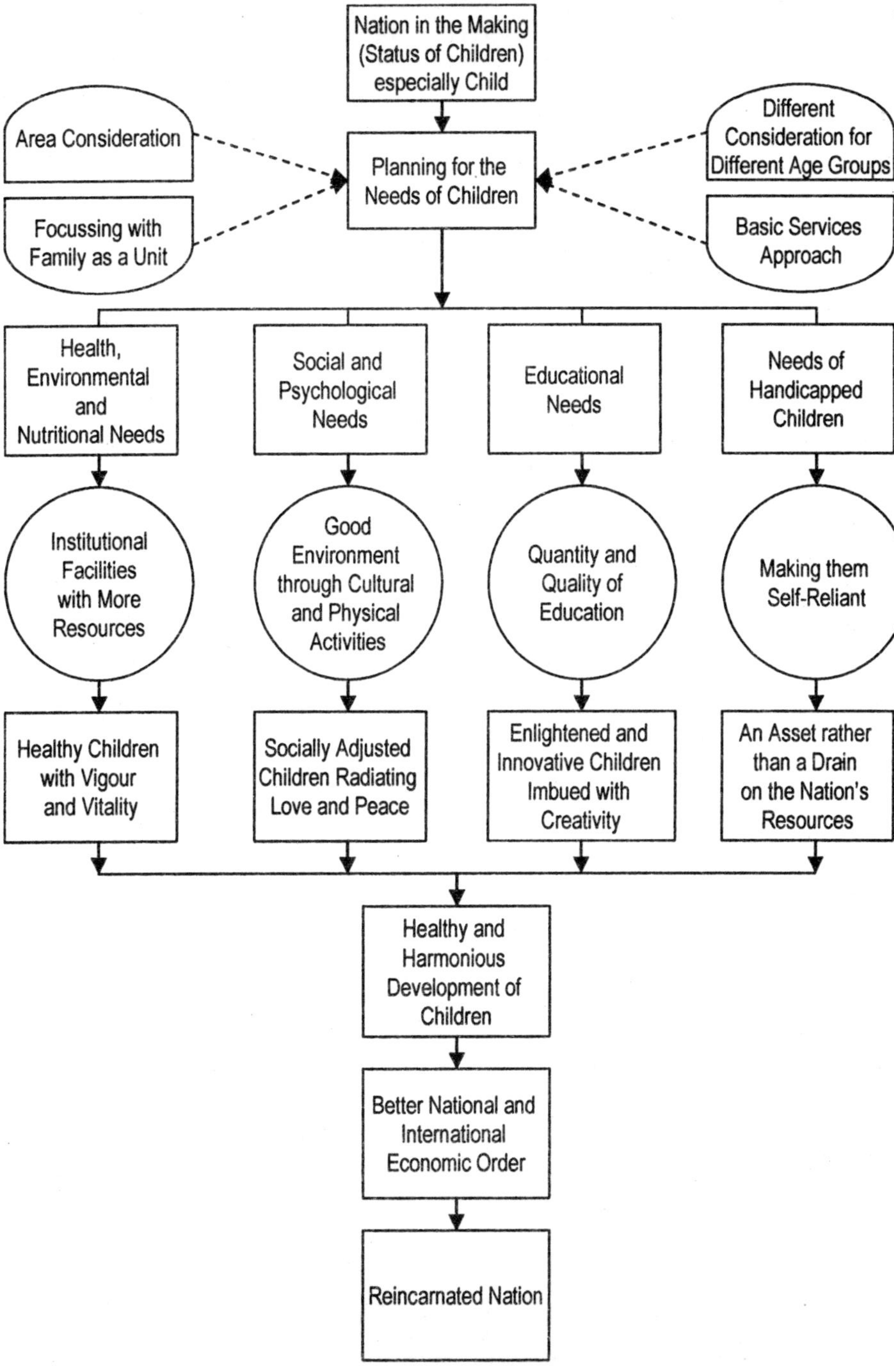
Nation in the Making (Status of Children) especially Child
Area Consideration
Focussing with Family as a Unit
Planning for the Needs of Children
Different Consideration for Different Age Groups
Basic Services Approach
Health, Environmental and Nutritional Needs
Social and Psychological Needs
Educational Needs
Needs of Handicapped Children
Institutional Facilities with More Resources
Good Environment through Cultural and Physical Activities
Quantity and Quality of Education
Making them Self-Reliant
Healthy Children with Vigour and Vitality
Socially Adjusted Children Radiating Love and Peace
Enlightened and Innovative Children Imbued with Creativity
An Asset rather than a Drain on the Nation's Resources
Healthy and Harmonious Development of Children
Better National and International Economic Order
Reincarnated Nation

important reasons for this neglect is that the children are considered a weak and vulnerable group. In the words of Gabrietla Mistral, the Noble Laurate of Chile: We are guilty of many errors and many faults, but our worst crime is abandoning our children, neglecting the fountain of life. Many of the things we need can wait, the child cannot. To him we cannot answer "tomorrow." His name is "today."

Hence top priority should be given to planning for the needs of children. An oriental proverb rightly stresses the need of planning for children.

> "If you are planning one year ahead, sow rice, if you are planning five years ahead, plant trees, but if you are planning for a generation ahead, you must grow men."

To quote Dr. H. Mahler: "There is a need to understand that while the task of safeguarding the health of today's children is urgent, it cannot be accomplished through conventional means. What is required is a radical new approach emphasizing the just distribution of health resources, mobilisation of national and international resources, imaginative use of traditional medicine and its practitioners, research and development of appropriate health technologies relevant to local needs; and close cooperation among the nations of the world."

The newly created Ministry of Women and Child Development has taken charge of child protection programmes transferred from the Ministry of Social Justice and Empowerment. In addition to its nodal function on all policy issues related to children and the implementation and monitoring of CRC, the Ministry now has the primary responsibility for planning, implementation and coordination of child protection services. However, child protection is not the exclusive responsibility of the MWCD; other sectors have a vital role to play. The Ministry is therefore looking at child protection holistically and examining how to rationalize programmes and approaches for creating a strong protective environment for children, diversify and provide essential services for children, mobilize inter-sectoral response for strengthening child protection and set standards for care and services.

The Constitution of India recognizes the vulnerable position of children and their right to protection. Therefore, following the doctrine of protective discrimination, it guarantees in Article 15 special attention to children through necessary and special laws and policies that safeguard their rights. The right to equality, protection of life and personal liberty and the right against exploitation enshrined in Articles 14, 15, 16, 17, 21, 23 and 24 further reiterate India's commitment to the protection, safety, security and well-being of all its people, including children.

The Chapter on Directive Principles of State Policy in the Constitution of India enjoins that the State shall, in particular, direct its policy towards securing:

(1) that the health and strength of workers, men and women, and the tender age of children are not abused and the citizens are not forced by economic necessity to enter avocations unsuited to their age or strength;
(2) those children are given opportunities and facilities to develop in a healthy manner and in conditions of freedom and dignity and childhood and youth are protected against exploitation and against moral and material abandonment; and
(3) that the State shall endeavour to provide early childhood care and education to all children until they complete the age of six years.

India's National Policy for Children 1974 provides a framework for policy and planning for children. In 1992 India acceded to the United Nations Convention on the Rights of the Child (UNCRC), committing to take measures to ensure the survival, protection, participation and development of its children. At the World Summit for Children in 1990 India adopted the World Declaration for Survival, Protection and Development of children. Additionally, India ratified the Optional Protocols on the Use of Children in Armed Conflict and the Sale of Children, Child Prostitution, and Child Pornography in 2005. It also reaffirmed its commitment to children by adopting the Millennium Development Goals and a World Fit for Children. Moving towards its commitments, the Government of India introduced the national Charter for Children, 2003, which stipulates the duties for the State and community, followed by a National Plan of Action for Children in 2005, which ensures collective commitment and action towards the survival, development, protection and participation of children by all sectors and levels of government and civil society. India has also signed the SAARC Convention on Combating Trafficking and Commercial Sexual Exploitation of Women and Children, 2002, the SAARC Convention on Regional Arrangements for the Promotion of Child Welfare in South Asia, 2002 and is signatory to the SAARC Decade on the Rights of the Child, 2001-10, decided in Rawalpindi Resolution on Children in South Asia in 1996.

The National Common Minimum Programme specifically states that, "The UPA government will protect the rights of children, strive for elimination of child labour, ensure facilities for schooling and extend special care to the girl child."

Despite such clear commitment to child protection enshrined in the Constitution of India and the UN Convention on the Rights of the Child ratified by India in 1992, and the two Optional Protocols ratified in 2005, and the various national and international commitments made children continue to remain vulnerable with the number of those needing care and protection is ever increasing.

More than decades of planned development has indeed failed to address the critical issue of 'Child Protection'. And in these many years a lot has changed in the lives of people, particularly children that calls for *a re-examination of the understanding of 'Child Protection' itself.*[2]

India is home to more than one billion people, of whom one-third are children under 18 years of age. Although we have made considerable economic and social progress since independence, a large number of our children are still living in inhuman conditions. Despite clear commitments to child protection enshrined in the Constitution of India and the UN Convention on the Rights of the Child ratified by India in 1992, and the two Optional Protocols ratified in 2005, and the various national and international commitments made, children continue to remain vulnerable with the number of those needing care and protection is ever increasing in the country.[3]

TABLE 15.1

Crime Against Children

Crime Head	*Year*					
	1999	*2000*	*2001*	*2002*	*2003*	*2004*
Foeticide	61	91	55	84	57	86
Infanticide	87	104	133	115	103	102
Murder of Children	NA	NA	1042	1073	1212	1304
Kidnapping and Abduction	6882	6561	5589	1986	2571	3196
Kindapping and Abandonment	593	660	678	644	722	715
Procuration of Minor girls	172	147	138	124	171	715
Buying of Girls for prostitution	5	53	6	9	24	21
Selling of girls for prostitution	13	15	8	5	36	19
Child Marriage Restraint Act	58	92	85	113	63	93
Immoral Trafflicking Prevention Act	75	82	125	49	48	47
Child Rape	3153	3132	2113	2532	2949	3542
NDPS Act	9	16	52	56	62	54
Importation of girls	1	64	114	76	46	89
Grand Total	11,109	11,018	10138	6,686	8,064	9,473

Source: Crime in India, 1999-2004, National Crime Records Bureau.

The Department of Health and Family Welfare is implementing several important programmes and schemes to address the issue of high infant and child mortality in the country. Notable amongst these are the (i) Universal immunization programme (UIP), where immunization of children is carried out against six vaccine preventable diseases, (ii) control of deaths due to acute respiratory infections (ARI), (iii) control of diarrhoeal diseases, and (iv) provision of essential newborn care to address the issue of the neonates. In addition to the above, the Department implements programmes for the prevention and treatment of two micronutrient deficiencies relating to (i) Vitamin A, and (ii) iron.

Under the second phase of the RCH programme, the activities being undertaken to achieve the goals of the NRHM are:

- (i) Integrated management of Neonatal and Childhood Illnesses (IMNCI),
- (ii) Home-based Newborn Care (HBNC),
- (iii) Promotion of breastfeeding and complementary feeding,
- (iv) Control of deaths due to Acute Respiratory Infections (ARI),
- (v) Control of deaths due to diarrhoea diseases,
- (vi) Supplementation with micronutrients: Vitamin A and iron, and
- (vii) Universal Immunization Programme (UIP).[4]

ANAEMIA AMONG CHILDREN

Iron Deficiency anaemia is widely prevalent in young children. The National Family Health Survey-II (1998-99) revealed that 74.3% children under the age of 3 years were anemic. There is a marginal difference in the prevalence in the rural and urban areas. While 75.3% of rural children were found to be anemic, the prevalence in urban children was 70.8%. The prevalence ranges from 43% in Kerala to 85.7% in Arunachal Pradesh. (NFHS III results are due out shortly)

Under the National Programme iron folic tablets containing 20 mg of elemental iron and 0.1 mg of folic acid are provided at the sub-centre level. Current programme guidelines instruct health workers to provide 100 tablets to children clinically found to be anemic.

PROMOTION OF INFANT AND YOUNG CHILD FEEDING (IYCF)

A Breastfeeding Partnership involving all the key partners has been formed under the auspices of the Hon'ble MOS. Revival of the Breastfeeding Hospital initiative has been approved and implementation shall be initiated.

BORDER DISTRICT CLUSTER STRATEGY

This is an initiative being implemented by UNICEF in 49 districts from 2003-07. It aims at providing focused interventions for reducing the infant mortality and maternal mortality rates by at least 50% over the next two to three years in the selected 49 districts in 16 States.

Under this project districts are being supported for:

- Development and training of Health and Nutrition Teams,
- Physical up-gradation of sub-centres and primary health centres,
- Additional supply of equipment and drugs,
- Organisation of outreach sessions,
- Support for mobility of staff,
- Development of local IEC for social mobilization,
- Training of medical officers, and
- Up-gradation of First Referral Units and filling of vacant posts through contractual appointments would be allowed.

This is a UNICEF assisted activity. UNICEF directly releases funds to the States.

IMMUNIZATION PROGRAMME

Immunization programme is one of the key interventions for protection of children from life threatening conditions, which are preventable. Immunization Programme in India was introduced in 1978 as Expanded Programme on Immunization. This gained momentum in 1985 as Universal Immunization Programme (UIP) and implemented in phased manner to cover all districts in the country by 1989-90. UIP become a part of Child Survival and Safe Motherhood Programme in 1992. Since 1997, immunization activities have been an important component of National Reproductive and Child Health Programme.

Under the Immunization programme vaccines are given to infants and pregnant women for controlling vaccine preventable diseases namely childhood Tuberculosis, Diphtheria, Pertussis, Poliomyelitis, Measles and Neonatal Tetanus. Except polio vaccine, which is administered orally all other vaccines are given as Injections.

To strengthen routine immunization Govt. of India under NRHM has planned the following which is a part of the State Programme Implementation Plan (PIP) part C:

- Support for alternate vaccine delivery from PHC to Sub-centers and outreach sessions.
- Deploying retired manpower to carryout immunization activities in urban slums and underserved areas where services are deficient.
- Mobility support to District Immunization officer and other officers as per State Plan for monitoring and supportive supervision.

- Review meeting at the State level with the districts on 6 monthly intervals.
- Training of ANM, cold chain handlers, Mid Level Managers, refrigerator mechanics, etc.
- .Support for mobilization of children to immunization session sites by Accredited Social Health Activist (ASHA), Women Self-Help Groups, etc.
- One Computer Assistant to State Headquarter and Districts.
- Printing of immunization cards and other' tools like tickler box, tally sheet, monitoring sheet, cold chain chart, vaccine inventory charts, etc.
- Implementation of routine immunization monitoring system software.
- Any other State specific issues.

In addition, the central support of the following will continue under immunization as supplies to States:

- Introduction of AD syringes for all immunization replacing the existing glass syringe and needles and supplies to the States has been stated from August 2005.
- Downsizing the BCG vial from 20 doses to 10 if doses in order to ensure that BCG vaccine is available in all immunization session site. The supply of 10 doses BCG has started from April 2005.
- Strengthening of cold chain system in the State.
- Cold Chain Maintenance.
- Supply of vaccines.
- Supply of vaccine van at the rate of one per district.

Significant achievement has been made under this programme. At the beginning of the programme in 1985-86, vaccine coverage level ranged between 29% of BCG and 41% for DPT. The recent household survey conducted in the year 2002-03 has indicated that he coverage levels in most of the districts have been declining with respect to district level coverage reported in the year 1998-99. The recent UNICEF survey conducted in 2006 indicated that the coverage at National level for BCG is 83.4%, DPT (3rd dose) -67.3%, OPV (3rd dose) -61.3%, Measles -68.1% and Full immunization at 54.5%. These coverage data indicates that the coverage of the immunization programme has improved over the previous years with strengthening of immunization programme under NRHM.

INTRODUCTION OF HEPATITIS-B VACCINE

A pilot project for the introduction of Hepatitis-B Vaccine in the National Immunization Programme was approved by the Government and launched by Hon'ble Prime Minister on 10th June 2002. Under this project Hepatitis-B Vaccine is being administered to infants along with the primary doses of DPT vaccine on 6th, 10th and 14th week. The project is presently being implemented in 33 districts and 15 metropolitan cities. Vaccine and syringes are being made available by Global Alliance for Vaccine and Immunization. Expenditure for IEC, training and monitoring budget is being incurred through the domestic funds.[5]

I. Special Programme for the Girl Child

Girl children continue to be killed off in their mother's womb through sex-selective abortions. The number of girls in the 0-6 age group is fast reducing, causing a red alert. World's highest number of child labourers is in India. To add to this, India has the world's largest number of sexually abused children, with a child below 16 years raped every 155th minute, a child below 10 children sexually abused at any point of time. Children are trafficked within and across borders for a number of reasons. Most subtle forms of violence against children such as child marriage, economic exploitation, practices like the 'Devadasi' tradition of dedicating young girls to gods and goddesses, genital mutilation in parts of the country, etc. are justified on grounds of culture, tradition and religion.[6]

SAARC declared 1990, "The Year of the Girl Child" and 1991-2000 as the "Decade of the Girl Child." During this period programmes are proposed to:

- Increase public awareness of the value of the girl child;
- Reach girls with basic services for their survival and development;
- Ensure their participation in programmes of child development, health, nutrition and education;
- Increase the age of marriage; and
- Create a positive environment to allow girls to develop into productive and confident young women.

A National Plan of action for the Girl Child for 1991-2000 A.D. has been drawn up by the Government. The Plan recognises the rights of the girl child to equal opportunity, to be free from hunger, illiteracy, ignorance and exploitation.

Towards ensuring survival of the girl child, the objectives are to:

- Prevent cases of female foeticide and infanticide and ban the practice of amniocentesis for sex determination;
- End gender disparity in infant mortality rate;
- Eliminate gender disparities in feeding practices, expand nutritional interventions to reduce severe malnourishment by half and provide supplementary nutrition to adolescent girls in need;

- Reduce deaths due to diarrohea by 50% among girl children under 5 years and ensure immunization against all forms of serious illnesses; and
- Provide safe drinking water and ensure access to fodder and drinking water nearer home.

Protection of the girl child is to be ensured through the following:

- Relief for those girls who are economically and socially deprived and belong to special groups;
- Intervention to sensitize various agencies on the need to protect the girl child and adolescent girls from exploitation, assault and physical abuse;
- Education and sensitization of male members of the family to the special needs of the girl child;
- Equal treatment, dignity and respect for girl children in the family and community as well as providing support and help in their day-to-day work so that they get time to avail of the opportunities for self-development;
- Rehabilitation services to reduce the growing instances of exploitation of girl-children and adolescent girls; and
- Protection of girl-children and adolescent girls from prevalent social evils such as dowry, child marriage, prostitution, rape, incest. molestation, etc. through appropriate legislation and proper enforcement.

Major Child Health Care Programmes

- National Prophylaxis Programme against Nutritional Blindness.
- Improve the coverage of all cases of massive dose Vitamin A administration.
- Health education to improve consumption of foods rich in B-carotene and improve their availability at affordable cost.

Child Survival Programme

Sustaining and strengthening the ongoing programmes of universal immunization, ORT, massive dose Vitamin A, Iron Folic Acid supplementation. Expanding the coverage of Acute Respiratory Infections (ARI) Control Programme and care of the newborn.

Let us mention here the special problems faced by girl child as given by South-East Asia Regional Office of WHO, in Regional Health Report, 1998 (Focus on Women). It is a common fact that girl children are less desired, largely for economic reasons and the roles they will play in adult life. Tradition does not consider them as future bread winners. In fact, they become an economic liability at the time of marriage, with large dowries expected from their families.

Under-nutrition is also more prevalent in girls. Inadequate feeding in childhood has serious health consequences. It can lead to impaired intellectual capacity, delayed puberty, possible impaired fertility and stunted growth, resulting in higher risks of complications during childbirth.

Child prostitution and sexual abuse of young girls including rape and incest are also issues of serious concern. Young girls, particularly in rural areas, contribute substantially to domestic chores and caring for smaller children in the family, and hence are often unable to attend school.

Causes of Child Mortality

Major causes of infant and child mortality are:

- prematurity;
- diarrhoeal diseases;
- acute respiratory infections;
- vaccine preventable diseases (in places where immunization coverage has not reached optimal levels); and
- about two-third of infant mortality is in the neonatal period.

2. Programme Intervention in Child Health

Universal Immunisation Programme

The Universal Immunisation Programme (UIP) was taken up in 85-86 and was given the status of a National Technology Mission in 1986. The Programme became operational in all the districts of the country by the year 1989-90 and became a part of the Child Survival and Safe Motherhood (CSSM) Programme in 1992. Under the Immunisation Programme, vaccinations to infants and pregnant women are given for the control of vaccine preventable diseases, namely, diphtheria. perptussis, childhood tuberculosis, poliomyelitis, measles and neonatal tetanus. Except vaccine for the Polio, which is administered orally, all the other vaccines are administered through injections. Significant achievements have been made under the programme.

The poor environmental factors are also reflected in the causes of the death of children in the developing world. If we examine the Table under shows we discern that the main causes of death of children in the developing world are diarrhoeal diseases and respiratory infections followed by communicable and preventable disease such as whooping cough and measles.

From the above statements about the health problems of children in the developing world, it is evident that no specific health measures and no single set of actions can remedy these problems. The real 'Iceberg' of which excessive infant mortality is but one visible tip consists of poverty, hunger, malnutrition, ignorance and many other socio-economic ills. In order to control this total 'iceberg', we must take care of the broad socio-economic development programmes directed at the root of these ills.

TABLE 15.2

Leading Causes of Child Deaths

Developed Country		*Developing Country*
Infants	Birth injuries Congenital anomalies Influenza, pneumonia Enteritis, diarrhoeal diseases	Enteritic, Diarrhoeal diseases Influenza, Pneumonia Bronchitis., etc. Whooping cough
1-4 years	Accidents Congenital anomalies Malignant neoplasms	Enteritis Diarrhoeal diseases Influenza, Pneumonia Bronchitis, etc. Measles
5-9 years	Accidents Enteritis, Malignant neoplasms Congenital anomalies Heart diseases	Diarrhoeal diseases Influenza, Pneumonia Accidents Measles
10-14 years	Accidents Congenital anomalies Heart diseases	Influenza, Pneumonia Malignant neoplasms Accidents Enteritis, Diarrhoeal diseases Meules

Source: Summarized from WHO Technical Report Series No 600.

Aspects of Child Health

Comprehensive, child health services including preventive, promotive and curative services are being provided to those who seek care in secondary and tertiary health care institutions. At primary health care level, the spectrum of services available is narrower, focus is mainly on essential new born care, essential child care including ARI and ORT programmes, immunisation, Vito A and anaemia prophylaxis programmes. Effective utilisation of available services for prevention and detection of under-nutrition in under five population is the aim of ICDS programme during the Ninth Plan period. Efforts are being focussed on improving quality of screening of children for early detection of health and nutrition problems and improving the referral services so that persons requiring care in secondary and tertiary level institutions receive them without delay.

Once the general policy has been determined, the problem is as to how can we devise programmes which ensure that this policy is implemented. Let us now discuss the various ingredients which can help in the effective formulation of the plan for fulfiling the health needs of children.

1. Change the Outlook of Planners

Planners and administrators should be enlightened to look upon the provision of health services for children as an investment in human resources, rather than a social welfare activity. The planners must be persuaded that a higher priority to the development of services for the young child would be beneficial to the modernization of the country. Secondly, the planners should not bother too much about the economic development in the narrow sense of increasing the GNP, but should talk in humanistic terms. There should be good communication between the health planners and the general planners.

Thirdly, while planning, we should allocate more resources to the development of children. When funds are cut for the children who need help the most, we mortgage the present to the future. Fourthly, the planners should understand that the benefits of child welfare programmes are being enjoyed by the urban children, who are already getting their needs fulfiled. The imbalance needs to be corrected and in future more resources may be invested for the development of the unprivileged children living in rural areas, urban slums and tribal areas.

2. Establish Objectives/Goals and Targets

On the basis of the gravity of the problem inferred from the statistical analysis, the objectives/goals and targets may be set-up for each area-national, regional and local; and activity health, nutrition, environment. On the basis of the present information, we may accomplish the goals of:

(a) Reduction in maternal, pre-natal, infant and childhood mortality;
(b) Reducing the child morbidity ensuring minimum maternal and child health services through proper cooperation with other developmental activities;
(c) Promotion of health through the provision of safe drinking water, primary health care, and nutritional services;
(d) Effective involvement of the community in delivering all these services;
(e) Ensuring proper knowledge and utilisation of family welfare services; and
(f) Promotion of wider community education or health and nutrition.

3. Adopt Basic Services Approach

The UN General Assembly in its Resolution 2.26 (XXV) has advocated the basic services approach for development. The main emphasis in this approach is on the involvement and active participation of the people of the communities; the use of responsible volunteers or part-time workers in providing services essential to the well-being of children; and the re-orientation of national structure to direct and support this approach.

using more para-professional workers. Through such thodology, the whole population can have access to services and not only better off people in better off areas. This approach would improve the conditions of family and community life. Improved mid-wifery, minimal preventive health measures, improved water supply and sanitation, cleanliness in the home, basic mother and child health care, knowledge on the part of the parents of family planning, better nutrition, campaigns for immunisation and distribution of Vitamin A to prevent blindness. All this can be carried out by basic village workers to help the small child grow to his full potential.[7]

Such services rapidly improve living conditions, they are labour-intensive, they demonstrate what community responsibility and self-reliance can achieve.

4. Adopt Family as a Unit

Healthy families make healthy people. The family can provide the most effective and socially appropriate milieu in which the physical and emotional development of children can be ensured. Family is a planning unit of health care, a front line in the sequence of education, prevention, diagnosis, treatment and rehabilitation of its members. According to Ihsan Dogramaci, Executive Director of the International Pediatric Association in Paris.

The integrated family unit is essential—all the experts in the field of child health, welfare and education agree—if today's children are to grow up healthfully and happily.[8] He further adds that, "This integrated family unit becomes the keystone of the healthy community in which it lives. And within such a family, this child emerges as a psychologically well-developed human being who is happy with herself or himself, with parents, relatives and the surrounding society. From such children and such families will one day evolve a world which leaves aggression behind and builds a future of peace. Let us all have the courage to face this challenge and do all in our power to ensure that what is known in theory is applied in reality for the benefit of all children."[9]

N.N. Mashalaba, Director of Maternal and Child Health Programme in the Ministry of Health of Botswana has rightly mentioned that, "Promoting better health for mothers and children and through them better health for the whole family, is the vital nucleus of action towards better health for all."[10]

5. Expand and Re-orient Health Care Services

The population covered by a PHC should be reduced to 25,000. One of the doctors at the PHC should have orientation in maternal and child health, and a community health nursing supervisor should be added to the staff. The sub-health centres should be made responsible for a population of 2,500 instead of 5,000 for better delivery of health services. Under 5-clinics or baby welfare clinics may be set-up in these centres. New born observation units should complement obstetric units at all levels.

Delivery of basic health services at the village level should involve the members of the village community. Training needs of all categories of health workers should be identified, and the relevant progress developed. The need to shift the emphasis in medical education from the narrow confines of hospital work to a broader social level should be given high priority. Training should be village-based. Neera Kuckreja Sohoni in an article, "Organisational Structure to Meet Children's Needs" concludes that:

> "It must be conceded that any effort to reorganise existing structures so as to have greater functional efficiency can only be attempted with great care and caution, and after careful study of all the procedural and programmatic ramifications. Equally, what needs to be acknowledged as hard core reality is that existing structures are deficient and in need of organisational overhaul. Unless this is undertaken, child welfare objectives and pursuits will remain at best platitudes and, at worst, a mockery."[11]

6. Meet the Challenge of Nutritional Deficiency

Nutritional deficiency has increased among lower income groups. There has been a rise in per capita income, however, the position of these groups has not changed, because the prices of basic commodities, especially food, have risen steeply. Nutrition education to improve utilisation, storage and consumption of locally available nutritive foods, should be launched allover the country. This should be done through projects like kitchen gardens, poultry and dairy units and fisheries. The community may be taught the right method of cooking and eating through demonstration projects. Para-professionals must carry out intensive nutritional monitoring of children.

7. Plan for Safe Environment

Potable water supply and its proper drainage must be provided. Sanitary latrines must be popularised. Health-related habits formed during childhood can play a crucial role in determining whether an adult will be destined to enjoy a long and healthy life. There is increasing evidence that many prevalent and disabling adult diseases are related to environmental and community factors. Exposure to pollutants and health-related habits formed during childhood can play a crucial role in determining whether an adult is healthy or is to suffer from cardiovascular or lung diseases, or cancer. The most appropriate motto to characterize those vital years of childhood is surely, "Sapines Qui Prospicit" ....he is wise who looks ahead.[12]

8. Plan far Health Education

Health Education must be provided to school children and the community. In schools, health, hygiene, nutrition environmental sanitation should be introduced. Yogic exercises may be made compulsory in schools. Games should be popularised.

The transfer of knowledge cannot be considered the final goal of. health education; the child has to learn how to use this knowledge and how to make the best choice in a given situation. Rapid changes in lifestyles, and the evolution of views of health and disease call for new departures in health education. A quick glance at health education material of even one generation ago will show how fast it tends to get out of date. Medical facts, it has been estimated, get outdated within a decade or so. Effective health education therefore requires a continuous stream of knowledge, development of the people's ability to absorb it, and decisions taken on the basis of a constantly changing body of information.

9. Plan for Educational, Psychological and Social Needs of the Child

Educational efforts should be geared to stimulate the child's intellect and creativity. According to Professor Piaget: The principal goal of education is to create men who are capable of doing new things, not simply of repeating what other generations have done—men who are creative, inventive and discoverers. The second goal of education is to form minds which can be critical, can verify, and not accept everything they are offered. The great danger today is of slogans, collective opinions, ready-made trends of thoughts. We have to be able to resist individually, to criticise, to distinguish between what is proven and what is not. So we need pupils who are active. Who learn early to find out by themselves, partly by their own spontaneous activity and partly through material we set-up for them; who learn early to tell what is verifiable and what is simply the first idea to come to them.[13]

All children should be covered by educational efforts. The education system should cater according to the needs of the children living in a particular area. Instead of a single entry point in schools, a multi-point entry should be introduced, and the sequential system should be removed, so that children can enter schools and complete their courses at their own pace, according to their age and ability. The search for talented students should start from the primary classes.

The idea of neighbourhood school suggested by the Education Commission should be implemented. Quality of primary school education should be improved by development of teachers through in-service training, and publication of attractive children's literature in regional languages.

10. Safeguard Children from labour

India has all along followed a proactive policy in the matter of tackling the problem of child labour, and always stood for constitutional, statutory and developmental measures that are required to eliminate child labour. India has ratified six ILO conventions relating to child labour and three of them as early as in the first quarter of the twentieth century. Legislative provisions have been made in various laws to protect children from exploitation at work and to improve their working conditions. In addition, a comprehensive law, namely, the Child Labour (Prohibition and

Regulation Act), 1986 prohibits employment of children in certain hazardous occupations and processes and regulates their employment in some other areas.

The National Policy on Child Labour was formulated in 1987 which apart from requiring enforcement of legal provisions to protect the interests of children, envisages focussing of general development programmes for the benefit of child labour and project-based plan of action in areas of high concentration of child labour.

Leisure and the chance to play are not luxuries for children, but essentials for normal health growth. Long hours of work have a stulifying effect on youngsters and may often cripple them emotionally. Children, our most precious resources, are literally the key to the future of our planet. Every effort should be made to provide the young of our species with the time to grow, to play and to learn during that period which we call childhood, to provide them from the beginning with the potential for leading better adults. The value we accord to life is affirmed in our treatment of our children.

Francis Blanchard, Director-General of the International Labour Office issued a declaration endorsing the aims of IYC. The declaration calls for action based on the following principles:

(a) a child is not a 'small adult' but a person entitled to self-fulfilment through learning and play so that his adult life is not jeopardized by his having had to work at an early age;
(b) governments should, in cooperation with all the national organisations concerned, take all necessary social and legislative action for the progressive elimination of child labour; and
(c) pending the elimination of child labour, it must be regulated and humanised.

These children are employed for various reasons. *The Tribune* editorial has rightly mentioned that:

> "The International Labour Organisation suggestion to ban child labour is obviously meaningless for this part of the World. The harshness that greets him at work can only be mitigated by accepting the fact that child labour cannot be wished away."
>
> "At the present moment, preventive legislation may be enacted to safeguard the health, safety and welfare of working children below 18 years of age. Such a legislation should cover working hours, rest periods, wages, leave, prevention of health and safety hazards and prevention of cruelty and exploitation of children in employment or apprenticeship training, Sufficient social security measures may be made for the children."
>
> "Until better laws are framed and public sympathy is evoked,

employment bureaus should be opened at the District level for children below 14. The employment Bureaus can at least create public opinion against employers who exploit children."[14]

Much of the legislation regarding child labour throughout the world is sound, and is certainly a necessary first step. The only trouble is that, given present circumstances, it is difficult to enforce in some of the poorer countries. It is all very well and good to pass laws insisting that children cannot work and must be in school, but in many areas there are simply not enough schools.

It is clear that child labour will never be fully eliminated until the conditions on which it thrives are eradicated. Child labour is the product of poverty and uneven development. Until development is seen, not in terms of higher gross national products but as a balanced growth leading to generalized adult employment and fairer income distribution patterns, it is likely to stay with us.

11. Emphasis on Prevention through Vaccination and its Integration with General Development

Health is wealth that can be preserved. Immunization protects children against infectious diseases such as measles, tetanus, diphtheria, whooping cough, polio limelights, and tuberculosis. Personal hygiene prevents many diseases, particularly diarrhoea. Breast feeding, followed by correct weaning and well-balanced nutrition, protects against malnutrition and strengthens resistance to infection. Day care activities, where play and exercise stimulate both body and mind, contribute to the harmonious development of the child.

Through vaccination and its integration with General Development, immunization provides a means of helping to break the vicious cycle of high infant and childhood mortality rates. By permitting more of a family's children to survive, it reduces the number of births desired by a family which, in turn, acts in strong synergy with family planning activities, and makes the further expansion of immunization services one of the best bargains available for primary health care and national development.

From a wider development perspective, immunization must go hand in hand with not only improvements in health services, water supply and sanitation, nutrition, family planning and education. But also economic development, which in the industrialized countries, virtually eliminated infectious diseases in recent history. Visionary initiatives like the CVI can have an enormous impact on human development within this larger picture.

It is the most opportune time to start planning effectively to meet the diverse needs of the children. Since the development of the children is the responsibility of many sectors and agencies at all levels, there is a need of coordinated planned efforts. The superiority of the integrated planning approach lies in that the various actions affecting the conditions and development of children are analysed and decided upon simultaneously and in relation to each other. "The interplay of inter-sectoral and intra-sectoral integration of services for children has assumed greater importance from plan to plan; it seems well accepted that inter-sectoral linkages cannot be disregarded in the formulation of policies and programmes for children and in carrying out the needed services for them in the most effective manner. Inter-sectoral linkages have to be established not only at the national and state levels, but about the field levels in order to obtain the best results."[15]

The problem of coordination must be worked out in detail to avoid conflicts and delay. Past efforts to attain such inter-developmental coordination have not been very successful at the field level. It would be necessary to review the present organisation and provide additional support if the goods and services are to be delivered to the needy children. Effective Planning for the health needs of the children require dynamic and integrated approach, which is capable of assessing the various backward and forward linkage effects that any programme of children development is found to have. Fanny Edeleman, Secretary of the Women's International Democratic Federation (WIDF) stressed while speaking in a seminar on "Child in Asia" held (from 30 January to 2 February 1978) in India that:

> "The problem of child development should be tackled by coordinating technical resources and know-how instead of taking isolated and *adhoc* action on individual issues and problems."

In this venture, a broad participation is crucial. Directorates of Health of Union, State and Union Territories, Medical and Nursing Colleges, autonomous institutions, universities, Social Welfare and Education Departments, and voluntary organisations must pool their expertise to make a rational plan for the all-round development of children. The foreign resources, wherever needed, may be tapped through the UNICEF and utilised judiciously.

Child welfare is to be planned and organised on a comprehensive basis by taking all aspects of the child's personality into account.

Some of the problems relating to child budgeting that have been identified over the years include:

- Gaps in budget estimates and expenditure;
- Problems in flow of funds from the Centre to the State;
- Inability of States to meet the matching grant requirement from the State in the case of Centrally Sponsored Schemes;
- Inadequacy of mechanisms to check misappropriation and misuse of funds;
- Dependence on external aid;
- Flaws in the very planning of various Ministries and Departments itself; and most importantly,

- Lack of meaningful communication and coordination between the Planning Commission, the Finance Ministry and the Ministries/Departments concerned with child protection issues at the stage of formulation of the five-year plan, mid-term review and final evaluation of the plan period.

The gaps and problems listed above have been brothering both Government and NGOs alike. Child Budgeting must be taken as a serious exercise and needs to be encouraged and undertaken at all levels of governance to identify and address the shortcomings for financing the social sector, particularly programmes relating to children. The exercise must begin at the very level of panchayats, the very basic unit of democratic functioning. For this to happen, the Eleventh Plan will have to focus on decentralised planning for all sectors. This will logically result in decentralized monitoring through analysis of allocation and spending by the panchayats against the plans they had made.[16]

CHILD PROTECTION IN FIVE YEAR PLAN

Child development has been a priority subject in the country's developmental planning right from **First Five Year Plan (1951-56).** The First Five Year Plan recognized the importance of promoting social services for maintaining and consolidating the gains of economic development, attaining adequate living standards and social justice. Accordingly, a comprehensive Social Welfare Programme that was developed during the First Five Year Plan included welfare of Women and Children, Family Welfare, Welfare of the Physically and Mentally Disabled.

In the **Second and Third Plans (1956-61 and 1961-66)** social welfare activities were extended to different sectors.

The Central Bureau of Correctional Services (CBCS) was set-up in 1961 for collection and compilation of national statistics and preparation of guide books and model schemes.

In the **Fourth Plan (1966-71)** all attempts were made to consolidate the initiatives taken in the previous plans. The activities of Central Social Welfare Board were further strengthened. In addition to the three National Institutes for the Blind, the Deaf and the Mentally Retarded, a National Institute of Orthopaedically Handicapped was set-up. For the placement of Disabled persons in employment, special employment exchanges were set-up.

The **Fifth Plan (1974-78)** proved to be the landmark in the field of child development through the adoption of a National Policy for Children (1974), and launching of the Integrated Child Development Services (ICDS) with a shift from welfare to development in the approach towards development of children.

The **Sixth Five Year Plan (1980-85)**, i.e. the early Eighties witnessed an effective consolidation and expansion of programmes started in the earlier Plans. The National Policy of Health adopted in 1983 set certain specific targets like bringing down the high rates of Infant and Child Mortality and take up universalisation of immunization, etc. by the year 2002 A.D.

The **Seventh Five Year Plan (1985-90)** continued the major strategy of promoting early childhood survival and development through programmes in different sectors, important among these being ICDS, universal immunization, maternal and child care services, nutrition, preschool education, protected drinking water, environmental sanitation and hygiene, and family planning. Under the maternal and child health services of the Ministry of Health and Family Welfare, the universal immunization programme to protect children from six major diseases which affect early childhood mortality and morbidity, viz. diphtheria, whooping cough, tetanus, polio, measles and childhood tuberculosis was strengthened for the development of children as a whole. ICDS continued to be the single nation-wide programme for early childhood survival and development during Seventh Plan. The Juvenile Justice Act (JJA) was enacted in 1986, to deal effectively with the problem of neglected or juvenile delinquents and provide for a standardized framework for dealing with such children. The Government of India enacted the Child Labour Prohibition and Regulation Act, 1986 and in 1987, the National policy on Child Labour was formulated.

During the **Seventh Plan and Annual Plans (1990-92)**, a significant expansion of programmes and services for the welfare of the Disabled took place. For education of the Disabled almost all the States implemented programmes to provide stipends and other incentives to the Disabled at the elementary schools stage. The Scheme to award scholarships to physically Disabled students to pursue general, technical and professional courses from Class IX onwards on the basis of means-*cum*-merit test, was continued. To provide technical support to 11 District Rehabilitation Centres for the disabled, 4 Regional Rehabilitation Training Centres (RRTC) were set-up for developing the training material and the manuals and for providing material to create community awareness through the use of different media. In addition to four National Institutes for Disabled, two other organisations, viz., the Institute for the Physically Handicapped (Delhi and the National Institute of Rehabilitation Training and Research (Cuttack) also offered a wide range of services for the rehabilitation of the Disabled and organized manpower training. The Science and Technology Project in the Mission Mode of Application of Technology for the Welfare and Rehabilitation of the Disabled was launched in 1988. Voluntary organisations were also assisted provide services to the physically handicapped in the areas of education, training and rehabilitation.

Human Resources Development being the major focus of the **Eighth Five Year Plan (1992-97)**, policies and programmes relating to 'child survival, protection and development' were accorded high priority with emphasis on family and community-based preventive services to combat high infant and under-5 child mortality and morbidity. Following the ratification of the 'Convention on the Rights of the Child', in 1992 the Government of India formulated two National Plans of Action (NPA)—one for children and the other exclusively for the Girl-Child.

The **Ninth Five Year Plan (1997-2002).** The strategy aimed at placing the Young Child at the top of the Country's Developmental Agenda with a Special Focus on the Girl Child; instituting a National Charter for Children ensuring that no Child remains illiterate, hungry or lacks medical care; ensuring 'Survival, Protection and Development' through the effective implementation of the two National Plans of Action—one for the Children and the other for the Girl Child; acknowledging that the first six years as critical for the development of children, therefore, greater stress will be laid on reaching the younger children below 2 years; continuing to lay a special thrust on the 3 major areas of child development viz. health, nutrition and education; universalizing.

It was recognized that the policy perspectives on Adolescents in the period up to the Ninth Plan have been piecemeal, with various sectors referring to this age group as part of the overall approach, and no specific focus was given in most cases.

The Draft National Youth Policy, 2001 provided comprehensive overview of youth issues and concerns and comes closest to a policy on adolescents. The draft policy "Working with youth and not merely for youth" highlighted several areas of concern for adolescents and youth in the country and emphasized an intersectoral approach. The policy laid stress on providing youth with 'more access to the process of decision making and implementation of these decisions'. The Draft Youth Policy actually made a distinction between the age of adolescence (13-19) and the age of attainment of maturity (20-30 years). By marking the age of adolescence, the policy facilitated advocacy efforts for focus on adolescents in government programmes.

Programmes for Adolescent Girls

Apart from the two schemes for Adolescent Girls implemented by the Department of Women and Child Development, Kishori Shakti Yojana and the Balika Samriddhi Yojana other departments were also Implementing programmes for adolescent girls, which had a bearing on their being and developmental opportunities. Nehru Yuva Kendras undertook activities for Health Awareness to educate and enable people to adopt health and family welfare programmes. The Ministry of Social Justice and Empowerment implemented a scheme for providing educational facilities including scholarships and hostels for tribal girls. The Department of Family Welfare provided for maternal care including safe motherhood and nutrition facilities, prevention of unwanted pregnancies, and safe abortion facilities to all women. The Directorate General of Employment and Training, Ministry of Labour facilitated registration in employment exchanges for job placements and career counselling and vocational guidance for adolescents.

Tenth Five-Year Plan (2002-07)

Women, Children and Development The Tenth Plan has set certain monitorable targets for women and children including all children in school by 2003; all children to complete five years of schooling by 2007; reduction in gender gaps in literacy and wage rates by at least 50 percent by 2007; reduction of Infant Mortality Rate (IMR to 45 per 1000 live births by 2007 and 28 by 2012; reduction of Maternal Mortality Rate (MMR) to 2 per 1000 live births by 2007 and to 1 per 1000 live births by 2012. The other objectives of the Tenth Plan include arresting the decline in the child sex ratio; increasing the representation of women in premier services and in Parliament; and universalisation of the Integrated Child Development Services (ICDS) scheme.

Some of the problems relating to child budgeting that have been identified over the years include:

- Gaps in budget estimates and expenditure;
- Problems in flow of funds from the Centre to the State;
- Inability of States to meet the matching grant requirement from the State in the case of Centrally Sponsored Schemes;
- Inadequacy of mechanisms to check misappropriation and misuse of funds;
- Dependence on external aid;
- Flaws in the very planning of various Ministries and Departments itself; and most importantly;
- Lack of meaningful communication and coordination between the Planning Commission, the Finance Ministry and the Ministries/Departments concerned with child protection issues at the stage of formulation of the five-year plan, mid-term review and final evaluation of the plan period. The gaps and problems listed above have been bothering both Government and NGOs alike. Child Budgeting must be taken as a serious exercise and needs to be encouraged and undertaken at all levels of governance to identify and address the shortcomings of financing the social sector, particularly programmes relating to children. The exercise must begin at the very level of panchayats, the very basic unit of democratic functioning. For this to happen, the Eleventh Plan will have to focus on decentralized planning for all sectors. This will logically result in decentralized monitoring through analysis of allocation and spending by the panchayats against the plans they had made.

In the Eleventh Plan (2007-12), Child Protection will be viewed as an essential component of the country's strategy of placing 'Development of the child at the centre of the 11th Plan'. Violations of the child's right to protection, in addition to being human rights violations, are massive, under-recognized and under-reported barriers or obstacles to child survival and development. Failure to protect children has serious consequences for the physical, mental, emotional, social development of the child; consequences for the loss in productivity and the loss in human capital for the nation.

The NPAC has identified twelve key priority areas for the utmost and sustained attention in terms of outreach, programme interventions and resource allocations.

These are:

- Reducing Infant Mortality Rate;
- Reducing Maternal Mortality Rate;
- Reducing Malnutrition among children;
- Achieving 100% civil registration of births;
- Universalization of early childhood care and development and quality education for all children achieving 100% access and retention in schools, including pre-schools;
- Complete abolition of female foeticide, female infanticide a child marriage and ensuring the survival, development and protection of the girl child;
- Improving Water and Sanitation coverage both in rural and urban areas;
- Addressing and upholding the rights of Children in Difficult Circumstances;
- Securing for all children all legal and social protection from all kinds of abuse, exploitation and neglect;
- Complete abolition of child labour with the aim of progressively eliminating all forms of economic exploitation of children;
- Monitoring, Review, and Reform of policies, programmes and laws to ensure protection of children's interests and rights; and
- Ensuring child participation and choice in matters and decisions affecting their lives. The NPAC 2005 has articulated clear the rights perspective and agenda for the development of children, and provides a robust framework within which to promote the development and protection of children.

It is therefore logical and imperative that the NPAC 2005 becomes the basis for planning for children in the Eleventh Plan in all sectors and the principles articulated in it guide the planning and investments for children. All budget for child protection schemes and programmes should be in the plan category and not in the non-plan category.

The Guiding Principles of the NPA are:

- To regard the child as an asset and a person with human rights;
- To address issues of discrimination emanating from biases of gender, class, caste, race, religion and legal status in order to ensure equality;

- To accord utmost priority to the most disadvantaged, poorest of the poor and the least served child in all policy and programme interventions; and
- To recognize the diverse stages and settings of childhood, and address the needs of each, providing all children the entitlements that fulfil their rights and meet their needs in each situation.[17]

Notes and References

1. Annual Report, Ministry of Health and Family Welfare, 2006-07, p. 55.
2. Ministry of Women and Child Development, Sub-Group Report on Child Protection, For the Eleventh Five Year Plan, 2007-12, pp. 2-3.
3. *Ibid.*, Preface.
4. Annual Report, Ministry of Health and Family Welfare, 2006-2007, p. 35.
5. *Ibid.*, pp. 58-60.
6. Ministry of Women and Child Development, Sub-Group on Child Protection for the Eleventh Five Year Plan, 2007-12, p. 14.
7. UNICEF, A Strategy for Basic Services. p. 14.
8. WHO, *World Health*, Feb.-March, 1979, p. 20.
9. *Ibid.*, p. 33.
10. *Ibid.*, p. 31.
11. Neera Kuckreja Sohoni, "Organisation Structure to Meet Children's Need" in *The Indian Journal of Public Administration*, Vol. XXV, No. (July-Sept. 1979), p. 50.
12. Frank Falkner, "The Vital years", *World Health*, March 1979, p. 11.
13. Professor Piaget: Report of the Jean Piaget Conferences at Cornell University and the University of California: Conference on Cognitive Studies and Curriculum Development, Cornell University and the University of California, 1964; Piaget Rediscovered; Richard E. Ripple and Verne N. Rockcastle, eds., p. 5.
14. *The Tribune*, Chandigarh, 29 August 1979.
15. UNICEF, Study of the Young Child: Indian Case Study, NIPECD, 1976, p. 93.
16. Ministry of Women and Child Development, Sub-Group in Child Protection for the Eleventh Five Year Plan, 2007-12, p. 93.
17. *Ibid.*, pp. 67-87.

ANNEXURE 15.1

The Integrated Child Protection Scheme concretises the Government/ State responsibility for creating a system to protect children in the country. Such a system is influenced by the nature of regulatory frameworks, structures, resources, professionals, and the relationships between them. When the child protection system functions in the best interest of the child, adequate state and voluntary institutions, services and structures are put in place, backed strongly by policies, laws and regulations. Professionals providing services for children are competent and bound by professional standards. Children's views are taken into account.

The Integrated Child Protection Scheme is based on the cardinal principles of "protection of child rights" and "best interests of the child." The ICPS aims to promote the best interests of the child and prevent violations of child rights through appropriate punitive measure against perpetrators of abuse and crimes against children and to ensure rehabilitation for all children in need of care and protection. It aims to create a protective environment by improving regulatory frameworks, strengthening structures protection issues and provide child friendly services at all levels.

1. Principles of ICPS

The following key principles underlie the ICPS approach:

(i) *Child protection a shared responsibility*: The responsibility for child protection is a shared responsibility of government, family, community, professionals, and civil society. It is important that each role is articulated clearly and understood by all engaged in the effort to protect children. Government has an obligation to ensure a range of services at all levels;

(ii) *Reducing child vulnerability*: There is a need for a focus on systematic preventive measures not just programmes and schemes to address protection failures at various levels. A strong element of prevention will be integrated into programmes, converging the provisions and services of various sectors on the vulnerable families, like livelihood support (NREGS), SHGs, PDS, health, child day care, education, to strengthen families and reduce the likelihood of child neglect, abuse and vulnerability;

(iii) *Strengthen family*: Children are best cared for in their own families and have a right to family care and parenting by both parents. Therefore, a major thrust will be to strengthen the family capabilities to care for and protect the child by capacity building, family counselling and support services and linking to development and community support services;

(iv) *Promote non-institutional care*: There is a need to shift the focus of interventions from an over reliance on institutionalization of children and move towards more family and community-based alternatives for care. Institutionalization should be used as a measure of last resort after all other options have been explored;

(v) *Intersectoral linkages and responsibilities*: Child protection needs dedicated sectoral focus as well as strengthening protection awareness and protection response from other sectors outside the traditional protection sector including in emergencies and HIV/AIDS programming;

(vi) *Create a network of services at community level*: An appropriate network of essential protection services is required at all levels for supporting children and communities;

(vii) *Establishing standards for care and protection*: All protection services should have prescribed standards. Protocols for key actions and should be monitored regularly. Institutionalisation should be for the shortest period of time with strict criteria being established for residential placement and all cases of institutionalization reviewed periodically;

(viii) *Building capacities*: Protection services require skilled, sensitive staff. Equipped with knowledge of child rights and standards of care and protection. Capacities of all those in contact with children require strengthening on a continuing basis, including families and communities;

(ix) *Providing child protection professional services at all levels*: There is a need for varied special services for the many situations of child neglect, exploitation and abuse, including for shelter, care, psychological recovery, social reintegration, legal services, etc. which have to be professional and child-focused;

(x) *Strengthening crisis management system at all levels*: First response and coordinated inter-sectoral actions for responding to crisis need to be established and institutionalized;

(xi) *Reintegration with family and community*: Systems to be put in place for efforts to reintegrate children with their families and community and regular review of efforts instituted;

(xii) *Addressing protection of children in urban poverty*: Children in urban poverty are at high risk/increased vulnerability; constantly under threat of eviction; denial or exclusion from basic services; social turmoil; and the stretched capacity of the adults to function as adequate caretakers due to their poverty. This indicates the need for developing a strong social support and service system;

(xiii) *Child impact monitoring*: All policies, initiatives and services will be monitored for their child impact and reports made public, including for children themselves through child-friendly reports.

2. The Approach

In order to reach out to all children, in particular to those in difficult circumstances, the Ministry of Women and Child Development proposes to combine its existing child protection schemes under one centrally sponsored scheme titled "Integrated Child Protection Scheme (ICPS)." The proposed ICPS brings together multiple vertical schemes under one comprehensive child protection programme and integrates interventions for protecting children and preventing harm.

It does not see child protection as the exclusive responsibility of the MWCD but stresses that other sectors have vital roles to play. The Ministry looks at child protection holistically and seeks to rationalize programmes for creating a strong protective environment for children, diversify and institutionalize essential services for children, mobilize inter-sectoral response for strengthening child protection and set standards for care and services.

ICPS will function as a Government-Civil Society Partnership scheme under the overarching direction and responsibility of the Central/State Governments. It will work closely with all stakeholders including government departments, the voluntary sector, community groups, academia and, most importantly, families and children to create a protective environment for children in the country. Its holistic approach to child protection services 3 and mechanisms is reflected in stronger lateral linkages and complementary systems for vigilance, detection and response. The scheme, visualizes a structure for providing services as well as monitoring and supervising the effective functioning of child protection system, involving:

Government: To hold primary responsibility for the development, funding and operation of the service covered under the scheme. In order to ensure effective functioning of the system, the Government shall provide flexibility by cutting down rigid structures and norms. To attract the best professional, talent and strengthen public-private partnership, the scheme proposes to hire services of professionals on a contractual basis;

Civil society organisations

- *Voluntary sector*: To provide vibrant, responsive and child friendly services for detection, counselling, rehabilitation for all children in need as well as provide technical support; these may be financially supported by the State;
- *Research and training institutions*: To carryout activities related to research and capacity building of existing manpower as well as support creation of a cadre of professional manpower;
- *Media and advocacy groups*: To promote rights of the child and child protection issues with sensitivity and promote child's dignity and worth;
- *Corporate sector*; and
- *Community groups and local leaders, youth groups, families and*

children: To provide protective and corrective environment for children, to act as watchdog and monitor child protection services as well as service providers, both Government and NGO functionaries.

3. Target Groups

- Child in Need of Care and Protection Means a Child Who is found without any home or settled place or abode and without any ostensible means of subsistence;
- resides with a person (whether a guardian of the child or not) and such person has threatened to kill or injure the child and there is a reasonable likelihood of the threat being carried out, or has killed, abused or neglected some other child or children and there is a reasonable likelihood of the child in question being killed, abused or neglected by that person;
- is a mentally or physically challenged or ill child or a child suffering from terminal diseases or incurable diseases, and/or having no one to support or look after him/her;
- has a parent or guardian and such parent or guardian is unfit or incapacitated to care for or exercise control over the child; does not have a parent/parents and no one is willing to take care of him/her, or whose parents have abandoned him/her or who is a missing and/or runaway child and whose parents cannot be found after reasonable inquiry;
- is being or is likely to be grossly abused, tortured or exploited for the purpose of sexual abuse or illegal acts;
- is found vulnerable and is likely to be inducted into drug abuse or trafficking;
- is being or is likely to be abused for unconscionable gains; and
- is victim of any armed conflict, civil commotion or natural calamity.

Children in conflict with the law is one who is alleged to have committed an offence. Children in contact with law is one who has come in contact with the law either as victim or as a witness or due to any other circumstance.

Any other vulnerable child including, but not limited, to: Children of potentially vulnerable families and families at risk. Children of socially excluded groups like migrant families, families living in extreme poverty, lower caste families, families subjected to or affected by discrimination, minorities, children infected and/or affected by HIV/AIDS, orphans, child drug abusers, children of substance abusers, child beggars, trafficked or sexually exploited children, children of prisoners, and street and working children, would also be covered under the scheme.

4. Objectives of the Scheme

- (i) To create a safety net for children in need of care and protection and children in conflict with law by building a protective environment for them, keeping their best interests in mind;
- (ii) To promote preventive measures to protect children from falling in the situations of vulnerability, risk and abuse;
- (iii) To promote preventive measure to address the vulnerabilities of families and build their ability and capacity protect their children;
- (iv) To supplement and strengthen the infrastructure established under the Juvenile Justice (Care and Protection) Act, 2000;
- (v) To build capacities of families, communities, and NGOs to strengthen care, protection and response to children;
- (vi) To create State and District Child Protection Units as well as State Adoption Cells;
- (vii) To promote in-country adoption and regulate inter-country adoption as well as ensure minimum standards;
- (viii) To provide services to the more vulnerable categories of children through specialized programmes;
- (ix) To establish linkages for restoration of children to their biological families and placement with adoptive families or foster families, where necessary;
- (x) To provide specialized institutional care to infants and children up to 6 years of age who are either abandoned or orphaned/ destitute;
- (xi) To check and end female foeticide and infanticide in the country;
- (xii) To provide services to street and destitute children, including child beggars;
- (xiii) To provide for care and support services for children affected by HIV/AIDS;
- (xiv) To establish CHILDLINE in every district, for creating access in emergencies by providing counselling, restoration and rehabilitative services to children along with linkages to other available services under various schemes of the Government of India/State Governments;
- (xv) To train and sensitize local bodies, police, judiciary and other concerned departments of State Governments to undertake related responsibilities;
- (xvi) To strengthen the knowledge base by undertaking research and documentation, resource mapping of services, the creation of a Management Information System (MIS) for tracking vulnerable children, and database management;
- (xvii) To carry out advocacy and spread awareness about child and family-related issues for supporting the family;

(xviii) To network with the Allied Systems, i.e. Government departments and Non-Government agencies; and

(xix) To initiate any other need-based specialized innovative services through families, community and panchayats/local bodies, including child guidance and counselling, especially to combat drug abuse, sexual abuse, child marriage, and discrimination against the girl child.

5. Strategies

The ICPS will be guided by the critical child protection strategies and priorities visualized under the National Plan of Action for Children, 2005. These strategies will be based on four major parameters, including:

Prevention

- Preventing destitution and exploitation of children through care, protection and developmental programmes;
- Achieving 100% registration of births, deaths and marriages by 2010;
- Establishing support services for families at risk;
- Eradication of harmful, traditional and customary practices that put children at risk.
- particularly of trafficking and sexual exploitation;
- Ensuring survival, development and protection of the girls child and restoring her dignity by eliminating harmful, discriminatory and unethical traditional practices, and providing legal, medical, social and psychological support services and opportunities for development of their full potential;
- Ensuring enforcement of all laws relating to children, particularly the Child Marriage Restraint Act, PNDT Act, ITPA, Juvenile Justice (Care and Protection of Children) Act, Child Labour (Prohibition and Regulation) Act, amongst others;
- Prevention of cross-border trafficking and creation of nodal authorities and other infrastructure to deal with all kinds of child trafficking;
- Adoption of a national law to deal with child trafficking, including ratification of the international instruments such as the UN Protocol on Trafficking in Persons;
- Ensuring access to mainstream education for all child labourers by 2012 and access to nutrition, clothing and protection from all forms of abuse and neglect;
- Elimination of child marriages;
- Eliminate disability due to poliomyletis by 2007;
- Creation of effective links and quick referrals between ICDS, Primary Health Centres, mother and child programmes and hospitals (paediatric units) for early detection of high risk babies and children with disabilities;

- Access to neighbourhood schools and inclusive education, accessible and disable friendly infrastructure, early childhood care for the disabled child, inclusion of children with mental illness in all existing schemes from children with disability, vocational training, capacity building of care givers, access to services, support and protection, implementation of the disability law;
- Prevention of mother-to-child transmission of HIV/AIDS;
- Requisite counselling, awareness generation; and support services for adolescents to prevent them for becoming vulnerable and protect them from harm;
- Contingency planning and emergency preparedness;
- Convergence with related Ministries/Department at Central and State levels;
- Enlisting support from the private sector; and
- Ensuring child specific interventions in all urban planning.

Protection

- Special measures for protection of children in urban and semi-urban situations;
- Special attention to certain categories of children requiring greater focus such as, child beggars, child labour, street children, children in need of care and protection and children in conflict with law as covered by the juvenile justice act, trafficked children, child victims of sexual abuse and exploitation, children affected by natural and man-made disasters, children of sex workers and prisoners, children affected by armed conflict and civil disorders;
- Ensuring a supportive and enabling environment for care and protection of children affected by HIV/AIDS;
- Quality health care and services, including free Anti-Retroviral therapy for children infected with HIV virus;
- Development of special packages for children abandoned on account of HIV/AIDS;
- Promoting community-based care and rehabilitation for all children in difficult circumstances;
- Childline and other necessary support service, infrastructure, referral for children in emergency situations;
- Promotion of quality institutional and alternative care;
- Up-gradation of standards of existing services;
- Infrastructural support to NGOs for destitute, orphan children through in-country adoption;
- Combating trafficking of narcotic drugs, psychotropic substance to prevent the use by children and creating Mechanisms for rehabilitation of child substance abusers;

- Drop-in-shelters which encourage children's voluntary attendance and participation in activities such as music, theater, yoga and meditation, computers, games and other creative activities so as to ensure their overall development, care and protection and to reduce social deviance;
- Implementation of juvenile justice law;
- Creation of child-friendly judicial and administrative procedures for dealing with children;
- Free legal aid and advice for children in conflict with law;
- Assistance to child victims of abuse and exploitation for their full physical and psychological recovery, development and social reintegration;
- Institution of a rights-based uniform definition of child labour and bonded labour;
- Elimination of all forms of child labour by linking it with ensuring right to education for all children;
- Convergence with related Ministries/Department at Central and State levels;
- Enlisting support from the private sector. Awareness and Capacity Building;
- Public awareness, sensitization and mobilization of parents, caregivers, community and other actors in civil society;
- Professional counselling services for children in psychological trauma and establishment of accredited training courses/ institutions for creating a cadre of trained counsellors;
- Large-scale investment in capacity building of all caregivers and service providers;
- Sensitize allied systems to the problems of children;
- Convergence with related Ministries/Department at Central and State levels; and
- Enlisting support from the private sector.

Research and Documentation

- Development of a system of identification, investigation, reporting, follow-up and referral of children at risk within and outside homes/institutional care;
- Maintaining disaggregated data-base for all categories of children in difficult circumstances, including child labour, child marriage, disabled children, etc. through census and programme specific management information system MIS;
- Convergence with relating Ministries/Departments at Central and State levels;
- Enlisting support from the private sector.

Source: Ministry of Women and Child Development, Sub-Group Report on Child Projection for the Eleventh Five Year Plan, 2007-12, pp. 178-84.

16

CHAPTER

Health of the Elderly

For many people, living longer is not living better. Adding years to life is important. But adding life to the added years is even more important.

Population ageing has become a global phenomenon. The population of older persons in India is increasing at a fast pace. Because of the general improvement in the health care facilities over the years, there is a continuous increase in the life expectancy. This has resulted in the fact that more and more people are now living longer. As such, India became the second largest country in the world in respect of the population of older persons. As per Census 2001, the total population of older persons in India is 7,66,22,321. Projection studies indicate that the number of 60+ in India will increase to 100 million in 2013 and to 198 million in 2030. The special features of the elderly population in India are: (a) a majority (80%) of them are in the rural areas, thus making service delivery a challenge, (b) feminization of the elderly population would be women and (c) increase in the number of the older persons (above 80 years) (*Source*: Registrar General of India).[1]

"Active Ageing makes the difference" was the World Health Day Theme for 1999., By the year 2020 more than 1000 million of the world's population will be over 60 years old. To help promote a global response to this major societal concern, WHO, in 1995, restructured its programme of health of the elderly and gave it a new name-Ageing and Health. This area of health care is becoming a dominant concern as the next millennium approaches.[2]

By the year 2020 more than 1000 million of the world's population will be over 60 years old. To help promote a global response to this major societal concern, WHO, in 1995, restricted its programme of health of the elderly and gave it a new name—Ageing and Health. This area of health care is becoming a dominant concern as the next millennium approach. The main perspectives which guide the programme activities in the Region are:

- Approaching ageing as part of the life cycle rather than compartmentalizing health care of the elderly;
- Promoting long-term-health—increasing awareness of the need of focus on the process of healthy ageing;
- Observing cultural influences;
- Adopting community-oriented approaches;
- Recognizing gender differences; and
- Strengthening inter-generational links.[3]

AGEING LEADING TO LONGEVITY

Ageing has become the leading demographic issue as we approach the new millennium. As such, it is an achievement to be celebrated. At the beginning of the 20th century, life expectancy at birth even in the richest countries was no more than 50 years. Today, it has risen to more than 75. Let us look at the example of Japan the country that today shows the highest life expectancy at birth in the world for both men and women. In the 25 years upto 1996, the percentage of people in Japan aged 65 and over doubled from 7% to 14%.[4]

In 1980, the proportion of elderly people (60 years of age and above) was 6.12% of the total population in the Region. It is estimated that this proportion will increase to 7.41% by the year 2000 and to 12.44% by 2025. By the year 2000, the South-East Asia Region will have approximately one in five of the world's 603 million elderly persons.

The projected level of expectation of life at birth is shown in Table 16.1 It is obvious that over the next three decades India will be facing a progressive increase both in the proportion and number of persons beyond 60 years of age. It is noteworthy that women out number men in the 65+ age group; it is expected that over the next two decades longevity in women will substantially increase. Increasing longevity will inevitably bring in its wake increase in the prevalence of non-communicable diseases. The growing number of senior citizens in the country poses a major challenge; the cost of providing socio-economic security and health care to this population has to be met; currently several region and culture specific innovative interventions to provide needed care to this population are underway; among these are efforts to reverse the trend to break up the joint families. If these efforts succeed, it will be possible to provide necessary inputs for the care of rapidly increasing senior citizens population in the subsequent two.

India had 12 million old in 1901, 10 million in 1951, and 17 million in 2001; by 2025 numbers will be 177 million, 90 per cent of old are from unorganised sector, with no social security at 60. 30 per cent are below poverty line, 33 per cent marginally over it. 80 per cent live in rural areas; 73 per cent are illiterate. 55 per cent women over 60 are widows, many without support. India has 200,000 centenarians, right now. Most severely isolated are those over 75, particularly widowed older women.

Better medical care and low fertility have made the aged the fastest-growing section of our society, so much so that while in France it took 120 years for the gray population to double from 7 to 14 per cent; in India it doubled in just 25 years.

As India grays at a rapid pace, its senior citizens bear the burnt of the changing socio-cultural scenario. Many face isolation and lack the resources for a better quality of life. To ensure that senior citizens get their due, the Maintenance and Welfare of parents and Senior Citizens Bill, 2007, will be introduced in the winter session of Parliament, Aditi Tandon examines the provisions of this legislation.[5]

A relatively high proportion of elderly people in countries of the Region work. However, only 34% of rural elderly and 29% of the urban elderly are reported to be economically independent in India. A five country study on elderly care shows that arthritis, high blood pressure, foot problems, heart diseases and stomach ulcers were the most common illnesses among the elderly, along with visual and hearing impairments.[6]

Majority of the people in their sixties will be physically and psychologically fit and would like to participate both in economic and social activities. They should be encouraged and supported so that they do lead a productive life and also contribute to the national development. Senior citizens in their seventies and beyond and those with health problems would require assistance. So far, the families have borne major share in caring for the elderly. This will remain the ideal method; however, there are growing number of elderly without family support; for them, alternate modes for caring may have to be evolved and implemented. Improved health care has "added years to life." The social sectors have to make the necessary provisions for improving the quality of life of these senior citizens so that they truly add life to years.[7]

The Ministry of Social Justice and Empowerment is the nodal Ministry responsible for the welfare of older persons. The National Policy for Older Persons (NPOP) was announced with the objective of—

(a) To encourage families to take care of their older family members;
(b) to enable and support voluntary and non-governmental organisations to supplement the care provided by the family;
(c) to provide care and protection to the vulnerable elderly people;
(d) to provide health care facility to the elderly;
(e) to promote research and training facilities to train geriatric care givers and organizers of services for the elderly;
(f) to encourage individuals to make provision for their own as well as their spouse's old age; and
(g) to create awareness regarding elderly persons to enable them to become independent citizens.

TABLE 16.1

Percentage Distribution of Projected Population by Age and Sex 1996-2016, India

	1996			*2001*			*2011*			*2016*		
	M	*F*	*P*	*M*	*F*	*P*	*M*	*F*	*P*	*M*	*F*	*P*
0-4	12.6	13.0	10.6	10.6	10.8	10.7	10.1	10.2	10.1	9.7	9.7	9.7
5-7	13.2	13.3	11.3	11.3	11.6	11.5	9.4	9.4	9.4	9.3	9.3	9.3
10-14	11.9	11.5	12.0	12.1	12.1	8.9	9.0	8.9	8.7	8.7	8.7	8.7
15-19	9.9	9.5	11.0	11.0	10.5	10.8	9.7	9.9	9.8	8.3	8.3	8.3
20-24	8.6	9.0	9.0	8.7	8.9	10.4	10.3	10.3	9.0	9.1	9.0	9.1
25-29	7.8	8.5	7.9	7.9	8.2	80.0	9.4	8.9	9.2	9.7	9.5	9.5
30-34	7.0	7.2	7.2	7.2	7.7	7.4	7.8	7.3	7.6	8.7	8.2	8.7
35-39	6.2	6.0	6.4	6.4	6.6	6.5	6.7	6.9	6.8	7.2	6.8	7.2
40-44	5.3	5.0	5.6	5.6	5.5	5.5	6.0	6.5	6.2	6.2	6.4	6.2
45-49	4.4	4.2	4.3	4.7	4.5	4.6	5.3	5.4	5.4	5.5	5.9	5.5
59-54	3.6	3.4	3.9	3.9	3.7	3.8	4.6	4.6	4.5	4.8	5.0	4.0
55-59	2.9	2.8	3.1	3.1	3.0	3.1	3.7	3.6	3.6	4.0	4.0	4.0
60-64	2.4	2.4	2.4	2.4	2.4	2.4	2.9	2.8	2.9	3.2	3.1	4.0
65-69	1.7	1.8	1.9	1.9	1.9	1.9	2.0	2.1	2.1	2.3	2.4	2.0
70-74	1.3	1.2	1.3	1.3	1.3	1.3	1.4	1.5	1.4	1.6	1.6	1.0
75-79	0.5	0.5	.8	.8	0.8	0.8	0.9	1.0	1.0	0.9	1.0	1.0
80+	0.8	2.8	.6	.6	0.6	0.6	0.8	0.8	0.8	0.8	0.9	0.8
All Age	100.0	100.0	100.0	100.0	100.0	100.0	100.0	100.0	100.0	100.0	100.0	100.0

OPERATIONAL MECHANISM FOR IMPLEMENTATION OF NATIONAL POLICY ON OLDER PERSONS (NPOP) NATIONAL COUNCIL FOR OLDER PERSONS

The Government has re-constituted a National Council for Older Persons (NCOP) in 2005 under the Chairpersonship of the Minister for Social Justice and Empowerment to advise the Government on policies and programmes for older persons and also to provide a feedback to the Government on the implementation of the National Policy on Older Persons. The NCOP is the highest body to advise and coordinate with the Government in the formulation and implementation of policies and programmes for the welfare of the aged. The present number of NCOP member is 33. The NCOP's members are experienced and well-known individuals representing NGOs, citizen's groups, retired person's associations and from the field of law, social welfare and security, research, and medicine. The NCOP in their meetings held from time to time, reviews the policies for the welfare of elderly.

Inerministerial Committee

Ministry of Social Justice and Empowerment has an Inter-Ministerial Committee comprising twenty-two Ministries/Departments. The Ministry of or Social Justice and Empowerment has prepared the Plan of Action earmarking certain action points for implementation by the various Ministries/Ins. Departments concerned. Since the task ahead is vast, the Ministry of Social Justice and Empowerment envisages an annual phase-wise implementation of the Plan of Action. With this end in view, the Ministry of preparing Annual Plan of Action each and every year.[8]

There are no straight answers to many problems faced by the elders, given the complexities of elders' abuse in India. Bearing the burnt are 82 million elderly, so conditioned to subservience that they won't voice their pain. Four out of 10 elders in India reportedly face abuse, but only 1 case out of 6 is reported, says Help Age India, which recently interviewed 500 elders in Delhi and Mumbai.

It found that loneliness and isolation were the scourge of many old people's lives. The aged were overwhelmed by the new concepts of time and space and nuclear families and found it virtually impossible to cope with the "I-me-mys" generation they had —.

Help-Age —— only confirm the psychological pressures of urban existence the elderly face of the survey more than 12 percent said no one cared if they existed; 13 per cent felt trapped in their own homes; 21 per cent barely socialised. Most respondents, Help-Age found, were being mistreated by their children and spouses.

Adult children are the largest perpetrators of elders' abuse in India (47.3 per cent), followed by spouses (19.3 per cent), relatives (8.8 per cent) and grand children (8.6 per cent).

If one thought that disease was the most depressive factor in old person's lives, think again—neglect is the foremost form of exploitation the elderly face (48.7 per cent), followed by psychological trauma (335.4 per cent), financial exploitation (30.2 per cent), physical abuse (25.6 per cent cases) and abandonment (3.5 per cent).[9]

The Scheme of Integrated Programme for Older Persons is being implemented since November 1992 with an aim to empower and improve the quality of life of older persons. Under the scheme, financial assistance upto 90% of the project cost is provided to Non-governmental organisations for establishing and maintaining old age homes, day care centres, mobile medicare units and to provide non-institutional services to older persons. The scheme has been made flexible so as to meet the diverse needs of older persons including reinforcement and strengthening of the family, awareness generation on issues pertaining to older persons, popularization of the concept of life long preparation for old age, facilitating productive ageing, etc.

During 2004-05, an amount of Rs.15.68 crores was released to 444 Non-Government Organisations for running 338 old age homes, 241 day care centres, 45 mobile medicare units and 2 Non-Institutional Service

Centres benefiting 55,550 older person. Financial assistance of Rs. 5.53 crore has been given to 289 NGOs for running 223 old age homes, 151 day care centres, 31 mobile medicare units and 1 non-institutional service centre in different parts of the country during 2005-06 (upto 31.12.2005).

The Ministry has identified formulation of Central Legislation for promoting the maintenance, care and protection of older persons as one of the thrust areas of the Ministry. The objectives of the proposed legislation include provision of need-based maintenance, ensure minimum level of financial security, make a provision for adequate old age pension to meet basic needs of older persons, setting up a well equipped geriatric ward in each district and to provide mechanism for protection of life and property of older persons.[10]

PROBLEMS OF THE AGED IN DEVELOPING COUNTRIES

(1) Economically Dependent

Majority of the aged people depend on the family members. This creates a lot of problems. They do not get good facilities-food, clothing and shelter. Their life become highly miserable.

(2) Suffer from many Diseases

Old people develop large number of diseases like heart diseases, high blood pressure, depression, urinary problems, etc. A 1992 study in Thailand reported that the elderly (60 years of age and above) suffered most from back pain (17.7%), hypertension (13.9%), peptic ulcer (12%), arthritis (8.8%) and heart disease (6.1%). Mortality due to heart disease among elderly people in Thailand has increased sharply during the last decade, from 245 per 100,000 population in 1985 to 407.5 in 1996. Similarly, the mortality rate for diabetes increased from 28.8 in 1985 to 57.4 in 1996, and for cancer from 169.1 to 236.2.[11] (Refer Table 16.2). Same is true about India.

(3) Suffer Loneliness and Dejection

Family members being busy ignore the old people resulting in their isolation. Family members avoid them and allow them to suffer.

(4) Lower Status

Society and family members don't care for them. As in old times they were the leaders of the family while in modern times, they have become subservient to the family and society.

(5) Very Limited Medical, Recreational and Transport Facilities

Government have not provided good facilities to ensure dignity of life. The Government is trying to do for the aged people but because of limited resources is unable to provide decent services. Table 16.2 presents life expectancy in South-East Asian countries at the existing level. DPR Korea, Sri Lanka, Thailand have higher level of expectancy than India and

TABLE 16.2

Ten Leading Illnesses among the Elderly in Thailand by Sex, 1992-2000

	Total		*Male*		*Female*	
Illness	*Number*	*%*	*Number*	*%*	*Number*	*%*
Back Pain	1.040	17.7	443	17.5	597	17.8
Hypertension	820	13.9	308	12.1	512	15.3
Peptic Ulcer	705	12.0	359	14.1	346	10.3
Arthritis	520	8.8	202	7.9	318	9.5
Heart Disease	357	6.1	112	4.4	245	7.3
Diabetes	315	5.3	97	3.8	218	6.5
Asthma	224	3.8	129	5.1	95	2.8
Muscular Pain	146	2.5	50	2.0	96	2.8
Common Cold	123	2.1	50	2.0	73	2.2
Kidney Stones	104	1.8	71	2.8	33	1.0

Source: Thailand, Ministry of Public Health, Health in Thailand, 1995-96.

other country. South-East Asia Regional Office of WHO in its Regional Health Report, 1998 with focus on women enumerated the following special problems of elderly women. For many women, living longer is not living better. Adding years to life is important. But adding life to the added years is even more important. As life expectancies in women increase, so do the numbers of elderly females in the population. Longer life can be both a penalty and a prize. In the case of women it may be more of the former. As the World Health Report, 1998 states, "Many millions of women are made old before their time by the daily harshness and inequalities of their earlier lives, beginning in childhood. They experience poor nutrition, reproductive ill-health, dangerous working conditions, violence and lifestyle-related diseases, all of which exacerbate the likelihood of breast and cervical cancers, osteoporosis and other chronic conditions after menopause. In old age poverty, loneliness and alienation are common."

Although women in the world today live longer than men, their longevity is offset by a higher rate of illness. Elderly women face a number of significant medical problems. Depletion of hormones at menopause may influence cause-specific morbidity and mortality, including cardiovascular diseases and malignant neoplasms. Osteoporosis, Musculoskeletal diseases, cardiovascular disorders, diabetes, cancers and injuries seem to be the common health problems of older women. For example, the most frequent problems seen in elderly women in Myanmar are arthritis (35.9%), lung disease (24.7%) and hypertension (17.7%). Psychosocial problems are also of great importance to the health and welfare of the elderly. With increasing urbanization and the pressures that go with it, disintegration of the extended family structure, economic hardships and the like. The elderly may become disadvantaged. Already, in some countries, old peoples homes have appeared where there were none before.

TABLE 16.3

Trends in Life Expectancy at Birth

		Life expectancy at Birth (in years)		
Country	*Year*	*Male*	*Female*	*Total*
Bangladesh	1975-80	47.1	46.1	46.6
	1990-95	55.6	55.6	55.5
Bhutan	1975-80	41.6	43.6	42.6
	1990-95	49.1	52.4	50.7
DPR Korea	1975-80	62,4	68.8	65.8
	1990-95	67.7	73.9	71.0
India	1975-80	53.3	52.4	52.9
	1990-95	60.3	60.6	60.5
Indonesia	1975-80	51.5	54.0	52.8
	1990-95	61.0	64.5	62.7
Maldives	1975-80	55.9	53.2	54.6
	1990-95	63.4	60.8	62.1
Myanmar	1975-80	49.7	52.9	51.2
	1990-95	56.0	59.3	57.6
Nepal	1975-80	47.0	45.4	46.2
	1990-95	55.1	54.1	54.6
Sri Lanka	1975-80	65.0	68.5	66.8
	1990-95	69.7	74.2	71.9
Thailand	1975-80	59.3	63.2	61.2
	1990-95	66.4	71.7	69.0

Source: UN, World Population Prospects, The 1996 Revision.

Precautions

Some simple precautions in daily life will reduce the risk of falls and therefore of injuries, just a driving carefully in a well-maintained car and wearing a seatbelt can minimze the risk of an accident and injury on the roads.

- Keep fit by exercising your muscles, your balance and your mobility, all of which are vital to be self-reliant. Joining a gymnastic group ensures your physical well-being and keeps you socially active. Take care of your diet too, which should be both sufficient and varied; if you are losing weight, it's better to consult a health professional.
- It doesn't cost much to eliminate the dangers in your home. Loose carpet; can be fastened down with adhesive, the bathtub can be fitted with handles and a non-slip rubber mat, you can install proper lighting and an easily accessible telephone, and make sure that stairs have banisters and that each step is clearly

marked. Improvements like these can make it safer to move about.

- Avoid dangerous behaviour such a climbing on a stool if you are not very steady on your legs or are subject to vertigo.
- Cut out or limit to the minimum sleeping pills and tranquillizers. Experience shows that in many cases these drugs are a habit rather than a necessity and that people can easily manage without them.
- Learn how to pick yourself up after a fall. You might lie for hours after a fall if you cannot get up (because of a fracture or simply through some temporary incapacity). .
- Plan how to alert somebody if you live on your own. Make sure that you can easily call a neighbour and if there is a telephone, that it is accessible from floor level.[12]

SUGGESTIONS

For older persons to continue to be a resource for their families, their communities and the economy, it is essential that they be active—physically, socially and mentally. The best possible foundation on which to build a long and fulfiling life is good health. In many developed countries, large numbers of older persons are already enjoying a healthy prolonged life and seeking ways to continue to contribute to their society. In developing countries, healthy ageing is even more important. In the absence of universal social security and within severe socio-economic constraints, a longer and more productive life will depend on vigour, vitality and health throughout childhood youth and middle age.

I. Family Support for the Elderly

Many elderly are being left in villages to fend for themselves at a time when they most need care. Emphasis on the nuclear family and the ever increasing burden of providing accommodation, food, clothing, education and health care for children pose a problem. Not only for the parents of the self-isolating family, but also for the ageing women. This is at a time when their waning strength and ability to earn make it difficult for them to obtain basic necessities of life, and deprive them of the help and company of those who under the traditional extended family system would have seen to all their needs. The plight of ageing women in the urban centres may even be worse. So if both ageing men and women in the urban centres may even be worse. So if both ageing men and women need certain services in common. Women have some unique needs as a result of being more dependent and more lonely.[13]

Experts who work in the field of ageing constantly underline the importance of strengthening the capacity of the family to prevent and cope with the problems of the elderly, and to provide them with economic, psycho-social, emotional or psychic security and other care support. This is true in both developed and developing societies.[14]

2. Aged People should remain Active as well as useful to Family and Society

What is important is that in extreme old age, people should not loose interest in the joys of life. It is equally vital that they should still do intellectual and physical work within their capacity, and that society should continue to benefit from their experience.

3. Establish Biological Age Rather than Calendar Age and Provide Medical Aid Accordingly

Since the frequency of many diseases increases with age. Many scientists speak of cancer, atheroscerosis and diabetes as pathological conditions typical of old age. We do not think so, and we do not regard ageing as a disease in itself. It is a physiological process which causes greater instability, more sensitivity and more susceptibility to pathological processes. At the same time, certain compensatory mechanisms start working in elderly people.

Without a profound knowledge of the process of ageing and of the diseases suffered by elderly people, the modern physician often makes mistakes in both diagnosis and treatment of patients, and of course is inhibited from taking radical prophylactic measures. The biology of ageing not only allows us to comprehend how and why the main human diseases develop, but also sets us on the road towards the prolongation of human life.

Studies made by the genetics laboratory at the Institute of Gerontology of the USSR Academy of Medical Sciences suggest that people grow old as two different population groups—one with a tendency towards a long life and the other towards a short one. The establishment of a biological rather than a calendar age will make it possible in the future to determine to which of the two groups a person belongs, and to choose the necessary preventive measures and methods of treatment.

4. Analysis of Epidemiology of Ageing

A wide ranging comparative epidemiological investigation of the position of old people and their need for medical and social aid is at present being conducted in a number of European countries, under the guidance of WHO's European Regional Office. The planning of similar investigations in the developing countries too will undoubtedly prove of value to those countries in the years to come. South-East Regional Office of WHO has also given Guidelines to Promote Healthy Ageing.

The main perspective which guide the programme activities in the Region are:

- approaching ageing as part of the life cycle rather than compartmentalizing health care of the elderly;
- promoting long-term health-increasing awareness of the need to focus on the process of healthy ageing;

- observing cultural influences;
- adopting community-oriented approaches;
- recognizing gender differences; and
- strengthening inter-generational links.

MEASURES TAKEN BY GOVERNMENT OF INDIA TO PROMOTE WELFARE OF ELDERLY PEOPLE—SENIOR CITIZENS

Welfare of the Aged

The Ministry of Social Justice and Empowerment is implementing a Central scheme of assistance to voluntary organisations for the programmes relating to the aged from November 1992. Under the scheme, financial assistance is provided to voluntary organisations for setting up and continuance of day-care centres, old-age homes, mobile medicare units as well as for supporting and strengthening non-institutional services for the aged. Under each of these programmes, the organisations are required to contribute 10 per cent of the expenditure (five per cent in case of organisations functioning in tribal areas) and remaining 90 per cent (95 per cent in case of organisations functioning in tribal areas) being met through the Government of India's grant-in-aid.

Old-Age Homes

The Old-Age Home is a residential unit for at least 25 poor destitute aged persons of 60 years and above. Aged persons coming from low-income groups and middle-income groups of society, in desperate need for shelter can also be considered for admission in these Homes, subject to thorough inquiry and discretion of voluntary organisations concerned. Under this programme, the physical and psychological well-being of the aged inmates is taken care of by way of provision of part-time medical officer and trained social workers' counsel. Medicines up to a limited extent are also provided.

Day-care Centres for the Aged

Assistance to voluntary organisations is given for maintenance of day-care centres for at least 50 persons in urban/slum/rural/tribal areas. The aim of this programme is to keep the aged integrated with their respective families and to supplement the activities of the family in looking after the needs of the aged. Both the well-to-do and the poor in the age-group of 60 years and above could benefit from the programme.

Mobile Medicare Services for the Aged

Under this programme, grant is provided to voluntary organisations which have experience and expertise in providing medicare services to the aged in rural/urban/slum areas.

Non-institutional Services for the Aged

Under this programme, a social worker is appointed to provide for services to the aged like legal counselling assistance for supplying pension, GPM, HRA, Income Tax, Bank Services, etc. The aged are also assisted towards medical examination of their eyes, for receiving spectacles, obtaining hearing aids and dentures, etc. The expenditure incurred under the scheme during the last six years (1992-93 to 1997-98) is Rs. 2,907.17 lakh. Expenditure during 1997-98 was Rs. 609 lakh.

The scheme of assistance to Panchayati Raj institutions/voluntary organisations for constructions of Old-Age Homes was launched during 1996-97. The scheme aims at providing at least one Old-Age Home per district for at least 25 persons over 60 years of age, preferably destitute (with 25 per cent of the capacity being reserved for scheduled castes/ scheduled tribes), in districts where no Government-aided Old-Age Home exists. The assistance under the scheme is a one time construction grant limited to Rs. five lakh.[15]

Enactment of Legislation

Introduced in the Lok Sabha in March this year, the proposed law draws upon the Himachal Pradesh Maintenance of Parents and Dependents Children Act, 2001, the Hindu Adoption and Maintenance Act, 1956 and the Criminal Procedure Code, 1973, which provides for partial maintenance to the elderly (Rs. 500 a month). This Bill, however, goes beyond CrPC by providing Rs. 10,000 as the maximum monthly maintenance to senior citizens. Born out of the need to remind children of their responsibilities towards the old, it also has built-in provisions for punishments for those who don't pay and those who abandon parents. The latter can face three month in prison or Rs. 5000 fine, or both.

By definition, the law seeks to "provide for more effective provisions for the maintenance and welfare of parents and senior citizens guaranteed and recognized under the Constitution."[16]

Senior Citizens Bill

- A senior citizen (60 years or above), including a parent who is unable to maintain himself, can claim maintenance from progeny.
- Parents can apply against children; childless senior citizens against relatives who are inheritors of the property.
- Children/relatives to maintain partners so that they can lead normal lives.
- Applications to be made to maintenance tribunals to be set-up by the state.
- Tribunals to have the power of civil court, decide applications in six months; provision of mediation before proceedings.
- District Judge to head Appellate Tribunal; sub-divisional officer to head maintenance tribunal.
- One-month jail for children who don't pay maintenance; three-month jail for children who abandon parents.

- Old age homes in every district, medical care of elderly in government hospitals.
- Tie-ups with police to ensure protection of life and liberty of the elderly.

Health of Elderly Women

For many people, living longer is not living better. Adding years to life is important. But adding life to the added years is even more important. "Active ageing makes the difference" was the World Health Day Theme for 1999. By the year 2020 more than 1000 million of the world's population will be over 60 years old. To help promote a global response to this major societal concern, WHO, in 1995, restructured its programme of health of the elderly and gave it as a new name—Ageing and Health. This area of health care is becoming a dominant concern as the next millennium approaches.[17]

As life expectancies in women increase, so do the number of elderly females in the population. Longer life can be both a penalty and a prize. In the case of women it may be more of the former. As The World Health Report, 1998 states, "Many millions of women are made old before their time by the daily harshness and inequalities of their earlier lives, beginning in childhood. They experience poor nutrition, reproductive ill-health, dangerous working conditions, violence and lifestyle-related diseases, all of which exacerbate the likelihood of breast and cervical cancers, osteoporosis and other chronic conditions after menopause. In old-age poverty, loneliness and alienation are common.[18]

In the South-East Asia Region, the number of women of 60 years and above increased from 37.5 million in 1985 to almost 51 million in 1995, and is projected to surpass 68 million by 2005. The health and other social needs of ageing women in the Region, however, have not yet been adequately studied. Although women in the world today live longer than men, their longevity is offset by a higher rate of illness. Elderly women face a number of significant medical problems. Depletion of hormones at menopause may influence cause-specific morbidity and mortality, including cardiovascular diseases and malignant neoplasms.

Musculoskeletal diseases, cardiovascular disorders, diabetes, cancers and injuries seem to be the common health problems of older women in the Region. For example, the most frequent problems seen in elderly women in Myanmar are arthritis (35.9%), lung disease (24.7%) and hypertension (17.7%).

Psychological problems are also of great importance to the health and welfare of the elderly. With increasing urbanization and the pressure that go with it, disintegration of the extended family structure, economic hardships and the like, the elderly may become disadvantaged. Already in some countries, old people's home have appeared where there were none before. For older persons to continue to be a resource for their families, their communities and the economy, it is essential that they be active physically, socially and mentally. The best possible foundations on which to build a long and fulfiling life is good health. In many developed countries, large number of older persons are already enjoying a healthy prolonged life and seeking ways to continue to contribute to their society. In developing countries, healthy ageing is even more important. In the absence of universal social security and within severe socio-economic constraints, a longer and more productive life will depend on vigour, vitality and health throughout childhood, youth and middle age.

CONCLUSION

Old-age values are changing-adverse economic force, the misallocation of resources, the yearning for material things, the struggle for self-esteem and status—all these factors are overtaking the traditional positive values as regards support for the elderly. What is important is that, in extreme old-age, people should not lose interest in the joys of life. It is equally vital that they should still do intellectual and physical work within their capacity, and that society should continue to benefit from their experience. For older persons to continue to be a resource for their families, their communities and the economy, it is essential that they be active physically, socially and mentally. The best possible foundations on which to build a long and fulfiling life is good health. In many developed countries, large number of older persons are already enjoying a healthy prolonged life and seeking ways to continue to contribute to their society. In developing countries, healthy ageing is even more important. In the absence of universal social security and within severe socio-economic constraints, a longer and more productive life will depend on vigour, vitality and health throughout childhood, youth and middle age.

Notes and References

1. Ministry of Social Justice and Empowerment, Annual Report, 2006-07, pp. 58-59.
2. *Ibid.*
3. WHO: Fifty Year of WHO, in South-East Asia, 1948-98, WHO, New Delhi.
4. WHO: SEARO: Fifty Years of WHO in South-East Asia, New Delhi, 1999, p. 90.
5. *The Tribune,* Nov. 4, 2007.
6. Fifty Year of WHO in South-East Asia, Highlight, 1948-98, WHO, New Delhi.
7. *World Health,* 51st Year, No. 2, March-April, 1998.
8. Ministry of Social Justice and Empowerment, Annual Report, 2005-06, pp. 58-60.
9. *The Tribune,* Nov. 4, 2007.
10. Ministry of Social Justice and Empowerment, 2005-06, pp. 61-62.
11. WHO: SEARO: Health Situation in South-East Asia Regions, 1994-97, New Delhi, 1999, pp. 177-78.
12. *World Health,* January 1993, p. 10.
13. Ninth Five Year Plan, *op. cit.,* p. 77.

14. Ministry of Social Justice and Empowerment, GOI, 2005-06, pp. 59-60.
15. Health Situation in South-East Asia Region, *op. cit.*, p. 178.
16. *The Tribune*, 4th Nov., 2007.
17. WHO: SEARO: Fifty Years of WHO in South-East Asia, New Delhi, 1999, p. 90.
18. Regional Health Report, 1988, *op. cit.*, p. 24.

BOOKS BY THE SAME AUTHOR

1. International Administration: WHO South East-Asia Regional Office (New Delhi, 1977), Sterling Publishers
2. Principles, Problems and Prospects of Co-operative Administration (New Delhi, 1979), Sterling Publishers (Co-Author Dr. B.B. Goel)
3. Administration of Personnel in Co-operative (New Delhi, 1979), Sterling Publishers (Co-Author Dr. B.B. Goel)
4. Health Care Administration: Ecology, Principles and Modern Trends (New Delhi, 1980), Sterling Publishers
5. Health Care Administration: Policy-making and Planning (New Delhi, 1980), Sterling Publishers
6. Health Care Administration: Levels and Aspects (New Delhi, 1980), Sterling Publishers
7. International Civil Service: Principles, Problems and Prospects (New Delhi, 1984), Sterling Publishers
8. Public Health Administration (New Delhi, 1984), Sterling Publishers
9. Public Personnel Administration (New Delhi, 1984), Reprint 1987, Sterling Publishers
10. International Civil Services—Principles, Problems and Prospectives (New Delhi, 1984), Sterling Publishers.
11. Social Welfare Administration: Theory and Practice (Vols. I and II) (New Delhi, 1988), Deep & Deep Publications Pvt. Ltd.
12. Hospital Administration and Management (ed.) Co-Author Dr. R. Kumar in 3 volumes (New Delhi, 1989), Deep & Deep Publications Pvt. Ltd.
13. Policy and Administration: Family Planning & Beyond (New Delhi, 1990), Deep & Deep Publications Pvt. Ltd.
14. Modern Management Techniques (Revised and Reprinted) (New Delhi, 1990), Deep & Deep Publications Pvt. Ltd.
15. Development Planning and Administration (ed.) S. Bhatnagar (Co-editor) (New Delhi, 1992), Deep & Deep Publications Pvt. Ltd.
16. Financial Administration and Management (New Delhi, 1993), Sterling Publishers
17. Advanced Public Administration (New Delhi, 1993), Sterling Publishers

18. Personnel Administration and Management
(New Delhi, 1994), Deep & Deep Publications Pvt. Ltd.
19. Educational Policy and Administration
(New Delhi, 1994), Deep & Deep Publications Pvt. Ltd.
20. Slum Improvement Through Participatory Urban Based Community Structures
(New Delhi, 1999), Deep & Deep Publications Pvt. Ltd.
21. Distance Education in 21st Century
(New Delhi, 2000), Deep & Deep Publications Pvt. Ltd.
22. Health Care System and Management: Organization and Structure
(New Delhi, 2000), Deep & Deep Publications Pvt. Ltd.
23. Health Care System and Management: Policies and Programmes
(New Delhi, 2000), Deep & Deep Publications Pvt. Ltd.
24. Health Care System and Management: Management and Administration
(New Delhi, 2000), Deep & Deep Publications Pvt. Ltd.
25. Heath Care System and Management: Primary Health Care Management
(New Delhi, 2000), Deep & Deep Publications Pvt. Ltd.
26. Management Techniques: Principles and Practices
(New Delhi, 2001), Deep & Deep Publications Pvt. Ltd.
27. Encyclopaedia of Disaster Management in 3 Volumes
(New Delhi, 2001), Deep & Deep Publications Pvt. Ltd.
28. Management of Hospitals: Hospital Core Services
(New Delhi, 2002), Deep & Deep Publications Pvt. Ltd.
29. Management of Hospitals: Hospital Supportive Services
(New Delhi, 2002), Deep & Deep Publications Pvt. Ltd.
30. Management of Hospitals: Hospital Preventive and Promotive Services
(New Delhi, 2002), Deep & Deep Publications Pvt. Ltd.
31. Management of Hospitals: Hospital Managerial Services
(New Delhi, 2002), Deep & Deep Publications Pvt. Ltd.
32. Public Personal Administration
(New Delhi, 2002), Deep & Deep Publications Pvt. Ltd.
33. Public Financial Administration
(New Delhi, 2002), Deep & Deep Publications Pvt. Ltd.
34. Urban Development and Management
(New Delhi, 2002), Deep & Deep Publications Pvt. Ltd.
35. Public Administration: Theory and Practices
(New Delhi, 2003), Deep & Deep Publications Pvt. Ltd.
36. Advanced Public Administration (Revised and Enlarged Edition)
(New Delhi, 2003), Deep & Deep Publications Pvt. Ltd.

37. Panchayati Raj in India
(New Delhi, 2003), Deep & Deep Publications Pvt. Ltd.
38. Encyclopedia of Higher Education in 21st Century: Organisation and Structure
(New Delhi, 2004), Deep & Deep Publications Pvt. Ltd.
39. Encyclopaedia of Higher Education in 21st Century: Quality and Excellence
(New Delhi, 2004), Deep & Deep Publications Pvt. Ltd.
40. Encyclopedia of Higher Education in 21st Century, Extension Education Services
(New Delhi, 2004), Deep & Deep Publications Pvt. Ltd.
41. Stress Management and Education: An Indian Perspective
(New Delhi, 2004), Deep & Deep Publications Pvt. Ltd.
42. Human Values and Education:
(New Delhi, 2004), Deep & Deep Publications Pvt. Ltd.
43. Public Health Policy and Administration
(New Delhi, 2004), Deep & Deep Publications Pvt. Ltd.
44. Administration and Management of NGO's: Text and Case Studies
(New Delhi, 2004), Deep & Deep Publications Pvt. Ltd.
45. Nursing Services: Management and Administration
(New Delhi, 2005), Deep & Deep Publications Pvt. Ltd.
46. Population Policy and Family Welfare Administration
(New Delhi, 2005), Deep & Deep Publications Pvt. Ltd.
47. Human Resource Development in 21st Century
(New Delhi, 2005), Deep & Deep Publications Pvt. Ltd.
48. Encyclopaedia of Disaster Management (3 Volumes)
(New Delhi, 2006) Deep & Deep Publications Pvt. Ltd.
49. School Health Education
(New Delhi, 2007), Deep & Deep Publications Pvt. Ltd.
50. Health Education: Theory and Practices
(New Delhi, 2007), Deep & Deep Publications Pvt. Ltd.
51. Good Governance: An Integral Views
(New Delhi, 2007), Deep & Deep Publications Pvt. Ltd.
52. Right to Information and Good Governance
(New Delhi, 2007), Deep & Deep Publications Pvt. Ltd.
53. Disaster Management: Text and Case Studies
(New Delhi, 2007), Deep & Deep Publications Pvt. Ltd.
54. Hospital Administration: Theory and Practices
(New Delhi, 2007), Deep & Deep Publications Pvt. Ltd.
55. Environmental Health Values and Education,
(New Delhi, 2008), Deep & Deep Publications Pvt. Ltd.

56. Administrative and Management Thinkers: Revelvance in New Millennium
(New Delhi, 2008), Deep & Deep Publications Pvt. Ltd.
57. Principles and Practices of Human Values
(New Delhi, 2008), Deep & Deep Publications Pvt. Ltd.
58. Distance Education: Principles, Potentialities and Perspectives
(New Delhi, 2008), Deep & Deep Publications Pvt. Ltd.
59. Educational Administration and Management: An Integral View
(New Delhi, 2008), Deep & Deep Publications Pvt. Ltd.
60. Women Health Education
(New Delhi, 2008), Deep & Deep Publications Pvt. Ltd.
61. Health Care System and Hospital Administration
Vol. 1 (Organizational Structure)
(New Delhi, 2008), Deep & Deep Publications Pvt. Ltd.
62. Health Care System and Hospital Administration
Vol. 2 (Resources: Human, Finance and Material)
(New Delhi, 2008), Deep & Deep Publications Pvt. Ltd.
63. Health Care System and Hospital Administration
Vol. 3 (Policy-making and Programmes)
(New Delhi, 2008), Deep & Deep Publications Pvt. Ltd.
64. Health Care System and Hospital Administration
Vol. 4 (Emerging and Thrust Areas)
(New Delhi, 2008), Deep & Deep Publications Pvt. Ltd.
65. Health Care System and Hospital Administration
Vol. 5 (Primary/Rural Health Care)
(New Delhi, 2008), Deep & Deep Publications Pvt. Ltd.
66. Health Care System and Hospital Administration
Vol. 6 (Secondary and Tertiary Health Care)
(New Delhi, 2008), Deep & Deep Publications Pvt. Ltd.
67. Health Care System and Hospital Administration
Vol. 7 (Management Techniques and Good Governance)
(New Delhi, 2008), Deep & Deep Publications Pvt. Ltd.
68. Education of Lifestyle and Lifetime Diseases
(Deep & Deep Publications Pvt. Ltd.)
69. Health Education Administration—From International Level to Village Level
(Deep & Deep Publications Pvt. Ltd.)
70. Education for Healthy Urban Cities
(Deep & Deep Publications Pvt. Ltd.)
71. Rural Health Education
(Deep & Deep Publications Pvt. Ltd.)

Bibliography

Acton Society Trust, Hospitals and the State: Hospital Organisation and Administration under the National Health Service Series, London: Action Society Trust, 1956, 54p.

Acton Society Trust, Hospitals and the State: Hospital Organisation and Administration under the National Health Service, London: The Trust, 1959, iii, 80p.

Andhra Pradesh, Health and Local Administration Department Panchayats Executive Officers Regulations relating to Recruitment, etc., Hyderabad: The Author, 1956, l6p.

Bannington, B.G., English Public Health Administration, 2nd ed., London: P.S. King, 1929, 325p.

Berkov, Robert, The World Health Organisation: A Study in Decentralized International Administration, Geneva Droz, 1957, 173p.

Better Health by Community Projects Administration, Planning Commission, New Delhi: Community Projects, Planning Commission, n.d., 32p.

Blum, Henrik L., Public Administration: A Public Health Viewpoint, N.Y.: Macmillan, 1963, 532p.

Hugh Flanagan and Peter Spurgeon, Public Sector Managerial Effectiveness: Theory and Practice in the National Health Service, Buckingham: Open Univ. Press, 1996, 128p.

Freeman, Ruth B., Administration of Public Health Services and Edward M. Holmes, Philadelphia: Saunders, 1960, 507p.

Goddard, H.A., Principles of Administration Applied to Nursing Service by H.A. Goddard, Geneva: World Health Organisation, 1958, 106p.

Goel, Rajneesh, Community Health Care, New Delhi: Deep & Deep Publications Pvt. Ltd., 2004, 403p.

Goel, S.L., Health and Care Administration: Policy-making and Planning, Delhi: Sterling, 1980, 288p.

Goel, S.L, Health Care Administration: Ecology, Principles and Modern Trends, Delhi: Sterling, 1980, 233p.

Goel, S.L., Health Care Administration: Levels and Aspects, Delhi: Sterling, 1980, 245p.

Goel, S.L., Health Care System and Management, New Delhi: Deep & Deep Publications Pvt. Ltd., 2004, 4 Vols.

Goel, S.L., International Administration: WHO South-East Asia Regional Office, Delhi: Sterling, 1977, 344p.

Goel, S.L., Population Policy and Family Welfare: Reproductive and Child Health Administration, New Delhi: Deep & Deep Publications Pvt. Ltd., 2005, 526p.

Goel, S.L., Public Health Administration, Delhi: Sterling, 1984, 472p.

Goel, S.L, Public Health Policy and Administration, New Delhi: Deep & Deep Publications Pvt. Ltd., 2005, 651p.

Graduate Study in Public Administration: A Guide to Graduate Programs by Office of Education, Department of Health, Education and Welfare, Washington: United States Government Printing Office, 1961, 158+p.

Greenfield, Margert, State-Local Service for Mental Health, Bureau of Public Administration, Berkeley: The Bureau, 1955, 93p.

Guangde, Sun, Health Care Administration in China, Westport: Greenport, 1993, pp. 53-62.

Handbook on Human Services Administration, edited by Jack Rabin and Marcia B. Steinhauer, New York: Marcel Dekker, 1988, 604p.

Health Policy Research in South Asia: Building Capacity for Reform, edited by Abdo S. Yazbeck and David H. Peters, Washington, D.C.: World Bank, 2003, 428p.

Heaver, Richard, Managing Primary Health Care: Implications of the Health Transition, Washington, D.C.: World Bank, 1995, 41p.

Health Status of the Underprivileged, New Delhi: Centre for Urban Studies, Indian Institute of Public Administration, 1991, 225p.

Indian Institute of Public Administration, Centre for Urban Studies, Urban Health System, edited by P.K. Umashankar and Girish K. Misra, New Delhi: Reliance and IIPA, 1993, 259p.

Institute for Training in Municipal Administration, Administration of Community Health Services, Chicago: ICMA, 1961, 560p.

Johnston, Timothy, Investing in Health: Development Effectiveness in the Health, Nutrition, and Population Sector, Washington, D.C.: World Bank, 1999, 69p.

Khandewale, Shreekant V., Health Administration and the Weaker Sections in an Indian Metropolis, Delhi: Devika, 1996, 231p.

Klinoubol, Kriengkrai, Public Health Development and Administration: A Study of Developing Economy, Delhi: Deep & Deep Publications Pvt. Ltd., 1989. 436p.

Local Self-Government Administration in States of India, 1956, New Delhi: Ministry of Health, 1956, 149p.

Local Self-government Administration in States of India, 1962, Ministry of Health, Delhi: The Manager of Publications, 1962, 161+p.

Legislature Committee on Local Administration by Health, Education and Local Administration Department, Madras, Madras: Health, Education and Local Administration Department, 1958, 5 Parts.

Morden, Margaret Gorsuch, Cooperative Health Administration in Metropolitan, Los Angeles: The Bureau, 1949, 52p.

Panchayat Manual, Madras: Health, Education and Local Administration Department, 1956, 368+p.

Papers in Public Administration, No. 6, Ann Arbor: The Bureau, 1950, 85p.

Public Services M.B.A. Induction Module: India-U.K. context (August-September, 1999: Indian Institute of Public Administration, New Delhi), Gender-related Issues (course material), New Delhi: Indian Institute of Public Administration, 1999, vp.

Report of the Regional Training Seminar on Social Security Administration, New Delhi: Regional Office for Asia and Oceania, 1979, 75p.

Rowbottom, R., Hospital Organisation: A Progress Report on the Brunel Health Services Project, London: Heinemann, 1973, 314p.

Survey of Research in Public Administration, 1980-90, edited by V.A. Pai Panandiker, Delhi: Konark, 1997, 631p.

Tebow, Hilda P., Staff-Development as an Integral Part of Administration, Washington, D.C.: Department of Health, Education and Welfare, 1959, 33+p.

The Indo-US Symposium on Community Mental Health at National Institute of Mental Health and Neuro Sciences, Bangalore: National Institute of Mental Health and Neuro Sciences, 1992, 520p.

Weaver, Jerry L., Conflict and Control in Health Care Administration, Beverly Hills: n.p., 1975, 197p.

Welfare Administration and Social Welfare Around the World, by Department of Health, Education and Welfare, United States, Washington: Government Printing Office, 1963, 9p.

Wishwakarma, R.K., Health Status of the Underprivileged, New Delhi: Centre for Urban Studies, Indian Institute of Public Administration, 1993, 283p.

Index